Irigaray

Key Contemporary Thinkers

Jeremy Ahearne, *Michel de Certeau*
Michael Caesar, *Umberto Eco*
M. J. Cain, *Fodor*
Rosemary Cowan, *Cornel West*
George Crowder, *Isaiah Berlin*
Maximilian de Gaynesford, *John McDowell*
Oliver Davis, *Rancière*
Reidar Andreas Due, *Deleuze*
Chris Fleming, *Rene Girard*
Andrew Gamble, *Hayek*
Neil Gascoigne, *Richard Rorty*
Nigel Gibson, *Fanon*
Graeme Gilloch, *Walter Benjamin*
Karen Green, *Dummett*
Espen Hammer, *Stanley Cavell*
Christina Howells, *Derrida*
Fred Inglis, *Clifford Geertz*
Simon Jarvis, *Adorno*
Sarah Kay, *Žižek*
Valerie Kennedy, *Edward Said*
Moya Lloyd, *Judith Butler*
James McGilvray, *Chomsky*
Lois McNay, *Foucault*
Dermot Moran, *Edmund Husserl*
Stephen Morton, *Gayatri Spivak*
Harold W. Noonan, *Frege*
James O'Shea, *Wilfrid Sellars*
William Outhwaite, *Habermas, 2nd Edition*
Kari Palonen, *Quentin Skinner*
John Preston, *Feyerabend*
Chris Rojek, *Stuart Hall*
William Scheuerman, *Morgenthau*
Severin Schroeder, *Wittgenstein*
Susan Sellers, *Helene Cixous*
Wes Sharrock and Rupert Read, *Kuhn*
David Silverman, *Harvey Sacks*
Dennis Smith, *Zygmunt Bauman*
James Smith, *Terry Eagleton*
Felix Stalder *Manuel Castells*
Geoffrey Stokes, *Popper*
Georgia Warnke, *Gadamer*
James Williams, *Lyotard*
Jonathan Wolff, *Robert Nozick*
Ed Pluth, *Badiou*
Stacy K. Keltner, *Kristeva*

Irigaray
Towards a Sexuate Philosophy

Rachel Jones

polity

First published in 2011 by Polity Press

Polity Press
65 Bridge Street
Cambridge CB2 1UR, UK

Polity Press
350 Main Street
Malden, MA 02148, USA

ISBN-13: 978-0-7456-5104-0 (hardback)
ISBN-13: 978-0-7456-5105-7 (paperback)

A catalogue record for this book is available from the British Library.

Typeset in 10.5 on 12 pt Palatino
by Toppan Best-set Premedia Limited
Printed and bound in Great Britain by the MPG Books Group

For further information on Polity, visit our website: www.politybooks.com

Contents

Full Contents

Acknowledgements

I would like to thank my colleagues in Philosophy and the 'Women, Culture and Society' Programme at Dundee; the students from those programmes who took the time to read and discuss Irigaray with me; and Nicholas Davey and Stephen Houlgate, who provided valuable encouragement and perspective at key stages of the project.

The feedback from the anonymous readers was invaluable in the development of this book; I would like to thank them for their comments and hope I have responded adequately to their thoughtful suggestions here. My thanks also to Oneworld for the impetus that led to this publication and to Mike Harpley in particular for his generous advice. My editor at Polity, Emma Hutchinson, provided excellent and timely guidance, particularly during the final stages of writing. David Winter's patient editorial assistance and support was greatly appreciated.

Special thanks to Christine Battersby, who first introduced me to Irigaray's work and who has taught me so much about reading (and writing about) philosophical texts; and to my friends – who were often my readers – for their philosophical insight and generosity with their time and support, especially Tina Chanter, Catherine Constable, Beth Lord, Aislinn O'Donnell, Johanna Oksala, Andrea Rehberg, Fanny Söderbäck, and Alison Stone.

With thanks to my mother, June, and my sisters, Beki and Naomi, for their constant love and support; and to Kurt, for reading and commenting on multiple drafts, for thinking with me, and for helping me to think further.

The publishers wish to acknowledge permission to reprint the following copyright material:

Material reprinted from Luce Irigaray, *Speculum of the Other Woman*, translated by Gillian C. Gill. Translation copyright © 1985 by Cornell University Press. Used by permission of the publisher, Cornell University Press.

Material reprinted from Luce Irigaray, *This Sex Which Is Not One*, translated by Catherine Porter & Carolyn Burke. Translation copyright © 1985 by Cornell University Press. Used by permission of the publisher, Cornell University Press.

List of Abbreviations

BEW *Between East and West: From Singularity to Community*, trans. S. Pluháček (New York: Columbia University Press, 2002). First published as *Entre Orient et Occident: De la singularité à la communauté* (Paris: Grasset, 1999).

DBT *Democracy Begins Between Two*, trans. K. Anderson (London: Athlone, 2000).

EP *Elemental Passions*, trans. J. Collie and J. Still (London: Athlone, 1992). First published as *Passions élémentaires* (Paris: Minuit, 1982).

ESD *An Ethics of Sexual Difference*, trans. C. Burke and G. C. Gill (London: Athlone, 1993). First published as *Éthique de la différence sexuelle* (Paris: Minuit, 1984).

ILTY *I Love to You: Sketch for a Felicity Within History*, trans. A. Martin (London: Routledge, 1996). First published as *J'aime à toi: Esquisse d'une félicité dans l'histoire* (Paris: Grasset, 1992).

S *Speculum of the Other Woman*, trans. G. C. Gill (Ithaca, NY: Cornell University Press, 1985). First published as *Speculum de l'autre femme* (Paris: Minuit, 1974).

Sf *Speculum de l'autre femme* (Paris: Minuit, 1974).

TS *This Sex Which Is Not One*, trans. C. Porter with C. Burke (Ithaca, NY: Cornell University Press, 1985). First published as *Ce sexe qui n'en est pas un* (Paris: Minuit, 1977).

Introduction: Towards
a Sexuate Philosophy

This book seeks to guide the reader through Luce Irigaray's transformation of western thought, showing how her project – at once
critical and creative – generates the terms for a sexuate philosophy.
The approach taken thus involves positioning Irigaray primarily
as a feminist *philosopher*.[1] This immediately raises numerous questions: what kind of feminist is Irigaray? What makes her work
specifically philosophical? Why does it matter to position her as a
philosopher? Indeed, given the patriarchal bias that her own work
locates at the very heart of western philosophical thought, why
should feminists have anything to do with philosophy? Conversely,
why should philosophers not particularly concerned with feminism have anything to do with Irigaray?

In response, one of the aims of this book is to show that
Irigaray's sustained, if profoundly critical, engagement with
western thought has much to contribute to key philosophical
debates concerning metaphysics and ontology (questions about
reality and being) as well as epistemology and ethics (questions
about knowledge and value) – not least because she challenges the
very terms in which these debates are traditionally framed. At the
same time, the book aims to provide an in-depth guide to the
philosophical grounding of Irigaray's project for those drawing on
her work to address specifically feminist concerns or issues of sex
and gender. Such readers may approach Irigaray from a range of
diverse fields including gender and women's studies, queer theory,
social and political thought, geography, history, film, art, literature,
or architecture, as well as philosophy. The book seeks to offer an

opening onto aspects of Irigaray's work that may be less readily accessible for those without a prior training in the history of western philosophical thought. But perhaps more importantly, it hopes to show why it is worth undertaking the intensive philosophical work Irigaray demands of us, if our aim is to challenge and transform the inequitable gendered structures – as well as the gender blindness – that inform western thought and culture.

The reason for foregrounding Irigaray's work as a philosopher is not because feminist philosophy has priority over other areas of feminist thought and praxis. Irigaray herself has conducted her theoretical work alongside her ongoing practice as a psychoanalyst and teacher, as well as her involvement in the realm of practical politics. Nor should the importance of other discourses to Irigaray's own work be underestimated, most notably those of psychoanalysis and linguistics. Rather than a question of priority, the issue is one of specificity: this book aims to introduce readers to the specifically philosophical dimensions of Irigaray's feminist project along with the ways in which she transforms the terms of both traditional and contemporary philosophical debate.

In keeping with this aim, the book's guiding thread is Irigaray's groundbreaking analysis of the history of western thought, *Speculum of the Other Woman*. In many ways, *Speculum* is feminist philosophy's first *critique*. In the *Critique of Pure Reason*, Kant famously displaces sceptical doubts about whether our knowledge conforms to the reality of objects by showing how objects necessarily conform to our cognitive faculties.[2] He thereby revolutionizes thought by grounding knowledge in the human subject rather than the objects known. In *Speculum*, Irigaray sceptically re-examines the philosophical subject's dependence on the object and introduces new doubts about the supposed self-sufficiency and universality of that subject. She does so by showing how the subject's identity is typically secured against a material, sensible realm aligned with the figure of woman. The supposedly 'universal' rational subject thus turns out to be implicitly male, while woman is mapped onto the position of object and 'other'. This pattern of oppositional thinking means that woman is defined against a male subject, rather than in terms of her sexed specificity or as a subject in her own right. Despite his revolutionary approach, Kant is seen as repeating and reinforcing this pattern, together with the forgetting of sexual difference it implies. Indeed, according to Irigaray, western philosophy since Plato has failed to think sexual difference, in that it has failed to think this difference *positively*. Instead, it has reduced the difference between men and women to a specular structure in which woman is always the 'other' or mirror-image of the self-same (male) subject. By reminding philosophy that each human being is born from a mother who is also a woman, Irigaray asks us to remember that a human being is two: western thought must therefore make space for *two* (different) subjects by attending to the irreducible sexual difference between them. She thereby seeks a revolution in thought no less significant or transformative than Kant's.

Whether one agrees or disagrees with the details of Irigaray's analyses, what matters more is the dramatic shift in perspective *Speculum* endeavours to produce, re-attuning philosophy to sexual difference and opening the way towards a culture of two, irreducibly different, subjects. While *Speculum* is thus a key text for understanding Irigaray's project, it demands a familiarity with philosophy that some readers may initially find off-putting. Thus, a central aim of this book is to aid readers in engaging directly with *Speculum* itself; in turn, *Speculum* will serve as a frame through which to trace key aspects of Irigaray's critical and transformative encounter with the philosophical tradition. The following chapters thus offer in-depth analyses of specific sections of *Speculum*, while pointing ahead to connections with Irigaray's later work.

These connections will be particularly foregrounded in Chapters 6 and 7; however, the purpose of this book is not to give a descriptive summary of Irigaray's extensive body of work, nor even of all her key texts. Rather, its aim is to provide readers with a way of approaching Irigaray – of 'following her trajectory', as one commentator puts it – that will aid them in reading and engaging with her texts for themselves.[3] In particular, it seeks to equip readers to approach Irigaray's writings with an attunement to their philosophical dimensions as well as to the ways in which philosophy is transformed via what Irigaray calls the '*interpretive lever*' of sexual difference (*TS*, 72). This lever operates not only by drawing critical attention to the specific claims western philosophers have made about women, but by revealing the gendering that marks the fundamental conceptual structures of their thought. As Irigaray shows, this gendering is paradoxically dependent on a blindspot regarding sexual difference. It is this blindspot that her work seeks to expose and to overcome.

Sexuate Subjects, Sexuate Others

A further key aim of this book is to show that, right from the start, Irigaray's project is never merely critical. While the intricate textual

fabric of *Speculum* undoubtedly seeks to reveal and displace the
blindspots of the tradition, it also contains many of the ideas which
Irigaray will go on to elaborate more fully in her later works so as
to cultivate ways of thinking, writing and living which are attentive
to sexual difference. Among the keys to this project is Irigaray's
notion of the 'sexuate', a neologism used in English translations of
her work (for the French *sexué*) as well as by Irigaray herself when
writing and speaking in English. Although it already appears in
the English translation of *Speculum*, this term becomes increasingly
prominent in Irigaray's later texts where she writes of the need for
sexuate rights, sexuate identity, and a sexuate culture characterized
by two (sexuate) subjects. In many ways, the notion of the sexuate
captures Irigaray's distinctive approach to the question of sexual
difference; thus, one of the central tasks of this book is to unfold its
significance. For now, however, it is worth noting that the 'sexuate'
refers neither to a mode of being determined by biological sex nor
to a cultural overlay of gendered meanings inscribed on a 'tabula
rasa' of passively receptive matter. The 'sexuate' does not separate
the becomings that shape our bodily being from the production of
social and cultural meanings or behavioural dispositions. Rather,
it signals the way that sexual difference is articulated through our
different modes of being and becoming, that is, in bodily, social,
linguistic, aesthetic, erotic, and political forms. In this book, I will
move fairly fluidly between the 'sexuate' and 'sexual difference' (as
does Irigaray). Broadly speaking, however, I understand sexual
difference to be that which western culture has forgotten and which
Irigaray seeks to recover, while the sexuate involves taking up a
positive relation to sexual difference by acknowledging it as the
irreducible difference which inflects every aspect of our being.

One reason why it is important to emphasize that the 'sexuate'
maps neither onto pre-discursive biological differences nor onto
gender understood as a purely discursive construct is because of
the pervasiveness (and importance) of this kind of sex/gender
distinction in much Anglo-American feminist debate. According to
this distinction, 'sex' is generally understood as referring to our
bodily existence as male or female, that is, as a matter of biology
and anatomy, while 'gender' is used to refer to masculinity and
femininity as cultural and social constructions. Many feminist
thinkers have – for good reason – sought to privilege the (change-
able) cultural constructions of gender and been suspicious of
attempts to root social and political structures in appeals to the
body: such appeals illegitimately make human structures seem

'natural' and hence *un*-changeable in ways that have all too often been used to legitimate discrimination against women. At the same time, others have been more suspicious of the normative power invested in the sex/gender distinction itself, and hence the supposed 'naturalness' of this very distinction has in turn been called into question, notably via the work of Michel Foucault and Judith Butler.[4] Indeed, part of the subversiveness and originality of Butler's position lies in the way she so thoroughly problematizes any sustainable distinction between (biological) 'sex' and (socially constructed) 'gender'. However, for the purposes of reading Irigaray, the most important point is that the sex/gender distinction which has been so important to Anglo-American feminist debates does not map neatly onto direct French equivalents:[5] the terms *'masculin'* and *'féminin'* have a broader significance than their English counterparts, while *'mâle'* and *'femelle'* are used in a much narrower, more strictly biological sense (e.g. when determining the sex of animals). For this reason, the work of thinkers like Irigaray, as well as others who came to be aligned with the 'new French feminisms', is not structured around a clear sex/gender divide.[6] Thus, when Irigaray uses the French *'féminin'*, this needs to be heard not as a direct equivalent to the English concept of the 'feminine' (understood as a culturally scripted set of attitudes, gestures and roles), but as encompassing women's bodily existence as female, as well as the social and cultural significances of that bodily mode of being.

As others have noted, this absence of a clear-cut sex/gender distinction is to some extent an advantage, given the ways in which this distinction can trap feminist theory back into a mind/body or nature/culture divide that it typically seeks to escape.[7] Moreover, one of the unfortunate effects of re-imposing a sex/gender distinction onto Irigaray's work is that this tends to lead to the charge of 'essentialism': read through this frame, Irigaray's appeals to female specificity are reduced to references to an unchanging and unchangeable body (women's 'sex') that determines what women are as well as how they act and think. I agree with many other readers of Irigaray that the charge of essentialism is misplaced, an issue I return to more fully in Chapter 6. For Irigaray, while biological features undoubtedly set certain limits on our modes of being, this is far from saying that we are simply determined by our biology. On the contrary, Irigaray makes it repeatedly clear that what is at stake is how biological differences are represented and what kinds of social and cultural value they are given. Indeed, the best evidence that biological differences are defined *through* their social and cultural representations is found in the historically pervasive image of women's sex as the inverse, lack or absence of a male sex organ. However, as will be shown in later chapters, it is crucial to Irigaray's position that we not only recognize the ways in which bodies are informed by their cultural representations. This needs to be matched with an acknowledgement of the active power of matter to shape and give form: the female body cannot simply determine women's being because bodies themselves are not unchanging and fixed, but active, animate, and generative. Thus, while the issue of Irigaray's supposed essentialism is by now well-trodden ground in Irigaray scholarship,[8] I have risked returning to it because I hope to add to the arguments against this reading by emphasizing the link between Irigaray's deployment of images of the female body and her re-working of philosophical understandings of form and matter.

The absence of a clear-cut sex/gender distinction in Irigaray's work is thus not merely a linguistic accident, but reflects a deep commitment to undoing the traditional oppositions between mind and body, nature and culture, form and matter, in ways that are central to Irigaray's project. Instead of the sex/gender distinction then, we need to sensitize ourselves to the notion of 'sexuate difference' which is neither grounded in nature nor imposed by culture, but articulates both nature and culture, and the relations between them. The question Irigaray poses is whether – as individuals or collectively – we seek modes of being which cultivate the sexuate, or whether we obliterate the articulations of sexual difference under the demand of sameness. This book will show why Irigaray thinks that the history of western philosophy is one of obliteration (what she calls 'dereliction') that has been especially damaging for women; at the same time, it will seek to show how Irigaray begins to elaborate the terms for a philosophy of difference that would allow women to become subjects themselves, without sacrificing their sexuate specificity.

Given her critique of the way the subject has traditionally been constituted via the exclusion of a (female) other, Irigaray also has to allay the concern that *any* notion of the subject, sexuate or not, risks reinscribing a logic of identity that inevitably depends on the exclusion of difference. Thus, just as important as the question of how women can become subjects is the question of how to think men as 'other' to women without defining male otherness as the negation of female subjectivity – that is, without positioning men

as lacking something women have or are. Such a reductive definition would repeat the very logic of the same which Irigaray is
seeking to displace. This is where Irigaray's distinctive approach
to the question of irreducible otherness (or alterity) plays a crucial
role. The claim that the so-called 'universal' subject is in fact implicitly male is well established in feminist philosophy (not least due
to Irigaray's own work), as is the idea that this subject has been
constituted against woman who has historically been ascribed the
position of man's 'other'. However, it is less often noted that this
means that the project of undoing the supposed neutrality of
the subject must be accompanied by undoing the supposed neutrality of the 'other'. If the subject is never neutral, neither is the
'other'. In place of the myth of undetermined, amorphous otherness, Irigaray seeks to recover the specificity of singular and always
sexuate others, for it is by attending to the specificity of an other's
alterity that I prevent myself from judging them only on my own
terms, as 'more' or 'less' different from me. Such modes of judging
continue to adhere to an ideal of sameness and cover over the possibility of relating to the other *as* other: that is, as irreducible to my
terms. Hence, in addition to a culture of two sexuate subjects, we
need to recognize the sexuate specificity of 'the other', so that
instead of being defined in relation to a single male subject, otherness can be approached by both sexuate subjects, male or female.
It is the ethical responsibility of each of these subjects to cultivate
ways of relating to others without negating or assimilating their
differences. Thus, if finding a positive account of sexual difference
is 'one of the major philosophical issues, if not the issue, of our age'
(*ESD*, 5), then 'to positively construct alterity between [the sexes]
is a task for our time' (*ILTY*, 62).

Reading Irigaray: Shifts, Continuities, Criticisms

It is worth noting (as Irigaray herself does) that the concern with
alterity *between* the sexes is already present in *Speculum* (see *DBT*,
137). This is important because of the way Irigaray's work is often
characterized as falling into three broad periods – indeed, Irigaray
herself often describes her work in these terms. Thus, her early
writings (including *Speculum*, first published in French in 1974)
tend to be seen as primarily offering a critical deconstruction of the
tradition, and as leading into a second phase that focuses more
positively on the elaboration of a distinctively female identity; this

in turn is seen as preceding a further shift in the essays of the late 1980s and 1990s, away from female subjectivity per se and towards a greater emphasis on the political as well as the relation between the sexes. This emphasis on the cultivation of a sexuate social and political world continues into Irigaray's most recent work, though some of her key texts from 2000 onwards have also been marked by a return to a more extended engagement with philosophical texts and thinkers.

Such divisions are a helpful working guide to the development of Irigaray's thought; nonetheless, they tend to obscure the continuities which run through her work and, in particular, the extent to which the issues that occupy her later writings are already prefigured in the earlier texts, where her engagement with them is often well underway. Thus it is worth noting that when Irigaray describes her own work in terms of three distinct phases, her descriptions often highlight the continuity of concern underlying these phases as much as the shifts in emphasis. In 'The Question of the Other', for example, the first phase of her project, which critiques woman's reduction to the 'other' of man, is also described in terms of *'free[ing] the two from the one'*; the second, which foregrounds the cultivation of a female subject, is described as returning to 'the reality of the *two*'; while the third, which attends to how this feminine subject might relate to *her* other, explores the alterity between the sexes required for a genuine culture of two (*DBT*, 129; 131; 137–9). Thus, through the shifts in emphasis, there is a continued focus on the need to substitute 'the *two* for the *one* in sexual difference'. This organizing thread is, for Irigaray, the 'decisive philosophical and political gesture', a gesture 'in favour of *being-two* as the necessary foundation of a new ontology, a new ethics and a new politics in which the other is recognized as other and not as the same' (*DBT*, 141).

In keeping with this, my overall approach in this book will be to read Irigaray's work against the backdrop of this continued concern with creating a culture of sexuate difference, or of *'being-two'*. The latter has itself been the subject of criticism in recent debates. Thinkers sympathetic to Irigaray's project of recognizing female specificity have nonetheless been uneasy with her emphasis on *'being-two'* because of the way this can seem to reinforce the normative heterosexism of the very culture she critiques. Others are equally uneasy about Irigaray's explicit privileging of sexuate difference above other kinds of difference (including race), at least in terms of its metaphysical and ontological significance: the worry is that while Irigaray may not be a biological essentialist, she seems close to being an ontological one. I will return to these criticisms in the final two chapters of this book. However, for now I wish to situate my approach in relation to that taken by Maria Cimitile and Elaine Miller in the introduction to their co-edited volume, *Returning to Irigaray*. While taking seriously the suggestion that there is a conceptual break or 'turn' between Irigaray's earlier and later writings, Cimitile and Miller also argue that 'although the shifts in Irigaray's later works may be more immediately striking to readers than their continuities, as scholars of Irigaray's thought we cannot read these writings out of context, but must foster a dialogue around the question of just *how* the political focus of Irigaray's recent thought emerges.'[9] This echoes a view already expressed in Margaret Whitford's *Irigaray Reader*, that the meaning of Irigaray's later texts 'depends on the complex analysis and infrastructure of the earlier work'.[10] Along similar lines, I would suggest both that the philosophical dimensions of Irigaray's thinking remain as important to her later work as its political focus, and that we cannot fully understand her later texts without taking into account the philosophical work already undertaken which informs and sustains them – work which some of her most recent texts, such as *The Way of Love* or *Sharing the World*, explicitly extend. As Whitford and others have also noted, the more direct style of some of Irigaray's later essays poses its own challenges: their apparent straightforwardness can belie the complexity of thought which has led to such distilled arguments, and which means that familiar terms (such as 'nature') are often being used in quite unfamiliar ways.[11]

Like Cimitile and Miller, I do not seek to take up a position on the question of the 'turn' as such; instead, this book aims to equip readers to approach Irigaray's later writings in ways that are more informed by an understanding of the key claims and commitments of her earlier work. In turn, my own approach has been centrally informed by the work of other interpreters who have explored the philosophical dimensions of Irigaray's project, particularly Tina Chanter, Elizabeth Grosz, Cathryn Vasseleu, and Margaret Whitford. As Carolyn Burke observes, it is thanks to the in-depth analyses offered by such thinkers that '[Irigaray's] rethinking of philosophy could be seen as the ground of her other forms of critique.'[12] Indeed, in many ways, this book seeks to take up a space opened by Whitford's *Luce Irigaray: Philosophy in the Feminine* and expanded by texts such as Chanter's *Ethics of Eros*. Together these works fulfil Whitford's aim of enabling us to see Irigaray not only as a philosopher, but 'as a *feminist philosopher* with the emphasis on *both* terms'.[13] Whitford's monograph also provides an initial answer to my opening questions: the specificity of Irigaray's approach lies in the way she does philosophy 'in the feminine'. In this book, I seek to expand our understanding of this distinctive mode of philosophizing and thereby to make a further contribution to the shared project of delineating 'the philosophical import of Irigaray's rereading of both philosophy and feminism.'[14]

This project has recently been expanded by the important – and very different – interpretations of Irigaray's later work offered by Penelope Deutscher, in *A Politics of Impossible Difference*, and Alison Stone, in *Luce Irigaray and the Philosophy of Sexual Difference*. These texts are exemplary insofar as they each show how Irigaray's thought can productively be taken forward in ways that are both generous and critically nuanced. My approach is influenced by both readings, though it also differs from both in some key respects. Thus, I agree with Stone that Irigaray's project involves a thoroughgoing rethinking of the form/matter distinction such that matter actively participates in a fluid generation of forms.[15] However, Stone argues that this rethinking of matter results in the emergence of a (more consistent) realist essentialism in Irigaray's later work; by contrast, in Chapter 6, I suggest that Irigaray's conception of active matter more fully displaces the essentialist charge, in ways that are connected to her claims about the ontological status of sexuate difference. Equally, I agree with Deutscher that sexual difference for Irigaray is that which has been foreclosed by the tradition and thus, is a difference which we are called on to anticipate, rather than to recognize as if it were something already in existence. However, where Deutscher suggests that Irigaray is at her best when she leaves both the ontological status and the specific content of the term 'sexual difference' completely open, such that it operates as a pair of 'empty brackets',[16] I would argue that sexuate difference for Irigaray *is* that which brackets our existence, insofar as it is the condition of possibility of our (coming into) being. The significance of sexuate difference can therefore be specified without treating it as a determinate object or thing. Thus, while I agree that a culture of sexuate difference is as yet only an anticipated possibility, I think Irigaray's philosophy positions this possibility as both less hypothetical and more realizable than Deutscher might allow.

By drawing on the philosophically informed readings offered by previous interpreters, I hope this book will take others to their work, as well as to the illuminating essays in both *Returning to*

Irigaray and the earlier collection, *Engaging with Irigaray*, co-edited by Whitford, Carolyn Burke, and Naomi Schor.[17] As many of these readings show, the more explicitly philosophical aspects of Irigaray's work remain inextricable from her concerns with psychoanalysis, politics, language, religion, and pedagogy. Thus, along the way, I will also refer to theorists who put Irigaray's thought to work in these and other fields – including architecture, art, queer theory, literature, film, and theology. Finally, however, this book aims not only to offer a guide to Irigaray's work as a feminist philosopher, but also to show why her work should be of particular interest to those engaged with the history of philosophy – whether from a specifically feminist perspective or not. Irigaray's relation to this history is complex: on the one hand, her readings of thinkers such as Plato, Descartes, and Kant provide support for her identification of a general pattern in western thought whereby woman has been treated as object and 'other' for a male subject, while her female specificity has been erased through a logic of sexual *indifference*. On the other, she does not claim that this pattern, powerful though it is, constitutes a complete account of the history of philosophy and is attentive to the potential within the tradition for approaching difference otherwise, as her readings of Plato and Descartes also show. Moreover, Irigaray never claims that her own readings are themselves 'indifferent'. They begin from the presumption that sexuate difference is worth cultivating. Her dialogues with the key figures in the western tradition should thus not be read as seeking to offer the 'true' interpretation of their texts; indeed, it is worth remembering that Irigaray's main aim is to find ways of rethinking sexual difference, not to add to the existing scholarship on canonical figures. Nonetheless, what is exciting is the fresh philosophical perspective that often emerges by re-reading canonical texts through the lens of sexual difference. Such readings tell us as much about the limits and possibilities for thinking sexuate difference as they do about the philosophies of Plato, Descartes, and Kant – but they also open up new possibilities for approaching central philosophical questions about human beings, our values, and the world we inhabit.

Chapter Outline

The first chapter of this book offers an expanded frame for approaching Irigaray, paying particular attention to her relation to the history of philosophy as well as to feminist philosophy and the challenges of doing philosophy as a woman. The emphasis will be on the transformative aspects of her approach, as well as on the crucial issue of her style for, as Burke notes, we should read Irigaray's work 'not only as thought *about* sexual difference but an attempt to bring that difference *into* language.'[18]

As indicated above, this book takes *Speculum of the Other Woman* as its guiding thread. Chapter 2 thus begins with a more specific introduction to *Speculum*, as well as to the Platonic roots of western thought which are so thoroughly and critically investigated in that text. The chapter focuses in particular on Irigaray's extended re-reading of Plato's Myth of the Cave. For Irigaray, this myth reveals the fundamental repression and appropriation of the maternal that lies at the origins of western metaphysics. The chapter shows how her reading both justifies this claim and works to destabilize Plato's grounding myth from within, opening the way towards a philosophy more capable of valuing both mothers and women.

Chapter 3 continues the analysis of Irigaray's engagement with Plato, drawing on her readings of other Platonic texts, such as *Timaeus* and *Symposium*. A key aim of this chapter is to show the extent of the transformation Irigaray is seeking, and why for her, the project of generating a philosophy of sexual difference is insep-arable from transforming the fundamental terms of western meta-physical thought, particularly those concerning the relation between form and matter. I show how Irigaray re-appropriates some of the terms for this transformative project from Plato's own texts, not only in *Speculum* but also in her later analysis of Diotima's speech from Plato's *Symposium*. In contrast to the Pla-tonic privileging of the eternal sameness of unchanging Forms, Irigaray re-assesses Diotima's speech to recover a fecund becom-ing nurtured in the relation between two who are irreducibly dif-ferent. Whereas the Forms are only accessible through the death of the body, this relational becoming acts as an affirmative repetition of birth.

In Chapter 4, I show how Irigaray's critical analysis extends beyond Plato and across the western tradition via the work of Aristotle, Plotinus, and – in particular – Descartes and Kant. The chapter explores the ways in which Irigaray deploys the perspec-tive of sexual difference to generate original and deepened critical readings of these well-known figures. Her analyses show how, in different ways, both the Cartesian self and the Kantian subject remain dependent on a female other while simultaneously disavowing that dependence. In contrast, Irigaray's writing continually makes visible her own project's dependence on her male forefathers, whose voices she explicitly draws upon and transformatively contests. She is thus able to acknowledge her debt to them without allowing them to determine her own project. It is in this spirit that, in her later text *An Ethics of Sexual Difference*, she takes up Descartes' notion of wonder. As Chapter 4 shows, for Irigaray, wonder allows for a non-appropriative relation to the other, and hence holds open a space in which the sexes might encounter one other in their irreducible difference.

Chapter 5 addresses the significance of Irigaray's engagement with psychoanalysis for her approach to philosophy. It focuses on the role of Freud and Lacan in her project, showing how she simultaneously deploys psychoanalysis to help reveal the gendering of western philosophy, while criticizing Freud and Lacan themselves for repeating and reinforcing woman's traditional position as 'other'. Contra Lacan, Irigaray seeks a space for an other woman, irreducible to the other of the male subject, and instead affirmed in her difference and specificity. Such a figure emerges as a possible subject when the (traditional) 'object' of male desire refuses her allocated role of passive complicity and begins to speak. Hence, this chapter also returns to the key issue of Irigaray's style, to explore both the risks it involves and the critical transformations it enables her to generate.

These issues are taken up again in Chapter 6, in the context of Irigaray's textual appeals to the female body in figures such as the two lips and the placental economy. These figures play a key role in Irigaray's quest for a female subject who is neither the same as, nor defined against, her male counterpart, but articulated in her own terms. In this chapter, I argue that such figural appeals to the female body are not reductively 'essentialist' as some critics have claimed. Far from positioning women as passively determined by their bodies and biology, these figures contribute to the project of articulating woman as a sexuate subject for whom materiality and agency are no longer opposed. The chapter suggests that for the transformative force of such figures to be fully appreciated, they need to be read in the context of Irigaray's thoroughgoing challenge to the traditional form/matter distinction as well as her re-working of the self–other relation.

Instead of reading her textual appeals to the female body as attempts to find 'true' representations of woman, I suggest that they are better understood in terms of an ethical relation; more specifically, drawing on Irigaray's relation to Heidegger, I position such appeals as an instantiation of an ethical poetics – or rather, of poetics as the potential site of a feminist ethics. The chapter concludes by examining the claim that Irigaray's later work betrays her emphasis on female specificity by succumbing to a form of heterosexism. While I suggest this criticism is largely (though not wholly) misplaced, there are important lessons to be learned from this debate. In the course of addressing it, I seek to clarify both Irigaray's notion of *genre* and her claims about the ontological status of sexuate difference. In turn, however, these claims lead to further concerns about the privileging of the sexuate over other kinds of difference, especially those of race, to which I return in the next and final chapter.

Chapter 7 takes up Irigaray's concern with the ethical, and in particular, with establishing an ethics of sexual difference. In a final reading of *Speculum*, the chapter begins by examining Irigaray's engagement with Hegel. Particular attention is paid to the ways in which she plays Hegel's reading of *Antigone* off against Lacan's so as to release woman from her entombment in the figure of the m/other of the male subject. This generative response leads to Irigaray's notion of a 'double dialectic' as well as her rethinking of the role of the negative. The chapter goes on to outline the continued significance of Antigone across Irigaray's later writings before pursuing the question of ethics via the critical yet fecund dialogue that Irigaray conducts with the work of Immanuel Levinas, whose notion of alterity becomes a key thread in Irigaray's later writings. I argue that, for Irigaray, rethinking woman's relation to herself in ways that acknowledge the irreducibility of sexual difference is a condition for acknowledging the irreducible alterity of others. In other words, according to Irigaray, an ethics of sexual difference is the condition of ethical relations in general. The implications of this view are critically examined in relation to both Irigaray's own comments on race and cultural difference, and the question of how an ethics of sexual difference that seeks to release woman from her role as man's 'other' might remain open – and hence, ethically responsive – to other 'others' in the western tradition.

The book concludes by returning to Irigaray's understanding of being (as) two. Far from trapping us within a fixed binary of male–female relations, I suggest that Irigaray's account of 'being two' opens onto a thinking of difference and sexuate specificity that cannot be captured in any dualism or opposition. The thought that (human) being *is* two makes it impossible to quantify (human) being(s) *as* two, and instead calls on us to nurture and protect an incalculable difference.

Note on Translation

As this book is designed for those working in an English-speaking context, I have used the standard English translations of Irigaray's work. While I have occasionally amended these to foreground a particular philosophical nuance, I am nonetheless indebted to the original translators, and in particular, to Gillian Gill for translating *Speculum*. Given the linguistic inventiveness of Irigaray's writings, some nuances are inevitably lost in translation, although others are often gained.[19] I hope that this book will encourage those who can to turn to the original French (or sometimes Italian) texts to rediscover Irigaray's words for themselves.

1

Approaching Irigaray: Feminism, Philosophy, Feminist Philosophy

Approaching Irigaray's texts is a complex matter, not least because of their extraordinary range. However, as this book seeks to engage with Irigaray primarily as a feminist philosopher, this chapter will offer a frame for approaching her work through her contested relations to both feminism and philosophy, drawing attention to the ways in which she seeks to transform both. Irigaray argues that the dominant theoretical and philosophical frameworks of western culture have continually positioned *woman* as object and other for a male subject. Her project is therefore to transform that theory and culture in ways that make it possible for *women* to take up a position as subjects in their own right. Negotiating the relations between (objectified, idealized) 'woman' and (singular, flesh and blood) 'women' is thus an integral part of her task. Irigaray challenges the reductive theoretical construction of *woman* as 'other' because of the ways this erases the sexed specificity of actual *women*. Instead, she is seeking to *parler femme*, a phrase that can be translated as both 'to speak woman' and 'speaking (*as a*) woman'. By way of a pun (*par les femmes*), the French also suggests that speaking (as a) woman is something that needs to be done 'by women', that is, among and between them.[1] *Parler femme* speaks of a way of articulating the female sex that would allow women to take up the position of speaking subjects themselves, and thereby to relate to one another as women, whose differences and similarities can be registered without mediation through a male voice.

Nonetheless, as she is acutely aware, Irigaray's own position as a theorist writing *about* women *as* a woman is problematic from the start, as the following passage indicates: 'We can assume that any theory of the subject has always been appropriated by the "masculine". When she submits to (such a) theory, woman fails to realize that she is renouncing the specificity of her own relationship to the imaginary. Subjecting herself to objectivization in discourse – by being "female"' (S, 133). How can a woman write about women without re-objectivizing them (or herself)? How might she theorize a female 'subject' if being 'a subject' means taking up a masculine position? And is it possible for her to theorize *as* a woman at all? If woman 'renounces her specificity' in submitting to theory, one of the challenges Irigaray faces is how to engage in theoretical analysis without subordinating herself to the masculine in the process. Thus, before we can begin to approach what Irigaray has to say, we need to examine how she negotiates the problems involved in producing theory 'about' women at all, especially as a woman.

In fact, the ways in which Irigaray negotiates this issue are inseparable from her transformative project. This is exemplified in the text through which we will approach Irigaray in this book. In *Speculum of the Other Woman*, Irigaray shows how woman has been excluded, appropriated, objectified, or otherwise devalued in western philosophical thought. To do this, she does not simply take up and work with the conceptual framework this philosophical tradition provides. Nor does she seek to re-accommodate woman within its terms. At the same time, she does not simply turn the tables on the tradition, distancing herself from masculine discourse in order to make it the object of her own analysis: such a reversal would continue to mimic the tradition by keeping the subject/object opposition in place.

Instead, Irigaray takes up key texts and voices from the tradition in ways that subvert their words from within. By asking questions and exposing blindspots, she twists their dense theoretical fabric around until it reveals its dependence on making woman both 'object' and 'other'. Given the oppositional logic on which such thinking relies, pitting subject against object and self against other, Irigaray's writing seeks to disrupt all such dichotomies:

Nothing is ever to be *posited* that is not also reversed and caught up again in the *supplementarity of this reversal*. To put it another way: there would no longer be either a right side or a wrong side of discourse, or even of texts, but each passing from one to the other would make audible and comprehensible even what resists the recto-verso structure that shores up common sense. (*TS*, 79–80)

Thus a key part of Irigaray's style lies in her disruption of conceptual oppositions such as form/matter, self/other, and of course, male/female. She achieves this partly by showing how in these conceptual couples, one side excludes and determines the other while nonetheless remaining dependent upon it. This undoes their apparent opposition along with the supposed self-sufficiency of the prioritized term. But it also shows how each term in a binary relation relies on the space *between*, which makes the distinction of one and another possible while resisting capture by a logic that insists on dividing everything up into 'one' (side) or the 'other'.

To avoid remaining trapped in such a logic herself, in *Speculum* Irigaray adopts a style in which she refuses to take up one position consistently against another, shifting instead between multiple voices and holding contradictory claims alongside one another. Nonetheless, this project of unsettling opposites is not merely negative. Rather, Irigaray is seeking to cultivate the passages and in-between spaces which resist such oppositional terms and thereby hold open the promise of a different, more fluid logic of relation. It is this positive dimension of Irigaray's project that distinguishes her from more strictly deconstructive approaches, despite the clearly deconstructive aspects of her work. Thus, Irigaray exploits the often contradictory representations of woman within philosophical texts not only to disrupt their apparent coherence, but at the same time to weave together a different voice, whose complexity slips between the accepted terms of philosophical discourse and can no longer be reduced to the mere opposite or other of a male subject. Such inventiveness results in a style that is at once deliberately disruptive and creatively constructive. It is nicely captured by Irigaray's own description of the language through which it might be possible to speak (as a) woman:

> Hers are contradictory words, somewhat mad from the standpoint of reason, inaudible for whoever listens to them with ready-made grids, with a fully elaborated code in hand. ... One would have to listen with another ear, as if hearing *an 'other meaning' always in the process of weaving itself, of embracing itself with words, but also of getting rid of words in order not to become fixed, congealed in them.* (*TS*, 29)

Seeking to write philosophy as a woman is one way of allowing woman to speak. *Speculum* is above all a performative text: what it says finds its fullest articulation in the way it is written. Thus, we will continue to pay attention to *how* Irigaray writes as well as to the ideas she seeks to convey.

The Importance of Style

In *Speculum*, Irigaray does not construct clearly defined arguments, or comment on the philosophical canon with a critically distanced voice. Instead, she weaves her own voice in and out of those of Plato and Freud, Lacan and Kant, quoting long passages verbatim, asking questions, and ironically taking up the language of her philosophical forefathers in a subversive mimicry that draws out its latent tensions and blindspots.

By remaining attentive to the multi-valence of Irigaray's voice and complexities of her style, this book will try to avoid giving an account of her project that simply reconceptualizes it in traditional philosophical terms. Indeed, one of Irigaray's most important claims is that forging the terms with which to think woman in her specificity is inseparably bound up with transforming the terms of western metaphysical thought. Hence the difficulty of writing 'about' woman: any such project will tend to get trapped back into a model that opposes a theorizing (masculine) subject to a theorized (female) object. To disrupt this framework so as to allow a woman to speak of and for herself (as well as to other women) without simply mapping her onto a male subject position, would mean answering Irigaray's central question: 'what if the "object" started to speak?' (*S*, 135). Such a possibility confounds the traditional framework by ascribing the activity of speaking to the object, rather than the subject, of discourse. At the same time, it displaces the traditional metaphysical oppositions between mind and body, reason and matter, by refusing to separate woman as a subject from her material, corporeal ('object-like') existence.

The double perspective such a project requires is exemplified in an essay from *This Sex Which Is Not One*, the volume that in many ways can be read as accompanying *Speculum*. In 'The Power of Discourse' Irigaray notes that: 'the issue is not one of elaborating a new theory of which woman would be the *subject* or the *object*, but of jamming the theoretical machinery itself' (*TS*, 78). Yet a few pages later, she asks what changes *would* be required for women to become speaking subjects themselves (*TS*, 85). On the one hand, this is a good example of the way that Irigaray puts theory into practice by not 'positing' something herself without almost immediately reversing it. As she says, when woman speaks, her words seem to overturn themselves in ways that are 'somewhat mad from the standpoint of reason'. On the other hand, such apparent contradictions are symptomatic of the radicality of the transformation required to speak (as a) woman. Read together, Irigaray's comments suggest that it *would* be possible for women to become speaking subjects so long as they were no longer trapped by a framework in which each was *either* a subject *or* an object. Such a subject would be more like a 'speaking object'. But in fact she could no longer be adequately theorized in terms of the subject/object dichotomy that has structured modern western thought.

We will return to Irigaray's critical analysis of this structure in the chapters that follow. For now it is worth noting that, whereas the masculine subject is reliant on an 'other' defined in his own terms, Irigaray often uses the same words to say several different things at once. Thus the difficulty of quoting her work to support a reading or interpretation. In so doing, one always runs the risk of identifying her text with a single meaning where there are several; in turn, this risks pulling her work back into the very conceptual framework she is resisting, where the quest for unity and identity privileges the 'one' at the expense of others who are thereby excluded.

This book will take the risk of quoting extensively from Irigaray, and in particular from her most multivalent work, *Speculum*. However, in working closely with her texts, it will seek to remain attentive to the ways in which several different things are often being said at once, in words that are almost always at least double in meaning. In so doing, I hope to at least mitigate 'the danger of every statement, every discussion, *about Speculum*', statements which, as Irigaray herself notes, run the risk of being just as reductive as 'every discussion *about* the question of woman' (*TS*, 78). Instead of reducing *Speculum* to one meaning rather than another, this book will seek to aid the reader in distinguishing some of the many different threads that run through Irigaray's work so as to be better able to hold them together. It will seek to develop an ear for those *other meanings* that are *always in the process of weaving themselves* and through which Irigaray forges a language both for thinking differently and for thinking sexual difference. The analysis will be necessarily incomplete, but in ways that I hope will leave openings for others to find further transformative layers of meaning as they read and re-read Irigaray's texts for themselves.

Irigaray and Philosophy

In approaching Irigaray as a 'feminist philosopher', then, what matters is the transformative effect each of these terms has on the other: both the way Irigaray's feminist project transforms philosophy, and the way her path through philosophy inflects her feminism. This inflection is not just a result of the conceptual resources that Irigaray manages to steal away from western philosophers to aid her feminist project. It is also a result of the position she forges as a feminist who wants to keep doing philosophy, despite its patriarchal or masculinist history.

In fact, Irigaray's negotiation of a critical yet non-oppositional relation to philosophy is indicative of the kind of feminism she espouses: one that seeks to make space for (sexual) difference without reinscribing a reductive logic of opposition and negation. Indeed, it is this logic itself that is the problem insofar as it generates dichotomies that are governed by only one of their terms, and thus by what Irigaray calls a 'logic of the Same'. Accordingly, it is this logic which defines woman in terms of her difference *from* a male subject, and hence positions her as the *other* of the Same.[2] As Irigaray repeatedly insists, merely reversing the hierarchical opposition between the sexes – defining man in terms of his failure to be a woman, for example, or replacing patriarchy with matriarchy – would not be a real solution, but merely a repetition of such oppositional structures of thought.

Irigaray's position is doubly risky: on the one hand, some feminists will be suspicious of the very act of engaging with the 'master discourse' of philosophy in anything but a thoroughly critical way. From this perspective, Irigaray's desire to '*have a fling with the philosophers*' looks suspiciously like complicity with her oppressors (*TS*, 150). On the other hand, Irigaray's explicitly feminist orientation will tempt some philosophers to claim that her own approach is 'biased' in ways that distort the philosophical texts with which she engages. Irigaray thus runs the risk of being the doubly undutiful daughter: mistrusted by the philosophers, yet regarded with suspicion by her feminist sisters because of her passion for philosophy.[3]

I do not wish to deny that Irigaray's position is risky – but the stakes, as she would be the first to concede, are high: they concern nothing less than the question of being, and thus, the nature of human being. The question, for Irigaray, is whether we think being in terms of any kind of oneness, unified essence or identity, or whether we allow that being – and thus, human being – is two. Moreover, we should not presume we already know what this *'being-two'* means, for as I discuss in the Conclusion, Irigaray suggests that it resists normal systems of calculation by being irreducible to 'two times one'. Instead, the 'being' of *'being-two'* is found *in-between*.

Rather than deny that Irigaray's thought is biased by her feminism, we should look more closely at what is at stake in that so-called bias. Irigaray interrogates philosophy from a critical feminist perspective because of a bias that she argues is *already* built in to the dominant forms philosophy has taken in the western tradition since Plato; thus, *her* bias is corrective. Moreover, the pre-existing masculinist bias she identifies is grounded on a series of blindspots and denials that protect philosophy's own self-image: thus it is hardly surprising that some philosophers respond to Irigaray defensively. By accusing her of introducing a biased perspective, they can continue to remain blind to the ways in which philosophy itself has been dependent on the denial of difference, and specifically, the difference that woman embodies.

However, there is another reason why Irigaray poses a genuinely disturbing challenge to the philosophers. Her 'corrective' feminist perspective does not aim to cancel out a historically contingent but 'improper' masculinism in the name of establishing a 'proper' universal, neutral, or objective mode of thought. Were this the case, her position really would be re-absorbed by a model of philosophy that is the product and symptom of the very perspective she critiques. Rather, her aim is to challenge a masculinism that masquerades as universal, and an ideal of universality that masks an inadequate articulation of the nature of (human) being. In response, Irigaray calls into question the very idea that a universal or 'neutral' way of thinking could properly do justice to human beings. Instead, what is required is 'an ontology founded on "being two"' (*BEW*, 101): an account of being that takes sexual difference as primary in ways that allow us to acknowledge two different (sexuate) subjects. Thus her irreverent approach remains properly 'improper': not only does she reveal philosophy's own pre-existing bias, but she denies that philosophy has the resources to correct that bias, unless it is prepared to change its own nature and give up its commitment to an ideal universalism.

Of course, there are many modes of philosophizing that critique or reject universalism. Indeed, this rejection is taken to characterize a cluster of philosophies with which Irigaray herself is sometimes aligned, namely, those commonly grouped together under the label of 'postmodernism'. Broadly speaking, postmodern thinkers can be described as rejecting the Enlightenment ideals of progress and truth by undermining its faith in a universalizing reason as well as a rational and autonomous subject. This has lent itself to an image of the postmodern philosopher as dissolving the modern individual in a celebration of desire and the non-rational that irresponsibly undermines the basis for moral and political values, culminating in a dangerous nihilism. Such an image, however, is little more than another defensive caricature, incapable of doing justice to the subtleties of (and differences between) thinkers such as Lyotard, Baudrillard, Cixous, Derrida – and Irigaray. Indeed, to the extent that her alignment with postmodernism is justifiable, Irigaray herself stands as an exemplar of the ways in which postmodern thinkers are not simply engaged in a reactive undoing of Enlightenment ideals. Rather, they challenge us to think otherwise: to find and *give* value without relying on universalizing judgements that themselves deny the value of difference.

Irigaray's alliance with postmodernism is far from straightforward however. Indeed, one of the remarkable aspects of the reception of her work is the way it has been seen as exemplifying both a particular brand of deconstructive postmodernism and an essentialism that treats sexed identity as biologically determined; two approaches that are profoundly at odds with one another. Like the figure of woman that sustains the operations of traditional philosophy, 'Irigaray' herself comes to be represented in multiple and contradictory ways. My presentation of Irigaray's thought will show that to characterize her work either as 'essentialist' or as entirely 'deconstructive' is to misrepresent it in important respects. Nonetheless, the fact that Irigaray's project can be characterized in such contradictory ways is a further indication of the complexity of the challenge that she poses.

This challenge is not only to philosophy but also to feminism. As a feminist, Irigaray challenges herself to respond critically to philosophy without becoming merely reactive, and to think philosophically without losing the specificity of a voice marked by sexual difference. From this perspective, it is telling that some feminist readers are tempted to divide Irigaray's project into a productively critical and de(con)structive relation to philosophy on the one hand, and a more positive but dangerous essentialism on the other.[4] Such a characterization assumes that the attempt to offer a positive philosophy of female sexual difference will inevitably

reinscribe the traditional masculinist categories of essence and
identity which the critical deconstructive approach undoes, and
from which it is thereby insulated.

However, this does not do justice to Irigaray's own approach,
which does not allow that the only choices are: either, to remain
resolutely critical of philosophy's inherently patriarchal and masculinist logic, and thus to abandon any attempt to philosophize
positively as a feminist; or, to be co-opted once again by philosophy's traditional terms, whether inadvertently, via the implicit re-
inscription of philosophy's central categories, or knowingly, in
explicit demands for inclusion, such as the insistence that women
be given equal status to men as rational and autonomous subjects.
Indeed, if Irigaray refuses to concede the ground of philosophy to
masculinist thinking, this is not because she seeks to prove that
women are 'just as rational' as men, but rather because – along with
a number of other feminists – she calls into question philosophy's
account of the rational, along with the way reason is typically
structured against the material, the bodily, and the affective, as well
as the 'female' and the 'feminine'.[5] Rather than abandon philosophy, Irigaray's irreverence refuses philosophy's identification with
patriarchal thinking, and seeks entry for women on their own
terms in ways that demand that the fundamental categories of
philosophy be re-thought. In Irigaray's work, the critical is inseparable from the creative: her project seeks to transform and renew
philosophical thought as much as to attack its historically dominant masculinist instantiations.

Transforming Philosophy as a Feminist Project

It is this renewal of philosophy through the transformation of its
fundamental categories which makes Irigaray's project so distinctive and far-reaching. One of the key aims of this book is to highlight the extent of the transformations such a renewal would
necessitate. The outcome of such change cannot be fully predicted
or imagined, but remains exciting open territory for further thought.
Nonetheless, Irigaray's project is guided by a number of key principles, which are rooted in an affirmation of sexual difference and
in the importance of recovering the value and significance of that
difference for the ways in which we live. More specifically, Irigaray
argues that as well as positioning woman as the object and other
for a male subject, western thought and culture has systematically

displaced the significance of our maternal origins, of the way we come into the world through birth from a mother. Thus, running through her project are two central concerns: the need to recover the significance of maternal generative power, and the need for women to be recognized as subjects in their own right, that is, in ways that do justice to their sexed specificity. A key aim of this book is to show how these two guiding threads re-emerge across Irigaray's work and shape her engagement with different philo-sophical thinkers.

As we will see, these two guiding threads are not only closely related, but mutually interdependent. To seek a subject position for women without rethinking the significance of birth would inevita-bly lead to the repetition of the failings of the tradition, which has been unable to take the sexed nature of human beings seriously because it does not adequately attend to the way our existence is rooted in material relations with the sexed body of the mother. Without attending to these relations along with our inescapably corporeal beginnings, the sexed specificity of human beings, and thus of woman herself, remains obscured. But at the same time, to focus exclusively on the recovery of our maternal origins is to risk perpetuating the wholesale identification of women with their maternal roles, especially within a western tradition which, as Irigaray herself shows, has tended to reduce women (and the generative power of birth) to no more than a reproductive function. Unless we find the terms with which to articulate a female subject position that is no longer defined as the other of the male, it remains impossible to acknowledge in a meaningful way that those who are mothers are also women, and thus fully fledged subjects in their own right, with lives that are not reducible to maternal roles or reproductive functions. As Elizabeth Grosz puts it in her account of Irigaray's key aims:

> The debt of materiality, life, existence, that both men and women owe to the mother *cannot* be paid back, it cannot be reciprocated. But in exchange for this life which comes from the mother's body, the child/father/culture must acknowledge that, beyond her maternal roles, the mother is also a woman, a subject, with a life, sex and desires of her own. The mother cannot be entirely consumed in/by maternity. The excess or remainder left over is her specificity as a woman.[6]

Irigaray shows that making space for this sexed specificity in our social, political and cultural forms of life means re-working the fundamental conceptual categories of western thought. As we will see in more detail in later chapters of this book, we cannot think woman as subject and free her from being reduced to an object of male desire without *re*thinking the concepts of subject and object, as well as our models of desire; we cannot think woman's sexed specificity as integral to her existence *as* a subject without *re*thinking the traditionally oppositional relation between mind and body, reason and the senses; and we cannot allow for the full significance of our beginnings in birth without reconsidering philosophical accounts of origin, as well as the way our natal beginnings challenge and transform traditional models for thinking about the relation of self and other.

In this book, I will argue that one of the most important philosophical distinctions which Irigaray challenges us to rethink is that between form and matter. Indeed, her work shows that rethinking the form–matter relation is a crucial feminist project. Despite the many variations between different philosophical systems since Plato, one of the relative constants of western thought has been the centrality of hylomorphism as a way of explaining how individuated entities come into being. On the hylomorphic model, such entities are the result of the imposition of form on otherwise unformed or disorganized matter; in contrast to active form-giving powers, matter is seen as receptive, passive, and inert. Philosophers such as Nietzsche, Bergson, and Heidegger – and more recently, Deleuze – have challenged the dominance of this mode of thinking, displacing the form/matter distinction in favour of other explanatory concepts (such as life or creation) and re-aligning matter with active processes of generation, emergence and becoming. What is distinctive about Irigaray's contribution to these debates is her extended analysis of the ways in which the hylomorphic tradition typically aligns sensible matter with woman while representing the active power to give this matter form as masculine and male. Her analyses show that it is not possible to offer a thoroughgoing critique of the form/matter divide without also critiquing its historical gendering: otherwise, this gendering – in which feminine matter provides the resources for active male creativity – will simply reinscribe itself elsewhere.[7] Equally, however, while feminist thinkers do need to challenge the alignments form/masculine/male and matter/feminine/female, this on its own is not enough. It is the form/matter divide itself which needs to be challenged: but challenged from a perspective attentive to sexual difference. Indeed, for Irigaray, sexual difference provides the most compelling reason for seeking to undo the form/matter divide: if we are to recognize sexed embodiment as playing an active role in shaping individual lives and cultural forms, and if we are to recognize the female body's capacity to birth as an active generative power, then it is essential that we re-conceptualize matter as both active and capable of *generating* form/s.

Irigaray and Feminist Philosophies: Equality and Difference

It is thus central to Irigaray's approach that women's position in western culture cannot be changed without changing the underlying conceptual framework that informs that culture. For this reason, she differs significantly from some other feminist thinkers with whom she may nonetheless share many immediate goals. This includes one of her most important feminist foremothers, Mary Wollstonecraft. Irigaray would undoubtedly endorse Wollstonecraft's view that women should not be stunted by an educative process that assumes them to be the less rational but charming helpmeets of male citizens. Moreover, Irigaray's rhetorical strategy of disruptively weaving her own voice through those of her philosophical interlocutors can be read as an extension of Wollstonecraft's approach to Rousseau in the *Vindication of the Rights of Woman* (1792), where she interleaves extensive quotations from Rousseau's *Emile* (1762) with sharp questions and comments of her own so as to parody and undercut his position. However, while Wollstonecraft turns Rousseau against himself to argue that women too should be educated as rational creatures, she does not sufficiently attend to the ways in which his views on education are grounded in his account of human nature and in particular, of the relations between nature and culture, reason and the passions. Without challenging this underlying frame, Wollstonecraft cannot challenge the public-private divide which it legitimates, together with a sexual division of labour that excludes women from full participation in the public sphere. Thus in the end, as Moira Gatens has shown, Wollstonecraft's critique falters.[8] Gatens sums up the underlying problem as follows: 'This tendency to assume the viability of altering what appears to be superstructural parts of a philosopher's work without addressing the foundational assumptions of that work has been common in the history of feminist criticisms of philosophy.'[9] This book hopes to show that Irigaray takes forward the feminist concerns of Wollstonecraft and others without succumbing to this tendency.

Examining Wollstonecraft alongside Irigaray is useful for a further reason: it helps to illuminate why Irigaray is so far from a feminist liberal tradition that seeks equality for women on the same terms traditionally accorded to men, that is, as autonomous rational subjects. Because Wollstonecraft defines human beings in terms of a gender-neutral and essentially disembodied capacity for reason, she seeks recognition that women are just as rational as men. Irigaray and others will argue that because we are neither disembodied nor gender-neutral, this approach not only fails to provide an adequate account of human beings. It also reinscribes the traditional model of the rational subject which only masquerades as gender-neutral, but which is in fact defined against woman and the feminine and thus remains normatively male. Calling for recognition on the same terms as men means calling for women to be (more) *like* men; it implicitly assumes men as the standard of comparison.[10]

For Irigaray, the demand for equality, when posed in these terms, only reinforces a pernicious double-bind: it condemns women to judgement in terms of a standard (that of the male subject) which they can never fulfil without sacrificing their specificity as women, while making it impossible for this specificity to be acknowledged or valued as in any way intrinsic to their status as subjects. Irigaray is thus often aligned with a group of theorists typically described as 'feminists of difference', in contrast to 'feminists of equality'. Such appellations need to be handled with care: it is not so much that Irigaray and others who seek to affirm sexual difference are not concerned with equality,[11] as that they seek to redefine what real equality might consist in: so for example, equal status under the law might mean the ratification of different rights for men and women in ways that take their sexed specificity into account.[12] More fundamentally, ensuring equality – in terms of both rights and opportunities – would mean facing up to Wollstonecraft's blindspot and challenging the sexual division of labour that has informed western socio-political life without assuming that this issue can simply be neutralized by pretending there are no (significant) differences between the sexes. For Irigaray, equal social, political and cultural status for men and women would mean recognizing them as two – *different* – subjects. Thus, the choice between equality and difference is a false one; instead, as Deutscher notes, Irigaray argues 'for an equality based in the affirmation of difference.'[13]

This affirmation is illuminated by Irigaray's comments on her relation to Simone de Beauvoir. To some extent, Irigaray is of course building on de Beauvoir's analysis of the way woman has been positioned as the Other of the male subject in western thought and culture.[14] However, while paying homage to women's debt to de Beauvoir,[15] Irigaray takes up a critically different stance on this issue. Whereas for de Beauvoir, the problem is woman's identification with the Other, for Irigaray, the problem is that woman has not been recognized as 'other' enough: 'Rather than refusing, as Simone de Beauvoir does, to be the other gender, the other sex, I am asking to be recognized as really an other, irreducible to the masculine subject' (*DBT*, 125). Thus for Irigaray, despite being framed in terms of freedom rather than reason, de Beauvoir's positive project (like Wollstonecraft's) still remains trapped by a claim to equality with men. By contrast, Irigaray argues that women's exploitation is based on the difference between the sexes, and thus, can only be addressed by re-valuing sexual difference affirmatively – hence her positioning as a 'feminist philosopher of difference' alongside other key French thinkers such as Hélène Cixous and Julia Kristeva.[16]

These thinkers share a profound wariness of feminisms which seek an identity for women equivalent to that of the unified male subject, and a commitment to reclaiming sexual difference – as well as difference more generally – in positive terms. This means not only refusing the harmful economy whereby *women* are defined wholly in relation to the male subject, but mobilizing the distinctive powers of the feminine to disrupt *any* mode of thinking which positions difference in terms of negation, opposition, or exclusion. In response to such destructive traditions of thought, Irigaray, Cixous and Kristeva insist on the constitutive role of sexual difference in the formation of all subjectivities, those of men and women. Instead of the appropriation and disavowal of difference, their work calls for the cultivation of a risky but transformative openness to the other *as* other.

Despite these shared commitments, the projects of these three thinkers are far from the same. There are as many productive tensions between them as productive resonances. Often they are closer in what they are critiquing – oppositional modes of thought that privilege sameness and deny difference – than in the alternatives they propose. This is entirely appropriate, not only because such alternatives involve projecting paths into the as yet undetermined future, but because it is intrinsic to the kind of future each of them is seeking that it should be open to differences *within*, and hence inclusive of very different ways of being and thinking. Thus, while all three draw attention to the constitutive repression of the maternal body and the feminine in western thought and culture, the ways in which they seek to reclaim this repressed otherness are very different.

To pinpoint these differences, we might think about the relation between Cixous' explorations of a mode of writing that affirms feminine corporeality and desire – what she calls *écriture féminine* – and Irigaray's project of allowing woman to speak (*parler femme*). Both thinkers celebrate the way that, despite the power of phallocentric norms, the feminine remains stubbornly uncontainable by them. However, for Cixous, because the feminine is that which refuses containment in binary oppositions, while it may in some ways be more approachable by women (not least because their bodies can bear the other within in pregnancy and childbirth), the feminine is open to men too. Repressed but irrepressible, the feminine returns to undo unified sexed identity in men and women, releasing them into a fluid bisexuality.[17] Irigaray also affirms the way the feminine resists and exceeds its position as other of the subject,[18] but she does not wish it to remain excessive; instead, her project involves cultivating the feminine into a different kind of subject position, where one might speak *as* a woman. To this extent, Irigaray is not so much seeking to recover a repressed femininity as to invert the position of the feminine *as* other in order to form an other (female) subject.[19]

Kristeva too seeks to mobilize sexual difference to rethink the very notion of the subject. Through her notion of the semiotic, for example, she explores the ceaselessly pulsing drives and energies that pre-exist the infant's awareness of itself as a distinct being, separate from the mother; such rhythmic pulsions provide the material from which symbolic structures are formed, but can also return to disrupt and redirect the structures which they animate.[20] By situating subjectivity as that which emerges and is continually re-emerging in this dynamic interchange, Kristeva works towards an account of the subject as a 'subject-in-process'.[21] As for both Irigaray and Cixous, on this account, the body of the mother is central and generative, providing a paradigm of a mode of being which can live with otherness within. Through the mother, and in particular, the pregnant female body that also gives birth, we can learn how 'the subject can relate to an other as other because she is an other to herself.'[22] Both Irigaray and Kristeva emphasize the ethical urgency of this lesson, which teaches us how to relate to others while neither denying nor assimilating their alterity. However, for Irigaray, the capacity of the mother's body to bear otherness within provides a starting point for thinking a different, and specifically female, subject position. For Kristeva, by contrast, the maternal body reminds us of the alterity that inhabits and unsettles any apparently unified identity; thus, attending to the body of the mother can lead to a deepened awareness of the constitutive heterogeneity of each and every subject, not least because each is seen as incorporating both masculinity and femininity.[23]

Thus, while the work of Kristeva and Cixous should not be conflated, one shared aspect of their thinking might well be a suspicion of the overall direction of Irigaray's project. The question their work points us to is: how can Irigaray call for a female subject position without inevitably reinscribing the exclusion of the other on which the identity of any subject has traditionally depended? This question is helpful because it enables us to see just how revolutionary Irigaray's project is: if she is to succeed, she will need to generate an entirely new way of thinking about the conditions for being (and becoming) a subject. One of the aims of this book is to show the extent to which she does succeed in this aim. As will be shown in later chapters, the first and pivotal claim that makes such a revolutionary shift in our thinking possible is that we cannot give *one* account of the conditions for being a subject: rather, there need to be two such accounts, for two different subjects, neither of whom can lay claim to the status of the universal. Instead, sexual difference itself is the universal which articulates human beings as two.[24]

This claim is simple, yet changes everything. If it is accepted, then there is no longer *one* subject constructed via the exclusion of *its* other, but two subjects, each of which requires an account of its constitution and its relation to otherness, as well as to both nature and culture, and the passage between them. And while of course there is always a risk that the logic of appropriation and exclusion may re-insert itself in one or other of these different processes of self-constitution, it is no longer the case that the very possibility of being a subject is grounded in the necessary exclusion of an other whose own possibilities for being a subject are denied. Instead, difference itself is primary. It manifests itself in the relation between two that means that any subject always already stands in a positive relation to another who offers a different articulation of the possibility of being (and becoming) a subject. The distinctiveness – and riskiness – of Irigaray's project thus lies in her claim that it is possible to develop a culture of two subjects without either being secured through the exclusion of difference.

Irigaray and the History of Philosophy

Subsequent chapters of this book will show in more detail how Irigaray develops the conceptual resources for a culture of two rooted in the recognition of human beings as sexuate. However, in keeping with her attentiveness to our beginnings in birth and concomitant dependence on others, Irigaray recognizes that such a culture cannot spring from nowhere. Her journey through the history of philosophy is a way of reclaiming the resources buried within the tradition for thinking sexual difference positively and thereby cultivating a place for woman as a sexuate subject in her own right.

Such a journey through our philosophical past has become a key resource for many feminist thinkers, allowing them both to generate critical perspectives on the tradition and to recover lost possibilities for thinking (woman) otherwise. In a helpful article, Genevieve Lloyd draws on Richard Rorty's characterization of two typical modes of engaging with the history of philosophy, before outlining a third approach that she suggests is more typical of feminist work. As Lloyd explains, Rorty distinguishes between a 'past-centred' approach, which seeks to understand philosophical work in relation to the specific historical and philosophical context in which it arose, and a 'present-centred' approach, which engages with philosophical texts or arguments in terms of that which remains universally justifiable and accessible to reason. The former emphasizes the differences between previous philosophies and the present of the historian of philosophy; the latter assumes a transhistorical rationality which operates as the ultimate arbiter of the philosophically valuable.[25]

Lloyd suggests that, because women philosophers typically stand in an 'uneasy' relation to the philosophical and institutional present in which they find themselves, they often turn to more historically distanced voices as alternatives to those which dominate contemporary debate.[26] Nonetheless, this is not a matter of seeking a return to a historically situated philosophical past, particularly as this remains a past from which women were often alienated and excluded. Rather it is a matter of seeking to activate the latent potential of past philosophies for thinking differently in the present. Such an activity is characterized by Lloyd as 'thinking with' a past philosopher in ways that often take their thought in directions they themselves could not have foreseen – and of which they would not necessarily approve.[27]

Much of Irigaray's work belongs with this third kind of approach – including her engagements with Plato and Descartes in *An Ethics of Sexual Difference*. However, as indicated above, Irigaray's earlier work, and *Speculum* in particular, is more typically seen as offering a critical deconstruction of the masculinist bias of western philosophy. Such work is often regarded as a necessary stage in feminist thought that both opens the way to, but is also superseded by, the more positive re-appropriations that characterize the third approach outlined by Lloyd. It is certainly true that, by showing how the repression of sexual difference is bound up with philosophy's most fundamental categories, Irigaray has played a crucial role in sharpening the critical gaze of other feminist thinkers. Her work has helped to make others more attentive to the dissenting voices within the history of philosophy that might aid feminist attempts to rethink concepts of form and matter, mind and body, subject and object, culture and nature. However (as should by now be clear), this book seeks to demonstrate the extent to which Irigaray's own positive project of cultivating female subjectivity and a sexuate culture of two is already present in *Speculum*, in ways that are sometimes underestimated. Even in the midst of *Speculum's* thoroughgoing critique, Irigaray is always thinking both critically and creatively, not only *against* but also *with* and *through* the philosophers with whom she engages.

This double approach has led to a double criticism, even from sympathetic feminist readers. On the one hand, some have argued that, despite the value and significance of her project, Irigaray's mode of feminist critique tends to unduly homogenize the history of philosophy. In other words, by focusing on the repeated pattern whereby sexual difference is occluded and woman excluded, Irigaray tends to cover over significant differences and inconsistencies *between* philosophical systems or even *within* texts and positions.[28] On this view, Irigaray's approach risks obscuring the resources that different systems may hold, despite themselves, for alternative feminist projects. On the other hand, as indicated above, others would argue that any attempt to positively re-appropriate philosophy for feminism results in a counter-productive compromise with the master discourse. Indeed, those who most wholeheartedly endorse Irigaray's critique of the history of philosophy

may also be those most likely to be suspicious of the value of philosophy's terms. Philosophical notions of the subject, identity,
nature, matter, knowledge: all may be regarded as hopelessly
ensnared in a logic of the same whose theoretical abstractions are
incapable of rendering justice to the lived, bodily specificities of
female experience.

Again, I do not wish to deny that Irigaray does indeed face such
risks, particularly where the first criticism is concerned; but I would
nonetheless argue that she negotiates these risks in several productive and inter-related ways. First, although her guiding thread is
the role of woman in philosophy, she remains attentive to the specific and often contradictory ways in which the figure of woman
operates in different philosophical contexts (at times becoming the
exemplar of a mute material passivity, at others, the face of terrifying and excessive nature). Second, through such attentiveness, she
shows how the figure of woman repeatedly exceeds a masculinist
logic in ways that both disrupt this logic from within and generate
possibilities for articulating woman differently. As Deutscher elo-
quently puts it, Irigaray shows not only how philosophers have
failed to address sexual difference, but 'how such failures themselves fail, thereby opening themselves up to the advent of the new:
the possibility of an alternative thinking of sexual difference.'[29]
Irigaray's approach thereby displaces the supposed authority and
unity of the 'master discourse'. Finally, while her project does
involve picking out repeated patterns that recur between thinkers
– particularly of course, where woman is concerned – it also
involves working closely with particular texts to re-appropriate the
specific resources they offer for articulating sexual difference
non-reductively.[30]

Thinking Other-Wise

An alternative way of defending Irigaray from the criticisms
outlined above is to position her approach as 'strategic' in certain
key respects. This line of interpretation fits with the claim that
Irigaray's project constitutes a counterbalance to philosophy's
pre-existing patriarchal bias: her own focus on the ways in which
philosophy occludes sexual difference can thus be positioned as
strategically necessary. Moreover, it can be argued that this critical
corrective does not preclude feminists from drawing on philosophy's resources themselves. On the contrary, it may be claimed,
insofar as we still inhabit a culture whose models of ethics, justice,

and politics are centrally informed by the western philosophical tradition, feminists have a duty to re-appropriate and re-deploy the terms of that tradition strategically and subversively, in order to ensure women's present needs and perspectives do not remain unrepresented. According to this line of argument, it is sometimes legitimate to focus exclusively on philosophy's exclusion of women, while at other times, it will be both appropriate and necessary to take up philosophical concepts for feminist purposes. Both are required, as long as we do both 'strategically', as a means to a (feminist) end.

Despite its appeal – for the banner of the 'strategic' allows Irigarayan feminists to be both critical and creative, philosophical and political at once – I think this answer is ultimately unsatisfactory. By legitimizing the use of philosophical concepts on strategic grounds, it implicitly accepts the view that philosophy's language is necessarily and essentially 'masculinist', and that the best feminists can do is subversively deploy its terms for their own ends. To this extent, such a position itself remains ensnared by the logic of the same and in its own way, continues to constitute a denial of difference. On the one hand, it refuses to allow that philosophy could become other to itself: by contrast, Irigaray's notions of a sexuate subject or 'being two' are not merely 'strategic' but integral to the development of an ontology and metaphysics rooted in a positive account of sexual difference. On the other hand, such radical transformations are only possible because philosophy never was wholly self-identical, but always already fissured from within.

Thus, Irigaray is attentive both to the dominance of certain masculinist patterns of thought, and to the fissures and cracks that nonetheless run through the history of philosophy, and that refuse the reductive equation of *logos* (discourse, reason/ing) with an all-encompassing and inevitable *phal-logo-centrism* (a discursive order taking the male form as norm and ideal). As her analyses show, the multiple figures of woman in philosophy both attest to repeated patterns of occlusion and exclusion, and simultaneously signal gaps and openings. Rather than closing the tradition down into a unified image of oppression, by remaining sensitive to the specificities of woman's role and image in different philosophical moments, Irigaray opens up multiple passageways towards a culture and philosophy of sexual difference.

Such arguments may help convince feminist thinkers of the value of Irigaray's philosophical engagements. Nonetheless, the claim that her work ought to be of interest to those concerned with

the history of philosophy more generally may still need some justification. This is especially so given that she is certainly not a
'good' historian of philosophy in either of the two senses proposed
by Rorty. That is, she does not seek to represent the thought of
Plato, Plotinus, or Descartes in ways that these philosophers would
readily recognize as reflecting their central concerns, whether these
are situated in their specific philosophical-historical contexts, or
approached from a (supposedly) trans-cultural rational perspective. Rather, Irigaray seeks to show how, whatever their explicit
philosophical and cultural horizons, both the central concerns of
western philosophy and the models of rationality deployed to
assess them are enframed and sustained by a blindspot concerning
sexual difference. Thus, at one and the same time, she shows that
neither the history of philosophy, nor approaches to that history,
can legitimately lay claim to a pure objectivity or rational neutrality. Rather, the very claim to a universal, non-perspectival reason
is shown to be both product and symptom of a mode of thinking
that is dependent on the repression of (sexual) difference.

Thus, precisely what makes Irigaray a good reader of the history
of philosophy is that she makes explicit both the (feminist) perspective that informs her own reading and the fact that no reading is
ever perspective-free or value-neutral. This is why it would be a
mistake to be overly apologetic for what might be described as the
polemical character of some of her writings, including much of
Speculum. Like Nietzsche, Irigaray writes polemically because she
is a philosopher of value more than of truth. This is not because
she thinks that – in any simple way – there is no such thing as
'truth', but because (again, like Nietzsche) she recognizes that what
is taken to be true confers value, and that what has been taken to
be true in western philosophical thought has tended to de-value
both the specificity of women and sexual difference. The value of
Speculum, and indeed Irigaray's work more generally, thus lies not
in the extent to which it offers a 'true' account of the tradition, but
in its power to make us re-examine what has been taken to be 'true'
so as to re-value our own, inherited values. As on the third model
outlined by Lloyd, then, for Irigaray the value of interrogating the
history of philosophy lies in the potential this holds for transforming our present, as well as our possible futures.

Perhaps in the end, it is better to think of Irigaray not so much
as doing the history of philosophy, as engaging with that history
so as to do philosophy differently. Thus it is as important not to
elide Irigaray's Plato with Plato as it is to distinguish Nietzsche's

Schopenhauer from Schopenhauer, or Heidegger's Nietzsche from Nietzsche. This is not, however, so as to be able to identify what 'properly' belongs to Plato in contrast to the 'new' thoughts that are Irigaray's (or Nietzsche's or Heidegger's) 'own'. It is true that by transforming the thought of others, each of these figures transforms their own ways of thinking (and ours). But it is not clear to whom the new possibilities that emerge belong, precisely because they change both the thinker and the thought of the one whom they have selected to 'think with' simultaneously. Hence it is vital to preserve the difference between them, in which thought moves and new ways of thinking take shape. As Irigaray herself teaches, it is not by identifying one with the other, nor by irrevocably separating them, but *in-between* two (or more) that the unique and singular is able to emerge. In the following chapters, we will see how new ways of thinking emerge as Irigaray applies the lens of sexual difference to the canonical texts and figures of philosophical and psychoanalytic thought.

2

Re-Visiting Plato's Cave: Orientation and Origins

How to begin? The question of beginnings – where we begin, how we come into the world – is at the heart of Irigaray's thought. In some sense, the answer is simple: each of us, every human being, is born of a mother. Yet Irigaray shows how much work has gone into denying and displacing the significance of this 'simple fact' in western thought and culture, and how this denial is bound up with a forgetting of sexual difference. Even more importantly, she shows how recovering sexual difference, together with the significance of the maternal, would transform the fundamental structures and values of that culture.

Unsurprisingly, this transformative project involves going back to the beginnings. Thus a significant proportion of Irigaray's first major work of feminist philosophy, *Speculum of the Other Woman*, is devoted to one of the foundational passages from one of the foundational texts of western thought: the Myth of the Cave from Plato's *Republic*. For Irigaray, this text is archetypal insofar as it inscribes the forgetting of the maternal, and consequently of sexual difference, into the foundational structures of western metaphysics.

In this chapter, I will introduce Plato's myth, and examine Irigaray's treatment of it in detail. Instead of offering counter arguments to prove Plato wrong, or developing an alternative thesis with which to oppose him, Irigaray works with his text to show how it works against itself. As we will see, her analysis suggests that while it may be designed to orient us towards the eternal Forms, the Myth of the Cave still testifies to our maternal origins, despite itself. Hence it offers an opening for thought to recover the significance of those origins. However, before turning to Irigaray's reading of Plato, I will begin with a more general introduction to *Speculum* itself, as the book's title and structure already have much to tell us about Irigaray's project.

Speculum

A speculum is a mirror. In particular, the term refers to the concave mirror used to examine the inside of bodies. It is also an instrument used in gynaecological examinations: a speculum penetrates a woman, turning her sex into an object for an enquiring scientific gaze (*S*, 144). The speculum can thus be read as representing the *specular* patriarchal economy that Irigaray critiques because of the way that it reduces woman to an object of the male gaze.

To make the inside of a woman's body visible, the speculum must be curved, like that body. Mimicking the body it mirrors, the speculum (as mirror, rather than dilating instrument) is thus concave. However, as Plato himself tells us, concave mirrors distort and invert. In a passage from his dialogue *Timaeus*, which Irigaray quotes directly, Plato observes that unlike flat mirrors, concave ones do not reverse the image left to right. Moreover, if turned vertically, they invert the image so that it appears upside-down.[1] As Irigaray notes, it is not just this second, inverted image that generates confusion: insofar as the unreversed image allows us to see ourselves as others see us, it makes us other to our selves rather than aligning us with our own self-image (*S*, 149).

Thus, insofar as it is a concave mirror, a speculum exhibits the 'distorting' effects that the western philosophical tradition has typically attributed to the female body. As Irigaray shows, in this tradition, woman has been aligned with the bodily and material, while the bodily and material has in turn been regarded as corrupting the purity of form, spirit, or soul. As Irigaray also shows, however, this 'distorting' power of female materiality has a double valence. Alongside a negative capacity to deform, it also suggests a more positive power to *transform*, which among other things, might generate new ways of seeing the relation between form and matter, as well as body and soul. The image of the speculum thus embodies the processes that turn woman into a passive object of the gaze and link female matter to the inversion or distortion of 'proper' form. Yet it simultaneously links the female sex to a more subversive power to produce new forms, and thereby hints at the possibility of transforming the ways in which woman herself is represented.

As we will see, it is not a coincidence that at the centre of Plato's myth we find a cave-wall that operates as a reflecting screen, and that Irigaray reads as a concave mirror, a speculum or distorting glass at the heart of metaphysics. For now however it is worth noting that the multiple valences of the image of the speculum is exemplary of Irigaray's mode of thinking and writing, which she describes as a subversive and productive *mimicry*.[2] If woman in the western tradition is represented in ways that reflect man's desire, Irigaray shows that reflection is never simply a passive matter. Indeed, it is the 'matter' in which the desires and discourse of a male subject are reflected which has the capacity to subvert and transform them – whether this matter is the female body, or the shadowy substance of images, or the materiality of words on a page. As we will see in more detail later, Irigaray's mode of writing, her subversive mimesis, not only 'jams the machinery' of patriarchal discourse but allows her to speak (as) woman in a different voice, to speak from 'elsewhere' (*TS*, 76–8).

Hence the second part of the book's title, 'of the other woman', is equally double in valence. Read negatively, it signals the ways in which woman is defined as the other of a male subject, and thus reduced to his terms. Read positively, it points to the ways in which woman is genuinely other to that subject, in the sense of being *irreducible* to his terms. It is this latter, positive figure of woman which Irigaray seeks to recover.[3] Finally, as Irigaray notes, the title of her book deliberately invokes the notion of a *speculum mundi*, a Latin term that literally means a mirror of the world, but that was used in the medieval period for works which sought 'not so much the reflection of the world in a mirror as the thought of the reality or objectivity of the world through a discourse' (*ILTY*, 60). Irigaray's *Speculum* seeks both to reveal the ways in which woman has been discursively constructed as man's 'other', and to find other discourses that speak positively of woman's irreducible difference and thus construct reality otherwise, as a world shared between two sexuate subjects.

Along with the title, it is helpful to situate Irigaray's reading of Plato in relation to the structure of *Speculum* as a whole. This is a book that most pointedly does not begin at the beginning. Instead, *Speculum* starts with a long section on Freud. This is followed by a middle section composed of ten self-contained chapters. The first of these condenses *Speculum*'s key claims and concerns by showing how 'Any Theory of the "Subject"' is dependent on woman as both object and other. The following chapters take the reader on a critical journey through the history of western metaphysics by focusing on key figures, including Plotinus, Aristotle, Descartes, Kant, Hegel, and Lacan. The section's concluding chapter, 'Volume-Fluidity', weaves together many of the voices that have come before, this time foregrounding the possibilities for figuring woman differently that Irigaray has disinterred from the tradition. By showing the unexpected transformations that reflection can produce, this chapter forms the counterpart – but not the simple mirror – of 'Any Theory of the "Subject"'.

There are two chapters in this central part of *Speculum* which focus on Plato: the first explores the role of light and mirrors in sustaining Platonic metaphysics; the second consists of direct quotations from Platonic dialogues which speak of woman and in which it becomes clear that she is seen as inferior to the male. Together these sections provide a useful context for approaching the third and final part of the book, which they prefigure, and in which Irigaray works through Plato's Myth of the Cave. Her analysis shows how woman's positioning as an inferior being is not merely a correctable surface feature of Platonic thought, but plays a foundational role in a metaphysics which seeks to appropriate the mother's generative power. At the same time, as we will see, Irigaray's text also shows how the economy of mirror-images on which Plato's theory depends is internally unstable to the point where it undoes itself from within.

As Irigaray herself points out, by starting with Freud and ending with Plato, *Speculum* seems to approach the history of thought backwards; but this order is itself reversed in the central section where the chapters progress chronologically again (*TS*, 68). Moreover, the final long section on Plato is replete with images that directly echo the opening reading of Freud. While these echoes carry the reader back to the 'beginning' – in which Irigaray addresses psychoanalysis as the 'end' or culmination of the western metaphysical tradition – they are not so tightly knit as to form a closed circle. Rather, in the echo-chamber *Speculum* becomes, psychoanalysis informs Irigaray's reading of Plato while her reading of Plato retroactively inflects the sections on Freud, making the implicit metaphysical commitments of psychoanalytic theory more readily discernable. Thus '[s]trictly speaking, *Speculum* has no beginning or end' (*TS*, 68).

By refusing to work through the tradition in a linear fashion – either wholly forwards or backwards – Irigaray displaces two tempting but dangerous models for feminist thought: on the one hand, an autonomous female identity is not to be found by moving beyond the tradition into a utopian future; on the other, neither is it to be recovered as a lost origin buried in the pre-patriarchal past. In this respect, the non-linear structure of *Speculum* already blocks the idea that there is any 'essential' feminine identity which has been lost and which must 'simply' be recovered. To borrow from her reading of Plato, Irigaray's project is not about recalling 'a truer truth', or a more real reality (*S*, 270). Rather, it demands we transform our understanding of the 'true' and the 'real' from a perspective informed by a re-valuation of sexual difference.

As Irigaray herself points out, nothing is to be gained by seeking simply to over-turn or reverse the order of the tradition for '[t]he reversal ... would still be played out within the same' (*TS*, 156). Irigaray's point here is not just that a reversal of the tradition (for example, by substituting matriarchal for patriarchal power) would not change its terms but merely repeat them in inverted form. More importantly, her point is that the terms of the tradition are those of 'the same': that the tradition has been governed by a logic that has taken one subject (the male) as norm and ideal, and defined others against and in the terms of this self-same subject. It is this logic of the same that has made it impossible to attend to sexual difference in any positive sense, for it reduces woman to the 'other' of a male subject rather than according her the terms appropriate to being a subject in her own right.

To escape this logic of the same, it is therefore crucial not to reinscribe it in reversed or inverted form. By neither mirroring nor simply reversing the history of western thought, the structure of *Speculum* is itself designed to help Irigaray escape the specular logic that she identifies and critiques.

Returning to Plato's Cave

Plato is generally taken to be the father of western metaphysics. It is thus all the more fitting that Irigaray takes him to task for establishing a metaphysics which obscures the originary and generative powers of the mother. Of course, the idea that western philosophy can be traced back to a single figure is itself a kind of fantasy – the kind of fantasy of unitary origin which Irigaray seeks to displace.

It is particularly ironic that Plato has come to represent such an origin as, famously, his philosophical theories have come down to us in the form of dialogues in which the key ideas are voiced through the character of Socrates. As the real Socrates was Plato's own teacher, it does not take long to see that the 'origin' of western metaphysics is complicated and far from unified. Things are further complicated by the fact that Plato himself is responding to other thinkers, such as Parmenides; moreover, as Plato wrote a large number of dialogues over many years, there are also significant shifts and tensions within his thought.

Nonetheless, it remains the case that Plato has come to stand for the origin of a particular way of thinking that we could broadly call 'western metaphysics', characterized by its separation of truth from appearances and being from becoming. On this view, what truly 'is' does not change or cease to be; it is beyond the ever-changing world that appears to the senses and instead can be accessed only by reason or the intellect. The Platonic devaluation of the world of the senses will be taken up and reworked both by Christianity, where it will inform the image of the Fall and the contrast between a transcendent heaven and an earthly realm of sin, and by the western philosophical tradition, which will typically divide mind from body and the senses from reason for at least the next two millennia.

This is of course a much reduced picture of the complexity of Plato's thought – but insofar as these are the strands of his thinking which are consolidated by the western tradition, it is this Platon-ism which Irigaray is seeking to work against. By taking his texts seriously as the supposed origin of this tradition, she is seeking to disrupt the originary status they have retrospectively acquired, and to reclaim openings for other modes of thought – for paths not taken and possibilities pushed to the margins.

If Plato's texts are seen as the origin of western metaphysics, then within those texts, the Myth of the Cave can be read as a dis-tillation of the metaphysical framework to which they give rise. This is how Irigaray positions the myth. More specifically, she pri-oritizes it because she sees it as exemplifying the originary appro-priation of the body of the mother on which, she will argue, western metaphysics depends. The original context of the myth is book seven of Plato's *Republic*, a dialogue that marries politics and philosophy by showing how the ideal rulers for the ideal state would be philosophers. The Myth of the Cave is an alleg-orical device designed to teach of the often painful process of enlightenment required to produce such rulers. It presents this process as a journey, through which human beings are re-oriented by being turned away from a captivating but deceptive world of the senses and towards a realm of reality and truth. In this way, human beings become lovers of wisdom, that is, philosophers.

Such is the power of this philosophical tale that its significance transcends its particular role in the context of the *Republic*. Plato's image of a journey from ignorance to wisdom and darkness into light has played a crucial role in orienting western thought in its on-going quest for philosophical enlightenment. In response, Irigaray's engagement with the Myth of the Cave is designed to re-orient her reader once again. In particular, she seeks to re-orient us in relation to our beginnings: both the beginnings of western metaphysical thought, and our individual beginnings in birth from a mother. As in Plato's original tale, this reorientation involves an often painful challenge to our habitual way of seeing the world, and is thus likely to meet with considerable resistance.

In the *Republic*, the myth is initially introduced by Socrates to his companion Glaucon as a metaphor for the effects of a *lack* of education. Glaucon is invited to compare human ignorance with the condition of being a prisoner, chained up in a cave and unable to see anything except the play of shadows on the wall opposite, which are mistaken for the true nature of things. The 'strange prisoners' in this 'strange image' are nonetheless 'like us': we too live in a condition of ignorance as long as we continue to regard the world of mere appearances as reality.[4] Thus begins a play of doubles which, as Irigaray will emphasize, runs through the entire mythic scene.

The shadows on the cave wall are created by a fire, located behind and above the chained prisoners. Between them and the fire some other men, also hidden behind the prisoners, pass along a path behind a low wall, holding up statues whose shadows make patterns on the back wall of the cave. Socrates asks Glaucon to imagine that one of these prisoners is suddenly freed and made to turn around. At first he would be confused, dazzled by the firelight, and reluctant to accept what he saw. The shadows would for a time seem more real and distinct than the men and artefacts who now emerge in the cave behind him.

Things get worse for the prisoner. Socrates instructs Glaucon to imagine someone dragging him forcibly up the path and out of the cave, into the even more dazzling light of the sun. By working his way up slowly from shadows, to reflections in water, to actual objects and then the heavens, this reluctant initiate would in the end be able to look at the sun itself, recognizing it as the true cause of all that is. By comparison with his knowledge of the real world outside the cave, he would realize the worthlessness of what passed as knowledge inside the cave; indeed if he returned, he would himself appear ignorant and ridiculous at first, as he would find it hard to see in the relative darkness and would no longer be able to identify the shadows with the same ease as his former companions who are still prisoners.

The shadowy world of the cave, Socrates explains, stands for the visible world, the everyday world of the senses and mere appearance. By contrast, the world outside the cave stands for the intelligible world and the true reality of the Forms or Ideas, the unchanging archetypes of all that exists in the ever-changing realm of appearances.[5] The Sun stands for the ultimate Form, the Form of the Good, which holds all the others in place and secures not only their reality, but the beautiful harmony of the good and the true. Thus, the ways in which the inside of the cave mirrors the outside – the fire is the double of the sun, the statues mimic 'real things' – maps onto the relation between appearances and Forms, whereby the former are imperfect copies of the latter.

It is worth pausing to note four further features of this relation between Forms and appearances which are important for Irigaray's reading. These are made explicit in a passage shortly preceding the myth itself. First, the Form of the Good is here metaphorically positioned as a 'father' of 'offspring' made in its likeness; second, this passage implies that there can be degrees of likeness to the Forms (Socrates offers to tell Glaucon of the offspring 'most like' the Good); third, though there are many visible things, Socrates confirms that there is only one Form for each kind of thing; and finally, as the intelligible Form makes each visible thing what it is, it is called 'the being' of each thing.[6]

Having encountered the radiance of the Forms, and thus the true nature of Being, the enlightened prisoner, Socrates suggests, will be reluctant to relinquish his knowledge of the real world for a life back in the shadows. Yet this is precisely why he ought to return to the cave. The true lover of wisdom – the philosopher – who has oriented himself towards the Forms will not only be the best placed to govern, as his decisions will be oriented by the Forms of the Just and the Good; he will also be the least susceptible to corruption, having no interest in merely worldly acquisition. Thus those who have made the difficult journey towards enlightenment should return to the cave, to share their wisdom with those who remain trapped in ignorance.

In her reading of the myth, Irigaray could be seen as tearing the story out of its specific context at the heart of the *Republic*, where it relates to the question of who should rule, and how rulers should best be educated. However, she does this to situate the myth in a still wider context, for as noted above, her concern is less with the way this mythic tale functions in the *Republic*, and more with the way it sets the scene for western metaphysics generally. This overarching concern is reflected in the way that Irigaray moves between the Myth of the Cave and passages from other Platonic dialogues without attempting to situate such passages in relation to the particular text in which they occur.[7] Such textual violence is far from unknowing. It is a deliberate re-appropriation of the images and conceptual structures through which western metaphysics is set up, and whose significance extends far beyond any particular dialogue. Instead, philosophy's founding narratives such as the Myth of the Cave are retrospectively inflected by the weight of the metaphysical tradition they help to establish – and which Irigaray seeks to displace. If the question of politics that informs the *Republic* concerns how we are best to live together (that is, to form a *polis*), then Irigaray's reading shows how, in the western tradition, the fundamental political issue has already been decided, prior to any explicit discussion of who should rule. According to Irigaray, the metaphysics that informs Plato's account of the ideal philosopher-rulers has already privileged sameness over difference, and one kind of being (the male, masculine, paternal) over an other (the female, feminine, maternal). Thus even before metaphysics is called upon to inform the ideal organization of the state, it has already decided who should rule – both in the state and in metaphysics. The 'violence' Irigaray does to the texts she reads is thus a deliberate counter to a violence already perpetrated by a mode of thinking that functions via the devaluation, exclusion, and negation of difference.

A Cave like a Womb

To re-orient our reading of Plato's myth, and hence the whole direction of our thinking, Irigaray deliberately dis-orients her reader. She shows how the images that represent the philosopher's journey fold and multiply in a dizzying play of doubles until all stable orientation is lost. She can thus be read as taking up a Socratic position herself, at least insofar as Socrates sought to re-orient his interlocutors by first making them unsure of everything they thought they knew, to the point where he is accused of numbing and confusing them like a stingray.[8] Such disorientation is thematized in the Myth of the Cave, in which the journey towards wisdom (the passage out of the cave) involves painful and initially confusing transitions. Irigaray shows how such confusion cannot be contained as a necessary but merely temporary stage on the way to truth. Instead, it seeps through the entire set-up of the myth, destabilizing its structures and with them, the horizon of metaphysical thought.

The origin of this confusion is a blindspot. More specifically, Irigaray shows that the metaphysical orientation of western thought both rests upon and is undermined by a blindspot concerning the way human beings enter into the world and receive their initial orientation within it via the mother. By positing the eternal Forms as the only true reality and the origin of all that is, Plato's metaphysics displaces our actual beginnings in birth. The ideal 'father' of visible offspring supplants birth from a mother. In this way, the horizon of metaphysical thought obscures the more primordial horizon that orients human beings in the world, namely, our relation to our maternal origins.

We can find a trace of this debt to maternal generative power in Socrates' appropriation of the image of the midwife. Famously, the Socratic philosopher is one who helps give birth to the thoughts of others.[9] Here again, Irigaray can be seen as miming the Socratic role to the extent that in *Speculum*, she seeks not so much to set out her own thesis as to allow others to come to see the blindspot of metaphysical thinking, and what it forecloses, for themselves. Nonetheless, Irigaray's re-appropriation of the role of philosopher-midwife is a subversive one, insofar as she seeks to return philosophy to the scene of actual pregnancy and birth. In so doing, she is not denying the value of giving birth to thought – indeed she seeks to regenerate philosophical thought via her own provocations. But she also aims to make philosophy confront the way that it has devalued the original act of generation on which the metaphor of the Socratic midwife is based.

This metaphorical appropriation lies at the centre of Irigaray's analysis of the Myth of the Cave. Her reading foregrounds the ways in which the central image of the myth derives much of its power from the obvious morphological resonance between the cave and the womb (in Greek, the *hystera*):

> Socrates tells us that men – *hoi anthrōpoi*, sex unspecified – live *under-ground*, in a *dwelling formed* like *a cave*. Ground, dwelling, cave, and even, in a different way, form – all these terms can be read more or less as equivalents of the *hystera*. ... As the story goes, then, men – with no specification of sex – are living in one, same place. A place shaped like a cave or a womb. (S, 243)

Just as human beings begin life in the darkness of the mother's womb, so the journey towards wisdom starts in the intellectual obscurity represented by the subterranean world of the cave. And just as human beings are born by passing through the mother's body into the world, so the prisoner is re-born by being forced up the passage and into the sunlit realm outside. Thus the figure of the cave appropriates the connotations of the womb to lend meta-phorical force to its story of (re-)birth.

Yet this birth is not a physical one: a substitution has already taken place. For while the womb-like cave recalls our corporeal birth from a mother, the journey undertaken by the prisoner is an allegory for an intellectual and spiritual passage that requires one to leave the body behind. As Plato reminds us in a dialogue centred not on birth but death (*Phaedo*), the body can only be a prison for the soul, tying it to the distracting demands of the senses as well as to the illusory realm of appearances.[10] True knowledge (of the Forms) can be attained only by untying the soul from the body, that is, by turning one's thoughts away from the sensible world (strug-gling out of the cave).

Thus, as Alison Stone notes, 'Plato is using the female body as the symbol of a state of ignorance and illusion. He implies that, in order to achieve knowledge and gain access to reality, one must leave the female body behind.'[11] Moreover, as Irigaray's reading continually reminds us, the appropriation of the womb in the image of the cave produces a dramatic inversion in perspective: 'the *hystera* has already been turned around' (*S*, 310). Whereas birth allows human beings to emerge *from* their uterine beginnings *into* the world outside, the passage out of the cave symbolizes the journey *away* from the sensible world of appearances and *back* to the origin. This inversion reflects the fundamental act of appropriation struc-turing the myth, whereby the originating power of the womb is projected 'outside' the cave and onto the Forms. Once secured, this appropriation produces a further twist, turning corporeal birth into its opposite. From the perspective of Platonic metaphysics, physical birth constitutes a passage into the world of becoming. As such, birth is not so much the beginning of a life, as the passage out of eternal being that condemns human beings to mortality and death. Thus, Plato's image of an intellectual re-birth feeds off the powerful connotations of the image of the womb, while simultaneously helping to secure a philosophical perspective that denies the value of bodily birth. Indeed, in a further strange inversion, the philosopher's journey towards intellectual re-birth becomes a practice for dying, as he struggles to untie the soul from the body so as to reorient it towards the eternal Forms.[12] Thus, instead of recognizing our beginnings in birth, the philosopher longs for a re-birth of the soul that depends on the death of the body.

In this way, the topology of the cave points us to the foundational appropriation, displacement and devaluation of the maternal that secures the ground of western metaphysics.[13] As Irigaray notes, by the time we find ourselves in the Platonic cave, set up in advance to orient us towards the Forms as origin, 'the inversion has always already taken place' (S, 363). The further reversals, projections and inversions that she will show to characterize the internal logic of the myth are secondary effects and symptoms of this primary '*détournement*' that makes metaphysics possible: the movement of turning away from the mother while metaphorically re-appropriating her generative powers (Sf, 301).

Irigaray's reading shows how the pattern of substitution and reversal that structures the myth also works to destabilize it. This can be seen in the logic of substitution and equivalence on which the allegory of the cave depends: 'Already the prisoner was no longer in a womb but in a cave – an attempt to provide a figure, a system of metaphor for the uterine cavity. He was held in a place that was, that meant to express, that had the *sense* of being *like* a womb' (S, 279). If the cave is 'like', or in some sense equivalent to, a womb, the journey from ignorance to wisdom is '*like*' a birth. Conjoining the Myth of the Cave with the familiar image of the Socratic midwife, Irigaray describes the anonymous 'someone' who releases the prisoner as leading him out of the cave 'as out of a womb, according to the techniques of childbirth' (S, 279). In this way, she shows how Plato's allegory privileges those elements that can be transferred from images of childbirth and a mother's womb to the story of enlightenment. In Socrates' interpretation of the story's true meaning, the elements that are 'the same' (the painful transition from one realm to another) are taken up, while those that are different (the bodily elements of physical birth) are conveniently screened out.

Yet matters are not so simple. For the image of the cave does not just transform the figure of the womb into a metaphor for the world of the senses, and physical birth into a metaphor for intellectual enlightenment. If 'the *hystera* is made metaphor'(*S*, 247), the cave is at the same time a metaphor *for* the womb. It represents precisely those physical origins which the myth seeks to transcend. Thus Irigaray's first, subversive instruction to the reader: 'The Myth of the Cave, for example, or as an example, is a good place to start. *Read it this time as a metaphor of the inner space, of the den, the womb or hystera, sometimes of the earth* – though we shall see that the text inscribes the metaphor as, strictly speaking, impossible' (*S*, 243; my emphasis). As a metaphor for the womb, the cave once again has a double valence. If the cave is *like* a womb, the womb by implication is like a cave. Plato's image produces a double of the mother's body that turns her into an inert container, a hollowed-out darkness of petrified matter. At the same time, and despite this, by evoking our beginnings in birth, the cave is also a morphological reminder of a maternal power to generate whose active life-giving powers cannot be captured in the deadening image of frozen rock.

Thus, if Plato's myth relies on transferring the powerful connotations of the womb onto the figure of the cave, Irigaray shows that this process of metaphorization is unstable and reversible: there is nothing to stop her (or us) reading the cave as a metaphor for the womb. Such a reading can lead us into a critique of the ways in which western thought has tended to represent the mother's body as a container and her active generative capacities as passively reproductive matter. At the same time, however, it can also lead us back through the myth, away from the ideality of disembodied Forms, and towards a revaluation of our corporeal maternal origins.

Forgetting We Have Forgotten

By insisting on the way the cave is a figure for the womb – the *hystera* – Irigaray makes visible the most fundamental substitution and reversal accomplished in the myth: that concerning the notion of origin. She does this via a complex mode of writing that turns passive mimicry into a productive kind of 'double-speak'. Crucially, this allows her to avoid repeating the logic of substitution herself. Instead of putting her own voice in place of Plato's, she writes in a way that allows both his voice *and* her own to resonate at once. Thus, instead of a doubling that reproduces the same, Irigaray allows (at least) two voices to speak together in ways that open up a new perspective.

One example of this subversive 'double-speak' is Irigaray's description of the men chained up in the cave. The prisoners, she notes, are 'Paralyzed, unable to *turn round* or *return* toward the origin' (S, 245), while the cave itself is:

> the representation of something always already there, of the original matrix/womb which these men cannot represent since they are held down by chains that prevent them from turning their heads or their genitals toward the daylight. They cannot turn toward what is more primary ... . Chains restrain them from turning toward the origin but/and they are prisoners in the space-time of the pro-ject of its representation. (S, 244)

This passage is typical of Irigaray's text for its dense multiplicity of layers and conjoined meanings. I will return later to the image of the matrix (which translates another ancient Greek word for womb, *metra*, derived from *meter*, mother); for now, however, I want to emphasize the way this passage speaks in a double voice. At one level, Irigaray here offers a relatively 'straight' re-telling of the Myth of the Cave, highlighting the prisoners' inability to turn towards the real world outside. This in turn represents the way that as long as human beings remain chained to the world of the senses, they remain incapable of recalling the Forms, whose unchanging being is the only true reality. The Forms pre-exist the world of appearances (they are 'more primary', 'always already there'), which are only 'pro-jected' copies or imperfect representations of these ideal archetypes. Unenlightened human beings, then, like the prisoners in the cave, have their backs turned 'to the origin, the *hystera*, of which this cave [the world of appearances] is a mere reversal, a project of figuration' (S, 249).

Nonetheless, this is a reading which pushes the role of the cave/womb as metaphor to the limit. Insofar as the Forms are positioned as the true origin of being, Irigaray suggests that it is not the cave, but the Forms themselves which are properly repre-sented by the metaphor of the 'womb'. By continually playing on the notion of 'origin' as both Forms and womb, Irigaray exposes the way that the Forms substitute for the womb. Read in this way, it is the Platonic metaphysicians who have turned their backs on that which is 'more primary' (birth from a mother), which they have supplanted with an alternative, non-corporeal and eternal origin (metaphorically aligned with the generative power not of the mother, but the father). Paradoxically, this ideal origin is a 'store of non-birth' (S, 312), as the Forms generate appearances without ever changing themselves.

This, then, is the founding act of western metaphysics: the appropriation of a maternal power to generate and its projection onto the Forms as the one 'true' origin of all that is. As Irigaray notes, '*Analysis of the projection seems never to have taken place*', something *Speculum* is designed to rectify (S, 310). If western philosophy, as is so often said, consists of footnotes to Plato, then on Irigaray's reading, it begins with this erasure of beginnings. Just as the prisoners in the cave are unable to turn towards the real world outside, and human beings struggle to recall the reality of the Forms, so Plato's own myth chains us in a metaphysics that prevents us from turning back to the significance of our maternal origins – even though the metaphorical power of the womb will continue to support the very myth that displaces those origins. Ever since this mythic-metaphysical structure came to determine our orientation in the world, human beings 'have been chained up within the project of making metaphor of the *hystera*' (S, 268).

For Plato, the journey of the philosopher, as represented in the Myth of the Cave, is one of recollection. By traversing his difficult path away from the seductive realm of appearances, he is returned to the true reality and the true origin of all that exists. If, however, we take up Irigaray's invitation to read the cave (both the dark cavern and the myth as a whole) in terms of the womb, we see how turning back to the Forms turns us further away from our maternal origins. Thus, while the forgetting of the Forms can be undone via recollection, to recover the Forms as origin depends on *continuing* to forget human beings' actual beginnings in birth. In other words, Platonic recollection depends not only on our having forgotten the Forms, but on forgetting that we have forgotten the maternal (S, 345).

Back to Front and Upside-Down

Irigaray's reading works to recover the maternal. She does this by destabilizing the Myth of the Cave so as to undo the logic of Platonic metaphysics from within. Her subversive re-telling draws our attention to the ways in which the founding substitution whereby the Forms replace our maternal origins is replicated in a whole series of doublings that both structure and destabilize the myth. These doublings are both spatial and temporal: they concern both the topography of the cave, and the prisoners' relation to origin.

To draw out this disorienting play of doubles, Irigaray shows how the Myth of the Cave relies on a specular logic in which inside mirrors outside, and images mirror reality. However, she also reminds us that, far from producing copies that are identical to their originals, flat mirrors reverse left to right, while concave mirrors invert top to bottom, turning the world upside-down. Such reversals characterize the topology of Plato's Cave, where the order of things is constantly being inverted and confused:

> The orientation functions by turning everything over, by reversing, and by pivoting around axes of symmetry. From high to low, from low to high, from back to front, from anterior to opposite, but in all cases from a point view in front of or behind something in this cave, situated in the back. *Symmetry plays a decisive part here* – as projection, reflection, inversion, retroversion – and you will always already have lost your bearings as soon as you set foot in the cave. (S, 244)

Thus, what first appears in *front* of the prisoners ('whatever presents itself before their eyes') is displayed on the *back* wall of the cave ('the back which is also the front, the fore') (S, 245). At the same time, the passage *behind* them turns out to be the *front* of the cave, at least from the perspective of someone in the world outside. Likewise, the fire and statues that are *behind* the chained men must in fact have existed *before* the shadowy reflections which the prisoners see first.

In time, the fire will be replaced by its own double, the sun, which is revealed as the true origin of the visible world. As source and origin, the sun must come first, yet is that which the released prisoner looks upon last, after the sky itself and other heavenly bodies. In this 'transposition of the anterior to the posterior, of the origin to the end, the horizon, the *telos*' (S, 245), the sun begins at the furthest remove behind the prisoners' backs, and ends high up in front of the released man as the ultimate goal of his journey. Thus the sun – and the Form of the Good for which it stands – doubles as both origin and end, source and goal, leading Irigaray to ask: 'Has everything been set upside down and back to front? But, in that case, where's the front? And the back? The only thing that remains constant is the retreat of what is behind. But it is at present

sent infinitely far in front. And up. Beyond the sky' (*S*, 363). Once again, the question of origins lies at the heart of this disorienting confusion: what should count as the 'front' in the Platonic Cave? What comes first? What is the proper order of primacy? Irigaray draws out the confusion via the Greek terms *hystera/hysteron* and *protera/proteron*. As we have seen, the men in the cave cannot turn toward what is more primary, 'toward the *proteron* which is in fact the *hystera*':

> Head and genitals are kept turned to the front of the representational project and process of the *hystera*. To the *hystera protera* that is apparently resorbed, blended into the movement of *hysteron proteron*. For *hysteron*, defined as what is behind, is also the last, the hereafter, the ultimate. *Proteron*, defined as what is in front, is also the earlier, the previous. (*S*, 244)

Part of the confusion here derives from a tension between the spatial and temporal connotations of these terms: as Irigaray notes, the *proteron* is that which comes earlier and is thus in front, while the *hysteron*, as well as being etymologically linked to the *hystera* or womb, also denotes that which comes later and is thus behind. But this means that what is behind us (spatially) lies ahead (temporally, for it comes later), while that which came first stands before us (spatially) even though it is (temporally) behind us.

Such confusions are exacerbated by the topography of the Cave, where as we have seen, the Forms which come first (temporally and ontologically, as the origin of all that is), are nonetheless at the furthest remove behind the prisoners' backs (spatially, as represented by the sun). Thus the men cannot turn towards the *proteron* – the origin, the sun, the Forms – which in the topography of the cave is the *hystera/hysteron*: the womb/origin that stands behind them.

At the same time, that which is ontologically and temporally secondary – the shadows, the appearances that are copies of originals – are projected onto the wall that lies opposite and ahead of the prisoners. This means the cave is an example of *hysteron proteron*, a Greek expression which can be roughly translated as 'putting the cart before the horse': in the topsy-turvy world of the cave, that which comes after/later (the shadows, the copies) has been misleadingly put up front. Thus it is not surprising that what lies in front of the prisoners turns out to be the back of the cave, and that what lies behind them as the ideal end of their journey turns out to be the starting point of everything. The myth is designed to effect this complete reversal in perspective that – supposedly – restores the proper order of things.

Yet, if we take up Irigaray's invitation to read the cave as a metaphor for the womb, matters become more complicated still. For if within the cave, the copies (as *hysteron*, that which comes later) are confusingly put up front (as *proteron*, that which comes earlier), this reversal in fact rightly positions the *hystera* (now read as womb) as that which comes earlier – as *protera*. From this perspective, the morphology of the cave directs us away from the Forms and back to our origins in the mother. Thus, the topography that from a Platonic perspective signals a disordering in need of correction, on Irigaray's reading becomes a reversal that returns us to the proper (maternal) order of things.

Origin and Offspring: A Disorienting Mimicry

As Irigaray's reading shows, the treatment of origins generates a confusion that concerns both space and time. This is unsurprising, as what is at stake here is not just the question of temporal primacy (what came first? the mother, the womb? or the Forms?), but the occlusion of the maternal space/place in which being begins. The question of temporal priority is further complicated by the tension between the temporality characterizing the journey of the released prisoner, who passes from cave to reality, and the temporal order of existence itself, whereby the sun comes first as the origin of the visible world.

Moreover, as origin, the sun – and the Form of the Good which it represents – is not just temporally but *causally* prior. Just as the sun's light and heat are the source of the visible world and changing seasons, the Form of the Good as pure Being is the cause of everything that appears to the extent that it participates in being (and thus, exists). On Irigaray's reading, it is via this *causal* priority that the Forms appropriate the generative, creative power of the mother. However, as she also shows, this foundational appropriation has after-effects which ripple through the entire myth, confusing the relation between origin and offspring.

Irigaray emphasizes how, both in the Myth of the Cave and in Plato's philosophy more generally, this relation is presented in terms of *mimesis*, understood as a process via which an original is copied or reproduced in its own likeness.[14] As indicated above, the

Forms (or Ideas) are thus the original archetypes which their off-spring (phenomenal objects) imperfectly replicate, creating a genealogical chain in which kinship is governed by degrees of sameness with the original (see *S*, 294). Thus, the images on the cave wall which the prisoners initially take to be real are revealed to be mere reflections, shadowy copies of the artefacts displayed in the light of the fire. The prisoners' ignorance in turn mirrors the way that human beings treat objects of the senses as real when, just like the shadows, they are in fact nothing but insubstantial copies of the original Forms.

Irigaray's reading shows that the relation between original and copy works on at least two levels in the Myth of the Cave. First, *within* the myth, not only are the shadows presented as mere copies of objects held up in front of the fire, but the whole space 'inside' the cave mirrors the 'real' world outside: the vault of the heavens corresponds to the ceiling of the cave; the sun corresponds to the fire (itself made in the image of the sun); and when darkness falls outside the cave, offering some relief to the released man's strained eyes, the night sky and gentle light of the moon double the dim light within the cave provided by the flickering flames (see *S*, 285). The shadows on the back wall are mirrored in the shadows and reflections in water that the released prisoner sees when he first emerges into daylight, while the objects casting the shadows outside the cave mirror the role of the statues within. In this way, the whole topology of the myth is organized according to a complex mimicry, where inside mirrors outside.

The second level at which the logic of copy and original operates is between the myth and what it represents. As we have seen, the inside of the cave is supposed to mirror the world of phenomena (that which appears to the senses), while the 'real' world outside the cave represents the reality of the Forms. To represent something is here to re-present it, to present its image or likeness. Thus, just as the inside of the cave mirrors the outside *within* the myth, so the myth as a whole mimes the relation between the world of appearances and the realm of the Forms.

Irigaray foregrounds the operations of this mimetic relation between original and copy to show how Plato's philosophy embodies a logic of the same (and hence substitutability): just as visible things are made in the likeness of the Forms, so the topology of the cave is organized by relations of likeness which allow one thing (the fire for example) to be substituted for another (the sun). In turn, to understand the myth, the good student must be able to work out what is 'like' what: that the world outside the cave is 'like' the reality of the Forms which transcends the shadowy realm of the senses, for example. This privileging of likeness might seem to be suspended when Glaucon notes the 'strangeness' of the subterranean prisoners; yet even here, Socrates immediately adds that this means they are 'like us', estranged as we are from the true reality of the Forms.[15]

Irigaray disturbs this logic of sameness by showing that the relation between original and copy is radically unstable. She hints at this in the passage cited above: if the night sky outside the cave mirrors the darkness within, is this because the cave's darkness is doubled by the night, or the night is the original which the subterranean darkness merely mimics? To the extent that the topography of the 'real' world seems to have been fashioned by duplicating key features of the cave, the problem of priority remains. Irigaray's point here is not to try and prove the so-called 'real' world (of the Forms) is in fact only a copy or projection based on the shadow-world of the senses. Rather, her point is that because of the way the cave's mythic topography pivots around an axis of symmetry that maps front onto back and inside onto outside (and vice versa), it is impossible to tell which has been made in the image of which: back or front, inside or outside, the realm of the senses or the realm of the Forms. The myth thus generates a fundamental confusion about where to locate the original that governs the operations of reflection and projection.

As we have seen, the logic of copy and original works at two levels, structuring the internal topography of the myth as well as the relation between the myth and what it represents. The confusion about what has the status of original and what is merely a copy thus impacts on both these levels. Irigaray can be read as commenting on both levels of confusion together when she notes that: 'if the cave is made in the image of the world, the world – as we shall see – is equally made in the image of the cave. In cave or "world", all is but the image of an image' (S, 246). If it is impossible to decide in any final way to what extent the world outside the cave is modelled on the inside (and vice versa), so too it is impossible to determine whether the image of the cave is modelled on our actual experience of the world of the senses, or our image of the sensible world (as no more than a seductive illusion) is itself modelled on Plato's seductive image of a subterranean world of shadows.

More seriously still, the reality of the Forms is represented in the myth by the realm of sensory objects outside the cave. But it is

precisely this 'reality' of sensory objects which the myth is supposed to show to be an insubstantial shadow world, like that *within*
the cave. Nonetheless, the highest Form of all, the Form of the
Good, is re-presented by the image of the sun: the 'real', fiery sun
that generates light. As Irigaray notes, 'This setup in which the
hystera is reversed fuels the confusion between a certain origin
defying representation and the daylight, the good clear light of
representation. The confusion between fire and light, the fire of
origin and the light of day' (*S*, 259). So, the (outside) world in the
myth is modelled on the (so-called) real world that we experience,
which is itself represented by the shadows inside the cave. But this
means that the myth models its representation of the Forms on the
very world that it teaches us to distrust.

On Irigaray's reading, then, the initial reversal of the womb
continues to produce further destabilizing effects. If the Forms are
modelled on the world of the senses, then the Platonic account of
origin is overturned. However, Irigaray does not seek simply to
reverse the structure of the myth to give the world of the senses
the status of origin. Rather, her reading suggests that the myth as
a whole is structured by a logic of mirroring which generates a
fundamental confusion between 'original' and 'copy', making it
impossible to tell where the true origin lies. Thus, in this *'topo-
graphic mime'* there is 'no possible recourse to a first time, a first
model' (*S*, 246). The apparently clear teleology of the myth, leading
us up and out of the cave in a straight line from illusion to truth,
is disrupted and undone.

The Wall Face that 'Works All Too Well'

The source of this confusion lies in the original act of representation: the image of a womb-like cave, and thus, a cave which
operates as a metaphor for the womb. As Irigaray puts it, 'this
cave is always already an attempt to re-present another cave, the
hystera, the mold which *silently* dictates all replicas, all possible
forms, all possible relation of forms and between forms, of any
replica' (*S*, 246; my emphasis). This originary substitution of cave
for womb must remain *silent* and unthematized: it 'prescribes
and overdetermines, in silence, the whole system of metaphor' (*S*,
259). If Socrates explicitly paralleled the cave with the womb as
the space/place where human beings begin, this would make it
impossible to posit the Forms as the one and only origin of

existence. Thus, the metaphorical operation whereby the generative powers of the mother are appropriated by the figure of the cave and projected onto the Forms must remain unacknowledged, or the status of the Forms themselves would be called into question: they would be revealed as projection rather than source, in ways that would compromise the whole trajectory of the myth. Hence, Irigaray argues, Plato's mythic account of origin depends on the success with which it 'conjures up a blindness over origin' – both human beings' origins in birth, and the origins of the image of the cave in the womb it re-presents (S, 294).

Yet, as we have seen, because the initial relation between original (womb) and metaphorical copy (cave) remains unacknowledged – as it must – the whole myth remains founded on an unacknowledged inversion: the passage leading *out* of the womb into the world becomes the passage leading *back* to the origin as the sun/Forms. Irigaray shows how this 'reversing projection' haunts the mythic structure (S, 259), generating a destabilizing confusion that cannot be resolved without turning back to address that first, silent act of inverting appropriation.

Her analysis shows that this appropriation is at least threefold: first, the womb is metaphorically taken up in the image of the cave to support an account of philosophical education as a kind of intellectual and spiritual re-birth; second, the myth ascribes the generative power of the mother to the Forms as origin; and third, it appropriates the materiality of the womb/cave in the service of the Forms, which require a material support for their productions. Just as the shadows can only appear on the back wall of the cave, which acts as a projecting screen, likewise, the archetypal Forms, as pure Ideas, must be materially instantiated if they are to appear at all. The cave/womb thus operates as the backcloth, the 'backdrop of representation' (S, 254).

Just as the generative power of the womb cannot be explicitly acknowledged but only silently appropriated, so in turn the power of the Forms to generate their own likenesses depends on the absolute passivity of the material in/on which they are reproduced:

> The feminine, the maternal are instantly *frozen* by the 'like', the 'as if' of that masculine representation dominated by truth, light, resemblance, identity. By some dream of symmetry that itself is never ever unveiled. The maternal, the feminine serve (only) to keep up the reproduction-production of doubles, copies, fakes, while any hint of their material elements, of the womb, is turned into scenery

to make the show more realistic. The *womb*, unformed, 'amorphous' origin of all morphology, is transmuted by/for analogy into a circus and a projection screen, a theater of/for fantasies. (*S*, 265)

If (phenomenal) copies are to mirror their (ideal) originals, then the mirroring material itself must remain inert and inactive: a 'frozen' and passive support of representation. It must add nothing new and make no real difference to what it reflects. At worst, the projected images might lose something of the originals, but providing the screen on which they appear stays still, they will remain recognizable – if less substantial – versions of the same. Thus the mimetic logic of the cave appropriates both the metaphorical power of the womb, so as to make its story 'more realistic', and its materiality, which supplies the necessary support for the shadow play of appearances.

In the Platonic metaphysics which the cave represents, the womb as a 'merely' material site of generation could not itself produce the form of that which grows within it. On this model, the womb is aligned with inert and formless matter (the frozen, bare surface of the rocky cave wall), as opposed to the generative reality of the Forms. It is the latter which actively in-form appearances and make things what they are. By showing how much the myth owes to the morphology of the womb, however, Irigaray exposes the deception involved in presenting the womb as simply 'a-morphous' or 'unformed'. The concept of 'morphology' is an important one for Irigaray, in ways we will return to in Chapter 6; for now, it is worth noting that this word is based on the Greek *morphē*, meaning shape or form. Significantly, form in this sense denotes the kinds of forms found in the sensible world, in terms of the shape, structure or configuration of organisms. The concept of morphology thus provides Irigaray with a language of sensible forms with which to counter both Plato's transcendent Forms or Ideas and the image of maternal matter as simply form-less. Instead, this matter gives the Forms a new form by allowing them to be translated into sensible configurations.

Irigaray's emphasis on the dizzying inversions between copy and original that characterize the cave's topography exposes the transgressive potential of the capacity of maternal-matter to turn (transcendent) Forms into (sensible) forms. Her reading constantly reminds us of the mirror's power to invert, multiply and transpose, rather than passively reflect and reproduce: 'The wall face works all too well. It multiplies all by itself' (*S*, 251). The maternal-matter that is appropriated as the support for visible representations thus refuses the passivity that would be required to adequately sustain the mimetic economy of the myth and the Platonic logic of 'the same'. In spite of the way the Myth of the Cave is designed to ascribe originary generative power to the Forms (and the Forms alone), the reproductive material on which the Forms depend continues to display its own active and transformative capacities.

The Artistry of Mirrors

If the cave wall functions as a reflective screen, it is not so much like glass, Irigaray notes, as the silvered back of a mirror, a speculum that has been introjected and incorporated in the very fabric of the myth (*S*, 255, 285). In a kind of morphological collapse, the cave/womb wall becomes a speculum, rather than being made visible in its mirrored surface. Once again, Irigaray shows that this introjection has complex effects. If the inside of the cave is a 'den of reflection' (*S*, 285), then the mimetic logic of copy and original that structures the relation of 'inside' to 'outside' is already in play *within* the cave. As Irigaray notes, within this subterranean space there are already *two* sets of men: the chained prisoners and those behind the wall. Yet already the instability of mimetic relations is suggested: although, as men, they are 'like' each other, they are not substitutible. The prisoners see the shadows but have no inkling how, or even that, that they are being manufactured. The 'magicians' behind the wall conjure up the shadows, but cannot see them: 'Hidden from the eyes they charm but equally kept away from seeing their own show, the effects of their own sorcery. ... They form artful attributes, eclipsing the light of the fire – the sun's image? – which etches their shadows on the back of the cave. Copy cats copied in their turn by reflections that steal out of reach of the miracle workers' (*S*, 250–1). The prisoners do not know what they are seeing; the magicians do not know what they are doing. Between them, the whole process unfolds, yet both are blind to what is really going on. The little wall that separates them allows objects to be held up in the firelight and multiplied as shadows without the mechanics of projection being seen.

Irigaray draws attention to the way that this little wall further destabilizes the structure of the myth, which opposes the shadowy darkness inside the cave to the sunlit realm outside. By dividing the cave in two, the wall means that the relation between inner and outer is already in play *within* the cave, making the relation of front to back even more unstable. Between them, the chained and unchained men '*uphold the process of mimēsis* from each side of a wall curtain in which their stratagems are lost in infinite regression. This facade doubles, redoubles, infinitely reverses the opposition of inner and outer, all within the symmetrical closure of this theater' (*S*, 251). On the one hand, the shadows are projected 'out' onto the wall by the fire; on the other, the prisoners' side of the wall is undoubtedly 'inner' insofar as it is deepest inside the cave. From another perspective, however, it is the space in which the fire is located that is 'inner', insofar as it is one step closer 'in' towards the Forms, while the back wall of the cave is the furthest 'out', as it is at the greatest distance from the sun.

Ultimately, it is of course the shadows themselves that make it most obvious that the mimetic logic of copy and original is already at play within the cave, long before the Forms make their (meta-phorical) appearance. In this regard, it is crucial that the objects projected above the wall are described by Plato as artefacts or statues: the shadows are thus copies of objects which are them-selves only imitations or copies, thereby reserving the status of the 'real' for the things 'outside' the cave.

Matters are therefore rather more complicated than they might at first appear. For as copies of copies, the shadows do not map directly onto everyday objects of the senses but onto the position Plato gives to works of art in Book X of the *Republic*. By re-present-ing what they see in the world around them, artists generate images that are at two removes from the truth: they make copies (art) of copies (phenomenal objects) of the Forms. On this view, works of art, like the 'artful attributes' projected onto the back wall of the cave, turn our gaze away from truth and ensnare us in a world of mere appearances.

Tellingly, when Plato describes the mimetic process via which artists produce their work, he uses the image of a mirror. The artist, Socrates notes, seems to be a remarkable craftsman, capable of making anything he wants: 'It isn't hard: you could do it quickly and in lots of places, especially if you were willing to carry a mirror with you, for that's the quickest way of all. With it you can quickly make the sun, the things in the heavens, the earth, yourself, the other animals, manufactured items, plants, and everything else mentioned just now.'[16] This image suggests that there is nothing genuinely creative involved in the production of art, no real work or activity at all. Just as a mirror cannot help but reflect what is placed in front of it, works of art passively mimic the surface appearance of things and are themselves no more than superficial images. In the context of the *Republic*, the passivity of the artist can be contrasted both with the active struggle of the philosopher to reach towards the truth, and perhaps more importantly, with the genuinely generative power of the Forms themselves as the true source of all that exists. Thus Socrates praises Glaucon when he remarks that although the artist can make an image of anything, he cannot 'make the things themselves as they truly are.'[17]

Likewise, the back wall in the Myth of the Cave can only reproduce insubstantial copies of statues that are themselves mere imitations of real things. Thus, as opposed to the Forms which generate the visible objects of the phenomenal world, the back wall does not really generate anything at all. Like artists' images, the shadows are only 'sham offspring' (*S*, 255), which do not directly reflect the reality of the Forms. And like the spinning mirror, the inside of the cave represents the danger of being ensnared in a seductive play of illusions.

By making the alignment between the cave and the womb explicit, Irigaray's reading presents Plato's myth as cementing a relation between the female sex and 'artful' appearances that will have a long and influential history. From the Bible to Film Noir, western culture is replete with images of deceptive seductresses whose superficial beauty lures the unwary man away from the Good and the True. More specifically, Irigaray shows how the image of the womb-like cave aligns the maternal-material capacity to generate with the deceptive powers of the artist:

> The mother. Place of conception of a still artful/artificial kind, haunted by magicians who would have you believe that what is at stake in (re)production can be executed by skilful imitators, working from divine plans. The cave gives birth only to phantoms, simulacra, or at best, images. One must leave its orbit to perceive the fake nature of such a birth. (*S*, 300; translation modified)

Despite its 'artfulness', it is crucial that this act of reproduction/representation is presented as nothing more than a passive mirroring, 'executed by skilful imitators'. Thus, strictly speaking, it is not an act at all but only a miming of reproduction: a fake birth that gives birth to fakes. On this model, insofar as the mother's power to birth belongs to the bodily realm of the senses, it is reduced to a capacity to reproduce sensible appearances in ways that are always already governed by the 'divine plans' provided by the Forms. Actual birth is thus a poor copy of the truly generative power that belongs to the Forms alone, and that ensures the proper mimetic relation between original and copy. The products of material reproduction must be made in the image of the Forms, however distantly related, while the Forms lend their imitations what little reality or 'being' they possess. As Irigaray notes, 'whichever way up you turn these premises, you always come back to *sameness*' (S, 263).

Irigaray's insistence on the way mirrors never simply passively reproduce, but always transpose and invert undoes Plato's image of artistic production as passive copying, as well as the mimetic logic that governs the Myth of the Cave. What Plato fails to account for sufficiently is the way in which both the method of projection, and the materiality of the projective surface, always make a difference to what appears. In the Myth of the Cave, this transforming power of reflective surfaces has to remain invisible for the 'proper' mimetic relation of Form and image, original and copy, to be established and preserved. This is why, Irigaray suggests, the magicians must remain blind to what they are doing and the mirror has to be introjected to become the back wall of the cave. The mirroring operations of mimesis must remain as invisible as possible, built into the very fabric of the myth, so that they need not be recognized as genuine activity at all.

Plato's cave is thus structured around:

> the inter-position of a certain *speculum* which, *naturally*, has already been enveloped. Everything on the inside here is already re-silvered. Closed up, folded back upon some kind of specular intuition. *A specularity of intuition that has yet to reflect its perspective and has yet to be interpreted into an intuition of specularity.* No mirror offers itself to be seen and read in this speleology. And the truth of what we see depends on this. (S, 255)

On Irigaray's reading, the unthematized role of the womb is matched by the necessary invisibility of a mirroring activity aligned with the cave's maternal-materiality. The silent appropriation of the mother's body is thus replicated in '*the disavowal of the mirror*' (S, 301). This mirror or screen, which supposedly reflects without making any active contribution of its own, in turn screens out the subversive possibility that maternal materiality might have its own capacity to form and transform.

In this chapter, we have embarked on a journey back towards the origins of western metaphysics whose aim is to question the metaphysical account of origin. As we have seen, Irigaray argues that the founding myth of this tradition borrows its resources from a maternal body whose generative powers it simultaneously disavows. By deliberately reading the cave as a metaphor for the womb, Irigaray seeks to make this appropriation visible and to reclaim the significance of our beginnings in birth. Much of her strategy lies in showing how the original appropriation on which the myth depends generates a logic of doubles and reversals that destabilize it from within and reveal that the cave's maternal materiality, far from operating as a meekly passive support, can work to actively distort and transform the representations projected onto it. As we will see in later chapters, it is this repressed possibility of an actively self-shaping matter that Irigaray seeks to recover so as to represent woman as a subject, rather than a metaphorical resource for matricidal philosophical myths.

3

The Way Out of the Cave:
A Likely Story ...

This chapter will examine Irigaray's reading of the birth of meta-physics as represented in the prisoner's transition out of the cave. As we will see, by linking the Myth of the Cave to key aspects of Plato's *Timaeus*, she deepens her analysis of the Platonic appropriation of the maternal. At the same time, however, this chapter will show that Irigaray's approach to Plato is never merely critical. Throughout her reading, she signals that which is forgotten and repressed within the myth. In so doing, she begins to find the terms with which to articulate an alternative philosophy of sexuate difference that recognizes our singular beginnings in birth.

The final section of the chapter will link Irigaray's reading of the cave to a later text in which she reclaims another Platonic figure: Diotima, the wise woman who reportedly teaches Socrates about love. Just as she seeks to recover the forgotten traces of the maternal from the Myth of the Cave, Irigaray reads Diotima's speech from *Symposium* against the metaphysical trajectory which it seems to support. Via this deliberately subversive reading, she recovers a lost teaching which privileges the relation between the sexes, rather than the relation to the Forms. Instead of a single and unchanging origin, then, Irigaray's Diotima teaches of a relation between two conceived as a mutual re-engendering that repeats and renews the fecundity of birth.

The Prisoner and his Shadow

Before turning to Diotima, it is worth following Irigaray as she tracks the prisoner's journey out of the cave, to see what this adds to her analysis. Given the reversal of the *hystera*, which turns the passage out into the world into a path back to origin, it is not surprising that the destabilizing confusions continue when the prisoner is led out of the cave. This primary reversal creates: 'hosts of symmetrical effects: from top to bottom, from outside to inside, from forward to backward. And vice versa. The transposition – or transpositions – at work in the project of the cave are repeated and redoubled, *both like and other*' (*S*, 289; my emphasis). As this last comment suggests, despite the play of mirroring effects, the inside and outside of the cave do not in fact map onto each other in any neat way. It is true that the fire is in the image of the sun, while the roof of the cave envelops the prisoner like the heavens which arch over the earth. But in the transition from inside to outside, not everything maps: 'What about the images in the water?' Irigaray asks, 'They correspond to *nothing* figuring in the grotto since all mirrors are banned there.' Likewise, there are 'no more magicians' outside the cave – 'or at least none under that name. No more instruments used to effect the magicians' enchantments, no more fetish-statues with fascinating reflections'. There is not even a path, 'merely a process, a progress of methodically forming the gaze' (*S*, 285). There are features of the scene outside that have no direct correlate inside the cave, and – more worryingly from a Platonic point of view – elements within the cave that are never translated directly into the scene outside.

This is problematic because outside and inside are not supposed to be disconnected. On the contrary, things on the outside are supposed to reveal the true nature of things on the inside, in the same way that the Forms reveal the true nature of that which appears to the senses. The fact that some elements remain *untranslated* on both sides not only shows that inside and outside do not map perfectly onto one another after all; it also suggests that there might be elements that are *untranslatable*, and that remain in reserve, resistant to the operations of symmetry. Despite initial appearances, then, it is not in fact possible to 'turn the scene of the womb or at least *its representation* back/over. As one might turn a purse, or a pocket, or a string bag, or even a wallet inside out' (*S*, 284). This is less of a problem with respect to elements on the outside that are not translatable into elements within the cave: that the Origin should exceed its weaker, poorer copies should not come as a surprise. But it *is* a problem if the supposedly derivative world of shadows includes anything that exceeds the Origin, for this suggests that the Origin might not, after all, be the cause of all that is.

The ways in which the topography of the myth turns out not to be fully reversible suggests that a risk remains of 'being over-whelmed by a surplus, a *remainder*, which (theoretically) has not been taken into account and which would go beyond all calcula-tion, all operation on/with already defined symbols' (*S*, 285). As we have seen, on Irigaray's reading, this 'remainder' is the female body, whose maternal and material aspects are appropriated by the myth while being denied any status or value of their own. Indeed, as we have also seen, this debt to the maternal can never be acknowledged: it constitutes a blindspot, a necessary repression, which is the condition of Platonic metaphysics.

Before we leave the details of the myth behind, it is worth noting several peculiar features that come into view when the prisoner leaves the cave, and to which Irigaray draws particular attention. For alongside the elements that do not translate at all from inside to outside, we find at least two which stay the same: the body of the prisoner, which travels up the passage from cave to world, and the shadows, which appear outside the cave as well as on its back wall: 'The shadows would correspond to the shadows. And effort will be made to convince you of this' (*S*, 285). This 'sameness' is a specific kind of untranslatibility that compromises the metaphori-cal structure of the myth. If the body of the prisoner and the shadows appear 'the same' both inside and outside, this means that they have no mirror images or analogical doubles. Thus, the mapping of one element onto an other cannot be all-encompassing or complete.

Nonetheless, it could be argued that the fact that the body of the released prisoner remains the same is not ultimately disruptive, but confirms a central feature of Plato's metaphysics. For if the body passes fundamentally unchanged between the inside and the outside of the cave, the mind or soul of the prisoner does not: indeed, the whole point of the myth concerns the intellectual trans-formation produced by the journey. Thus, this aspect of the myth can be read as confirming the Platonic division between body and soul, according to which the body is ultimately inessential to the philosophical journey towards wisdom.

In the case of the shadows, however, Irigaray's reading shows that things are more complicated. Just as the first thing the chained prisoner sees is the play of shadows on the cave wall, so shadows are the first thing the freed prisoner sees outside the cave. Instead of being analogically related to the realm outside the cave (as fire is to Sun), the shadows seem to simply re-appear there: there are shadows below and shadows above. Despite appearances, however, these shadows are not simply equivalent: they do not signify the same thing. The shadows *inside* the cave are copies of copies, and represent illusory appearances. The shadows *outside* the cave are reflections of 'real' objects (the Forms) and represent the lowest degree of reality that culminates in the Form of the Good. Thus, while all appearances are the same insofar as they are more or less imperfect copies of the Forms, there is still a hierarchy which distinguishes between them according to degrees of imperfection. As Irigaray's reading suggests, even where sameness seems to rule, there are still differences at work which prevent one thing from being mapped perfectly onto an other. So, 'The shadows are not the "same" shadows', after all (*S*, 286).

To complicate things further, Irigaray notes an odd omission where the shadows are concerned. For amidst all the shadows he does see, the prisoner never seems to see his own: 'The black shade spreading out over the earth at his feet' (*S*, 288). Hence, 'the relation between the prisoner and "his" shadow is never raised here. This is not the time for auto-reflection, much less for calculating its incidence upon the scene of representation' (*S*, 290–1). As with everything else, relations between men, and between man and his own image, are all regulated by the Forms, by:

> the search for more and more copies of the same, of the autos whose term is eclipsed by the domination of the Idea. Nothing, including man, therefore, can rejoice in its own image since 'own-ness' is dictated, commanded, monopolized by Truth. And Truth will in fact repeat, reproduce, represent only itself, in the shape of more or less good ideas, more or less faithful copies. Autogamous offspring of Truth. Thus man is a more or less good copy of the (more or less good) idea of man. (S, 291)

In the context of the mimetic logic that governs Plato's myth, it is telling that the relation between the prisoner and his own shadow is not explicitly thematized. This absence, Irigaray suggests, is symptomatic of the repressions that sustain Plato's metaphysical system in two ways.

First, were the myth to draw attention to the relation between man and his shadow – his projected outline – this might lead to questions about the extent to which other aspects of the cave are also made in man's image. It might make one wonder, for example, whose sensible forms might be tacitly reflected in the idealized realm projected over and above man's earthly home. It might lead one to notice that alongside and contesting the morphology of the womb/cave, another '*morphological impress*' marks the topography of the cave (*S*, 250): the straight line (the wall, the path), the vertical trajectory (up out of the cave), the erection (of statues and heavenly bodies). This morphological tendency culminates in the erection/projection of the Form of the Good as the Sun, high up above the earth. Such transcendence reflects the way that Platonic metaphysics privileges the intelligible over the sensible, the ideal and unchanging Forms over material becomings. Yet despite its devaluation of the sensible, this morphology of erection, Irigaray suggests, echoes and idealizes a specifically male – phallic – form (*morphē*). Read in this way, the myth stages an overcoming of the mother's body in favour of what Irigaray calls an '*ideal* morphology' (*S*, 317): ideal because of the ways in which phallic erection is idealized, but also because this morphology supports the erection of an ideal – metaphysical – realm.

The second way in which the absence of a relation between the prisoner and his own shadow is symptomatic of the repressions at work in Platonic metaphysics is in the lack of self-relation or auto-affection that it represents ('Nothing, including man, can rejoice in its own image'; *S*, 291). While Irigaray's key concern is with the way woman is defined in relation to the male subject, here she foregrounds this *male* subject's lack of relation to himself. If woman's relation to her own sex is mediated through man, within the context of Platonic metaphysics, man's self-relation is mediated through the (self-same) Forms. Because his gaze is turned away from his origin in the mother – away from the cave/womb – as well as away from his own body, he has no sense of himself as a singular being rooted in the uniqueness of his birth: no sense of himself as constituted 'within (an) origin and (as) an original' (*S*, 293).

Like the prisoner who emerges into the dazzling glare of the sun, the philosophical pupil who learns to focus his gaze on the Forms will be cut off: 'From everything that might remind him, bring him back toward, turn him in the direction of *his* beginning, an "origin" that is still inscribed within and also inscribes a singular history, "*properly one's own*" – one that re-marks itself in its projects, its projections, detours, returns, as well as in their metaphors' (*S*, 293; translation modified). Acknowledging one's bodily beginnings in the mother would permit each human being a sense of their own irreducible singularity, a singularity grounded in an originary relation to an equally irreducible other. This acknowledgement would also reinscribe itself in the ways in which human beings make sense of the world, leading them to invest in metaphors less appropriative of the m/other. Turning back to one's relation to a mother would thus transform the ways in which human beings project themselves onto the world and orient themselves within it.

More Mirrors

As shown in the previous chapter, the Myth of the Cave seeks to establish the proper order between origin and copy. By contrast, Irigaray shows how this project is destabilized from within because it is never acknowledged that the Forms themselves are already a copy: an idealized mimicry of maternal origins. Thus, despite the myth's orientation towards the search for Truth, Irigaray ironically praises its author for his own expertise in mimicry, aligning him with the production of fakes and imitations (*S*, 266). By reworking Plato's most famous image, Irigaray subversively mimes his mimicry.

That the Myth of the Cave is indeed governed by mimicry rather than truth is signalled by the proliferation of mirrors. Irigaray's reading suggests that not only is the back wall of the cave a speculum, so too is the Form of the Good. This is because, within the structure of the myth, there is more than one way to map inside onto outside, such that the Sun/Forms do not only correspond to the fire. Irigaray reminds us that a vertical axis also governs the relation of inside and outside: the prisoner travels from *down* in the cave *up* into the light. Thus we can pivot the image of the cave around the passageway that conjoins the two realms, mapping top to bottom and bottom to top. The Sun/Form of the Good would then map onto the same position as the back of the cave, where the shadow-play is reflected. Irigaray suggests as much when she positions the Form of the Good as a mirror:

> *But this source is already a mirror.* The enlightenment of the Idea makes flames just like a mirror that has concentrated the light. Of the Sun, of the Good. And, in a different way, of the eye, of the soul, of the eye (of the) soul. ... The same, (specifically) mirror, brings its reflections together and spawns a genealogy. It has to be the same if the hierarchy of ideas, their progression as well as their infinite regression, is to arise out of a certain order. A single one will reproduce itself differently in each, according to how clean, shining, polished

each may be, how apt it is for reflection. Descendence and ascend-
ence are degrees of perfection in the realization of the reproduction
of the Idea. Which is already, also, a speculum. (*S*, 294)

This passage shows how the Sun (the Idea or Form of the Good)
maps onto both the fire within the cave (the flames) and the back
of the cave as projecting screen (a mirror). The Sun/Form of the
Good concentrates the entire visible realm into a single origin
whose offspring are projected back into the world in an endless
succession of copies of the same. The Sun is thus not only a mirror
but a burning glass, a metaphor for the way the Forms consume
appearances, abolishing superficial differences between them by
grounding them all in *one and the same* origin.

   It is towards this burning origin that the prisoner's gaze is to be
re-oriented when he emerges from the shadowy depths of the
cave. Yet as Irigaray notes, this means the prisoner too becomes a
mirror: having been turned around to face the Sun, he is better
placed to reflect its light. Similarly, the eye of the soul must be
turned away from the material world and refocused on the realm
of the Forms if the educative process is to give birth to a philosopher. The student thus comes to reflect (on) the Form of which he
too is only a copy. He is both mirror and fake, a reproduction of
Truth, made (merely) in its image (see *S*, 291). Moreover, insofar
as any of us turns our gaze towards the Forms – as the myth
teaches we should – we are reduced to so many reflections of one
and the same origin, one and the same truth. Thus, on Irigaray's
reading, the myth reveals the way in which the metaphysical education that Socrates seeks to impart erases the singularity of individual human beings.

   Although Irigaray suggests that both the released prisoner and
the Form of the Good become mirrors, she also notes that in the
transition from inside to outside the cave, a crucial shift takes place
in the way the operations of mirroring are presented. On the one
hand, even though the wall of the cave operates as a reflecting
screen, Irigaray notes that there is nothing inside the cave that is
explicitly presented as a mirror. She suggests that within the cave,
mirrors must be banned to prevent too much reflection on the logic
of mimicry which organizes (and undermines) the myth as a
whole. On the other hand, once outside the cave, the prisoner is
presented with the reflective surface of the water, but now, crucially, the magicians who produced the shadows inside the cave
have disappeared. Instead of the obvious staging and trickery

inside the cave, shadows and reflections are now produced 'naturally': 'this time the reflections are guaranteed not by the cunning, the magic practices, the spells of the magicians – since these can result only in "opinions" – but by nature' (*S*, 289–90).

With the disappearance of the men who conjure up the shadows, the work that goes into producing a copy or image also ceases to be visible. The fact that such productions involve an activity of projection (the statues must be held up above the wall) as well as a gap between original and copy (marked by the little wall inside the cave) becomes more difficult to see. This in turn means that the difference between original and copy is occluded, along with the possibility that copying might involve active transformation rather than merely passive duplication. Instead, the production of copies is naturalized, 'within a *reduplication* that is more and more instantaneous, instantly masterable and mastered. More and more clear, luminous, evident. Or at least that's the idea.' (*S*, 289)

Indeed, not only is there no wall explicitly separating original from copy outside the cave, but as Irigaray notes, there is also no path leading the prisoner from objects possessing a lesser degree of being to those which are more real: 'No more *materialized* transition between the outside and the inside or noticeable separation between the entrance and the "back" of the cave' (*S*, 285). Once the prisoner is outside the cave, the remainder of his journey takes place not by following a path, but by methodically re-orienting his gaze. And while this still involves the body (Plato himself emphasizes the importance of turning the whole body towards the light of the Sun/the Good),[1] refocusing the gaze is nonetheless primarily an internal process, one that more readily lends itself as a metaphor for re-orienting the soul.

As Irigaray draws out, the disappearance of the explicit trickery that takes place inside the cave is one of the most deceptive ploys at work in the myth. The image of 'real' objects whose shadows and reflections are 'naturally' produced reinforces the idea that the relation between the Forms (the real) and their phenomenal copies is equally natural: that this is not only the way things *are*, but the way things *must* be and – as is 'natural' – *ought* to be. There is no visible trickery here: 'the hand-crafted contrivances of men on the underground scene have, supposedly, been suppressed' (*S*, 289). Yet just where things seem most 'natural' is precisely where the sleight of hand takes place.

According to the myth, Nature – material, physical nature – lacks the reality of the Forms, and is, at best, a necessary support for the shadow-play of appearances that constitute the phenomenal world. Like this shadow-play, nature is deceptive: by embodying the Forms, it corrupts their unchanging (non-material) 'nature' with the ever-changing world of birth, growth, decay and death. Thus, just as maternal generative power is appropriated in the name of the Forms, while material birth is degraded, so the legitimizing force of what is 'natural' is appropriated at the same time as nature itself is banished to a shadowy realm of deception.

The Maternal–Material: Blindspot of Metaphysics

Irigaray's reading shows how the traditional alignment of woman and nature is cemented in the figure of the cave, that womb-like space/place that represents both the maternal body and the material world, and opposes both to the ideality of the Forms. Maternal matter is frozen into the other of the Truth of Being – a dangerous yet necessary other. To elaborate this point, Irigaray draws on another Platonic dialogue which deals with the question of origins, namely, *Timaeus*. One of the advantages of this dialogue from Irigaray's point of view is that it makes the gendering of the metaphysical theory of Forms particularly explicit.

Timaeus offers an account of the origin of the universe, and of the natural world in particular. It is especially important in the western philosophical tradition because it is the first major text to offer an account of the world as the deliberate product of a creator–god who is seen as a kind of craftsman.[2] The question of origin makes this text powerfully resonant for Irigaray, as does its explicit presentation of the relation between the Forms and the phenomenal world as one of 'likeness'. Her reading of Platonic metaphysics as privileging a mimetic relation of sameness is in keeping with Timaeus' account of the creator–god who seeks to make the disorderly universe 'as like himself as possible',[3] and who thus organizes the entire realm of visible nature in the image of a perfect model: 'it must have been constructed on the pattern of what is apprehensible by reason and understanding and eternally unchanging; from which again it follows that the world is a likeness of something else.'[4] The visible universe mirrors the all-encompassing perfection of a model that 'comprises in itself all intelligible beings'. Thus there can be only *one* visible world, which in turn contains the phenomenal counterparts or copies ('ourselves and all visible creatures') of these original intelligible beings.[5]

What is especially telling from Irigaray's point of view is that in *Timaeus*, the creation of this single universe based on a single ideal model is clearly gendered. Not only is the creator–god both 'maker and father',[6] but the model from which he works is also metaphorically presented as the 'father' of the visible world.[7] *Timaeus* thus lends further justification to Irigaray's mapping of the Forms (and the Form of the Good in particular), onto the Father. In *Timaeus*, the universe is made in the image of a male divinity and male ideal. Men who fail to live up to such standards by living 'cowardly or immoral lives' are reincarnated as women.[8] On this model, both the female sex and sexual difference arise out of deficiency, in ways that are repeated and reinforced throughout the history of western philosophical thought.

The most significant aspect of *Timaeus* for Irigaray is the way in which it shows how the maternal principle aligned with woman remains a necessary resource for metaphysics, even as woman herself is presented as the result of a kind of deficiency or lack. *Timaeus* outlines a three level account of creation: there is the unchanging and intelligible model (the Forms); the visible and changing universe which is its copy (imperfect because changing); and what Timaeus calls the 'receptacle' or 'matrix' into and onto which the Forms impose their pattern so as to generate phenomenal objects. This threefold distinction is summarized as 'that which becomes [is in the process of generation], that in which it becomes [in which the generation takes place], and the model which it [the thing generated] resembles.'[9] Though the 'receptacle' receives the impress of the Forms, these do not mark it in any permanent way. The imprint of the Forms makes it *appear* differently at different times, but in itself, it remains always the same: that in which the Forms appear.[10] Timaeus suggests that the receptacle should thus be thought of as a kind of 'space, which is eternal and indestructible, which provides a position for everything that comes to be'.[11]

The parallel with the cave is already clear: both the cave and the 'receptacle' constitute the space/place of appearances. The link is strengthened when Timaeus refers to appearances as 'moving shadows' which need 'to come into existence in something else'.[12] But whereas the cave is *implicitly* gendered (as a metaphorical appropriation of the womb), the 'receptacle' of Being is *explicitly* compared by Timaeus to the mother: 'We may indeed use the metaphor of birth and compare the receptacle to the mother, the model to the father, and what they produce between them to their offspring.'[13] As Irigaray shows, this metaphor crystallizes an image

of sexual difference which will come to dominate the western tradition, in which active form-giving force is aligned with the father
alone, whereas the mother is an utterly passive receiver.

According to Timaeus, the receptive mother/matter must be
devoid of any features or activity of her own that could interfere
with the proper reproduction of the father's form:

> that which is going to receive properly and uniformly all the like-
> nesses of the intelligible and eternal things must itself be devoid of
> all character. Therefore we must not call the mother and receptacle
> of visible and sensible things either earth or air or fire or water, nor
> yet any of their compounds or components; but we shall not be
> wrong if we describe it as invisible and formless, all-embracing,
> possessed in a most puzzling way of intelligibility, yet very hard to
> grasp.[14]

The mother-receptacle is indeed a puzzle: like the Forms, she must
herself be eternally the same, yet it is impossible to say 'what' she
is: she embraces everything without being anything. Or, as Irigaray
puts it 'she is nothing, but shares in everything. ... Needed to define
essences, her function requires that she herself have no definition.
Neither will she have any distinct appearance. Invisible, therefore'
(S, 307). The mother-receptacle is the necessary support of the
visible realm, yet invisible herself; the necessary space/place in
which the Forms can appear to the senses, yet formless herself. It
is hardly surprising that Timaeus says we apprehend this necessary
receptacle 'by a sort of spurious reasoning'. Like the prisoners in
the cave, when we try and think about the mother-receptacle, we
get lost 'in a kind of dream'.[15]

As Irigaray notes, the philosopher's journey towards truth ought
to banish such dreams: 'all dreams, all fantasies, all fakes have been
condemned by him as childish nonsense' (S, 311). Once one learns
to reason properly, the illusions of the senses should be left behind,
just as the shadows should be left behind in the cave: such illusions
are like the fantasies that belong to infancy when one is still tied
to the mother. But as Timaeus suggests, and Irigaray emphasizes,
even once the philosopher begins to reason, his attempts to explain
the universe are haunted by a dream of the material-maternal
realm which the rational order of the Forms transcends, but on
which it depends nonetheless. For the Forms can only be materialized in the space of becoming, and yet, to protect the status of the
Forms as the sole origin of being, this space cannot itself contribute

anything to the being of that which becomes. This space is form-less: it cannot be articulated by reason, which is governed by the logic (*logos*) of the Forms, even though it is required for the articulation of Forms into beings. Irigaray's analysis shows that Platonic metaphysics depends on a necessary excess, an unrepresentable space/place which it gestures towards via an image: the image of the mother.

Metaphysical/Metaphorical Resources

If the mother serves as a figure for the necessary excess required to sustain metaphysics, this metaphorical alignment in turn reinforces a particular image of woman. On the one hand, it is only because the mother has already been represented as a passive receptacle for the father's form-giving force that she can be deployed as a metaphor for a space/place of becoming which lacks any form-giving force of its own. On the other hand, the alignment of the mother with this irreducible 'remainder' reinforces the image of woman as the necessary 'other' of rational order. The image of the mother and that of the 'receptacle of becoming' are thus mutually reinforcing: each strengthens the image of the other as a necessary but irrational excess defined in opposition to a rational form-giving force that is aligned with the father (human or divine).

Irigaray dramatizes this point by writing of both mother and receptacle together: 'She is always a clean slate for the father's impressions, which she forgets as they are made. Unstable, inconsistent, fickle, unfaithful, she seems ready to receive all beings into herself. Keeping no trace of them. Without memory. She herself is without figure or face or proper form' (*S*, 307). By collapsing the receptacle of becoming and the mother into a single female figure, Irigaray here mimes the ways in which Platonic metaphysics erases difference. Mother and receptacle are substitutable insofar as each is defined as 'other' to the Forms. There is thus no figure or form which represents the specificity of the mother's being as a woman.

On this model, woman is therefore left 'without memory'. As we have seen, for Plato, the philosopher's task is to recall the originary power of the Forms to engender beings in their own image. However, for this to happen, it is equally necessary that any active contribution made by the mother-receptacle is forgotten. Above all, Irigaray observes, it is crucial that woman herself does not recall her own role in this process: that she does not begin to examine the dependency of the Forms on a receptive maternal environment which allows them to appear, or to question whether maternal matter does not perhaps actively shape the Forms she reflects, especially as reflection always inverts and transforms. Likewise, if the primary inversion that attributes originary power to the Forms (or Ideas) is to be sustained, it is vital that this power to engender offspring does not remind woman of the generative powers of her own sex:

> And the receptacle, the place of becoming, remembers nothing. Otherwise it would – perhaps – bear witness to the irreducible inversion that occurs in specula(riza)tion and in the re-production of any imprint, any trace, any form, even ideal ones. If the process of the Idea's inscription is to be lost to consciousness, if the mirror that has always already reflected it is to be covered over, then it is obligatory to forget that the Idea once came into being. It must, absolutely must, not be known how much the procreation of the 'son', of the logos, by the father, owes to inversion. Nor that the mother is the place where that inversion occurs. That she is the one that makes it possible, practicable, that sustains it with/in her 'unconsciousness.' The mother, happily, seems to have no memory. She submits in all (new) projects, blind to all (new) projections. Screen-base, helping them to multiply. (S, 310)

In reminding the reader of what is supposed to be forgotten, Irigaray speaks in a disruptive female voice that refuses to forget and instead re-collects the specificity of maternal generative power and its role in sustaining metaphysics.

This alternative, non-Platonic act of recollection is exemplified in the way Irigaray analyses the relation between the receptacle and the Forms. Both the mother-receptacle and the Forms are invisible, but not in the same way. The receptacle is beyond representation because it underlies all visible appearances; the Forms by contrast transcend appearances as their engendering source. This means that, as Irigaray puts it, 'The "beyond" of the mother ... cannot be measured alongside that of the father' (S, 307). This comment not only suggests the way that the Forms and the maternal receptacle occupy different positions *within* Platonic metaphysics. It can also be read as suggesting that the maternal remains *outside* the standards established by the Forms in ways that cannot be accounted for in the father's terms. Read in this way, Irigaray's comment suggests that the maternal remains irreducibly other in ways that demand a quite different system of measurement: a different set of values to those embodied in Platonic metaphysics.

From Irigaray's perspective then, *Timaeus'* image of the receptacle reinforces the way that the body of the mother is appropriated to supply the metaphorical and material resources required by Platonic metaphysics: 'She is the reserve of "sensuality" for the elevation of intelligence, she is the matter used for the imprint of forms' (*S*, 141). But this image also helps us to recover a sense of the maternal as an irreducible excess that resists being fully comprehended within that metaphysical frame. *Timaeus* is also useful insofar as it makes explicit the more implicit role of the mother in the Myth of the Cave, where the cave/womb operates as the receptacle that receives the imprint of the Forms and thus as the screen or 'matrix' of appearances.

'Matrix' (*la matrice*) translates an ancient Greek word for womb (*metra*, from *meter*, mother), which is used in *Timaeus* alongside *hystera*,[16] and which has subsequently been overlaid with the Latin for both womb (*mātrīx*) and mother (*māter*). As others have noted, such etymologies mean that Irigaray's texts work to reveal and reclaim the *mater*-iality of matter, revaluing the maternal by rethinking the material, and acknowledging both as actively generative.[17] Irigaray uses the term matrix (*matrice*) repeatedly in her reading of the Cave, in ways that provide another good example of her style. By deliberately playing on the multiple meanings that co-exist within a single term, Irigaray encourages her reader to develop an ear for the multiple and often contradictory positions occupied by woman within western thought – as well as for the buried resonances of a forgotten maternal power. Both the original Greek word that can be translated as 'matrix' and its modern French correlate (*la matrice*) refer directly to the womb. The primary meaning of the modern English correlate – matrix as a material or environment in which something develops – foregrounds the parallel between the womb and the maternal space/place where Forms become appearances. The French and English terms also both signify a 'mould' (recalling the way the Forms impose their pattern on the receptacle),[18] as well as a lattice-like structure or a mathematical grid of quantities manipulated according to rules. This too is significant for Irigaray's multi-layered reading: the mother/matter both provides a frame for metaphysics, and is manipulated so as to fulfil the multiple functions required of her to sustain the system: screen, mirror, mould, receptacle; unstable yet inert; infinitely malleable yet utterly formless.

In this way, Irigaray's portrayal of the impressionable and undis-
criminating mother-receptacle draws out the contradictions which
mark woman's position as man's irrational 'other'. On the one
hand, she is positioned as unstable and ever-changing, impossible
to define or pin down. On the other, this instability never amounts
to activity; instead, she is blankly malleable and passive, incapable
of generating figures or forms of her own. 'Properly speaking, one
can't say that she mimics anything for that would suppose a certain
intention, a project, a minimum of consciousness. She (is) pure
mimicry' (S, 307). This passage again recalls the cave wall, which
sustains the flickering world of shadowy illusions while nonetheless operating as a supposedly mute and passive reflecting screen.
Thus, whether she is aligned with the space/place of becoming or
the material support of the Forms, woman is positioned as neither
having a form of her own, nor being capable of engendering forms.
Instead, she is reduced to the necessary 'other' to the Being, reason,
truth, and reality which orients the male philosopher.

By showing how Platonic metaphysics relies on a tightly woven
set of alignments between the mother, matter, the projecting/reflect-
ing surface, and the receptacle of becoming, Irigaray shows how
that metaphysics both reflects and reinforces a culture which reduces
woman to the other of a rational (male) order. At the same time,
however, she also shows how changing the position of woman –
that is, re-conceiving her in ways that do justice to her specificity
such that she is no longer reduced to a deficient male – will be
inseparable from rethinking the terms that inform the western
metaphysical tradition. If woman's bodily specificity as the sex
which gives birth is not to be aligned with an inert and irrational
materiality, then our model of matter (and indeed of reason) needs
to change just as much as the ways in which we represent the
mother.

The Forgotten Passage

A point not made explicitly by Irigaray, but in keeping with her
subversive reading, is that the account of origins given in *Timaeus*
is offered not by Socrates, but Timaeus himself, one of Socrates'
interlocutors and admirers. This rhetorical strategy in effect places
a question mark over the reliability of the text, underscoring the
necessarily mythic and speculative status of Timaeus' views.
Indeed, Timaeus himself reminds us that not only is he dealing

with events that occurred long before human beings existed, but with claims about the world of becoming which can never attain the status of (unchanging) truth. Thus, even though the contrast Timaeus draws between passively receptive matter and actively generative form will become the dominant model in western metaphysics, Timaeus' account is at best only 'a likely story'.[19] As Irigaray notes elsewhere: 'Things could be thought differently' (*ILTY*, 43).

Throughout her engagement with Plato, Irigaray works to recover the terms for a different story, and a different account of maternal matter than that offered in Platonic metaphysics. Importantly, Irigaray does not first critique Plato and then offer her own theoretical position. Such a linear progression would merely repeat the logic of the Cave by replacing (Platonic) illusion with a new (feminist) truth. However, the fact that Irigaray does not set out a clearly delineated theory of her own has tended to lead to an overemphasis on the critical aspects of *Speculum*. Irigaray is often described as 'deconstructing' Plato's metaphysics in ways that do not do justice to the manner in which she continually offers us the terms with which we could begin to think differently. She does this not by outlining an alternative theory, but by weaving a counter-voice through the text.

This voice exceeds the terms of Platonic metaphysics without straightforwardly opposing them. Instead, it emerges alongside and within Irigaray's re-presentation of Plato's thought. Thus, in her playful re-appropriation of the mother as 'matrix', Irigaray links the matrix (*la matrice*) to *matriciel* (see for example *Sf*, 368, 372). As a standard adjective, *matriciel* is generally used in mathematical contexts to refer to a mode of calculation. Irigaray makes the term resonate differently because of the way her text so strongly foregrounds its root in *la matrice* as womb. Thus, in *Speculum*, *matriciel* recalls *matricide*, linking 'matrix' with the metaphysical appropriation and obliteration of the mother's generative powers. However, *matriciel* also conjoins *la matrice* with the French for sky or heavens, *le ciel*. Even as she recalls a founding act of metaphysical matricide, then, Irigaray simultaneously invokes an image of the heavens as oriented by the mother rather than fathered by the Forms. She thereby invites the reader to imagine a different horizon, one oriented in relation to our maternal origins in birth.

Irigaray's deployment of the *matriciel* is another example of her productive 'double-speak', allowing her to speak of an order outside that of Platonic metaphysics by subversively miming and re-appropriating its terms. This mode of writing means that *Speculum* is never 'merely' subversive and critical. Instead, Irigaray's dense reworking of the Myth of the Cave shows that its fundamental terms can be re-thought in ways that recover our maternal-material origins as well as a non-reductive relation to sexuate difference. Like the wall face that works 'all too well', Irigaray's re-telling generates crucial differences that refuse to be wholly contained by the metaphysical horizon provided by the Platonic Forms.

To achieve this, Irigaray repeatedly draws attention to aspects of maternal morphology that the myth borrows yet cannot fully account for. In particular, she draws attention to 'the forgotten passage', between the cave/womb and the world outside. To say this is forgotten may seem odd, given Socrates' emphasis on the transition in which the released prisoner is dragged reluctantly up the passage in a painful journey into the world. In its mimicry of birth, this is an aspect of the myth that most obviously draws on the maternal metaphor (see *S*, 279). Yet in the opening pages of her reading of Plato, Irigaray insists that something has nonetheless been forgotten in the way the figure of the passage operates. In Plato's myth, once the released prisoner has passed out of the cave, what is emphasized is the difference between the darkness inside and enlightened world outside, between fire and sun, illusion and truth, appearance and reality, copy and original. In other words, as Irigaray argues, the myth foregrounds a set of oppositions 'that assume the *leap* from a worse to a better' (*S*, 247). The passageway is reduced to a pivot or axis of symmetry around which these oppositions revolve. As Irigaray puts it, its function is to 'subtend, sustain the hardening of all dichotomies, categorical differences, clear-cut distinctions, absolute discontinuities' (*S*, 246). The passage becomes the axis of reversal that secures the mimetic economy in which inside mirrors outside, and everything in the end is a reflection or inversion of the Same – the Forms.

What is thereby forgotten, Irigaray insists, is 'how to pass through the passage': it is the passage as transitional space *between* one and another 'that is neither outside nor inside, that is between the way out and the way in, between access and egress' (*S*, 246–7). Even within the topography of the Cave, Irigaray finds a trace of a different economy, one which does not function in terms of oppositions and reflections of sameness, but which is regulated by a space between which allows one and another to be conjoined while remaining distinct, to remain in touch without simply becoming one. Her reading reminds us that the birth canal is a passage that does not simply pass *between* inside and outside, but allows one to pass *through* another in a journey in which mother and child remain in intimate contact without being either the same or substitutable for one another. She thereby reminds us that the child begins life as an 'other within', in ways that cannot be mapped via the oppositional distinctions of inside/outside, same/other that structure the Myth of the Cave.[20]

Along with the passageway between the inside and outside of the cave, Irigaray's reading emphasizes the path within the cave that links front and back and allows the released prisoner to make the transition towards the fire that is the beginning of his enlightenment. By continually recalling the mother's body to the Platonic scene of representation, Irigaray's emphasis on this internal pathway provokes us to remember that other internal passage which the path within the cave both masks and recalls: the passage between mother and foetus made possible by the umbilical cord and placenta. As she develops more fully elsewhere, this 'placental economy' regulates the dis-symmetrical relations between mother and child in ways that allow them to co-exist in intimate contact without harming one another and without simply becoming one.[21] Instead of dividing one from another, such intimate proximity is characterized by relations of contiguity.

Across her reading of Plato, Irigaray continues to draw out further implications of the forgotten passage. Her re-telling positions the Myth of the Cave as breaking 'the genealogical contiguity' between mother and child and replacing it with a genealogy founded in the Forms (*S*, 293, translation modified; see *Sf*, 365: 'la contiguïté généalogique est tranchée').[22] The result is that individual human beings – male as well as female – lose touch with their singular and irreplacable beginnings. Instead, they are painfully re-oriented so as to reflect a single origin, whether this is identified with the Forms, or the undifferentiated maternal receptacle of *Timaeus*. Remembering the forgotten passage of birth permits each human being to recover a relation to the maternal, not as a homogenized origin, but a singular passage into the world for singular offspring. In turn, this allows each human being to enter into a genuine mode of self-relation, in which they are no longer reduced to merely another copy of the same original, but located within 'a singular history, "*properly one's own*"' (*S*, 293, translation modified; see *Sf*, 366: 'une histoire singulière, "*propre*"').

84 The Way Out of the Cave

As that which is 'between access and egress', the forgotten
passage is the condition of birth in another sense, in that it allows
for intercourse and copulation. Irigaray's reading plays on the relation between the copula ('is') and copulation: Platonic metaphysics
refuses to recognize that being – that which is – begins in copulation. Instead, everything that is, is dependent on its origin in the
Ideas. Hence, the copula that structures all definitions – 'x is y' – no
longer really joins different terms together, but expresses a series of
mimetic relations to one and the same origin of Being. For Plato, the
Forms, held in place by the single Form of the Good, constitute both
a single source of all beings and the unity of Being itself as One.

By contrast, the forgotten passage recalls the possibility that
human existence begins with an encounter between two 'whose –
sexual – difference will never have been considered as cause and
necessary condition for copulation' (*S*, 275). Thus, the Platonic
myth not only covers over the maternal origins whose power it
appropriates, it also forecloses the possibility of thinking sexual
difference in ways that would recognize the irreducibility of the
sexes, by making all beings reflections of one and the same Being.
In response, Irigaray seeks to remind us that being begins with two:
with the generative, copulative relation between the sexes. Moreover, these two are not two halves of the same (as Aristophanes
would have us believe),[23] but irreducibly different.

Contact and Contiguity

While Platonic metaphysics forecloses the irreducibility of sexual
difference, it does so in dissymmetrical ways. For as *Timaeus* makes
explicit, the generative power of origin is mapped onto the active,
form-giving force of the father, while it is the mother whose specificity disappears into inactive formlessness. Thus, if sexual difference is to be recovered, the generative power of the mother needs
to be reclaimed in ways that articulate her specificity, rather than
reducing her to a set of material-metaphorical resources. Once
again, the figure of the passage is crucial here, insofar as it suggests
the way in which the mother embodies a relation between one and
another that cannot be captured by the logic of oppositions and
instead is shaped by proximity, touch and contact.

Towards the end of her journey back through Plato's myth,
Irigaray emphasizes the significance of this mode of relation via
repeated references to contiguity (*contiguïté*):

when it comes down to it, *contact [contiguïté] between 'things' is of very little importance to the wise man. ... Contact [contiguïté] is lost in the analogy* that wraps it in its re-presentation, holding it paralysed on a one-way journey. And the sensible world always evokes contact [*contact*] as well as rupture, birth as well as death; yet here it suspends the alternation between its phases into one genealogy of images, of 'copies' whose closeness [*proximité*] to the model moves outside the time of generation, instead regulating itself according to the propriety of form (and) of name. (S, 348, 351; Sf, 437, 439–40)

It is relations of contiguity, Irigaray suggests, that are sacrificed by the mimetic logic established in the Myth of the Cave. This logic functions according to analogical substitutions of like-for-like: cave for womb, fire for sun, sun for Form. Each metaphorical image operates by simultaneously displacing and recalling its original. The attentive reader of such analogies has to move backwards and forwards between the terms which substitute for one another, and thus cannot appear side by side: '[T]hese two "terms" to the logic of discourse cannot/can no longer be related. A whole system of kinship – that is, in this case, of analogy – makes contact [*contiguïté*] between them impracticable. *The economy of metaphor that is in control keeps them apart*' (S, 346; Sf, 434). By contrast, as a relation of proximity, contiguity allows one thing to stand alongside an other. Like mother and foetus, contiguous beings touch on one another, without merging into one; their differences remain discernable, without their being completely separated from one another. Together, the related figures of the passage and of contiguity thus constitute starting points towards articulating metaphysics differently. Such a re-articulation would no longer be concerned with establishing a single truth and origin of Being, and would instead testify to Being-as-two by allowing different beings to co-exist without reducing either to a mere copy or substitute for the other. It would thus open the possibility of re-articulating sexual difference, in ways that neither occlude nor appropriate the mother's body, but instead do justice to her female specificity.

Irigaray's reading shows that the Platonic privileging of sameness is manifest both in the metaphysical logic of copies and original, and the metaphorical logic of substitution through which that metaphysics is represented. Likewise, an alternative metaphysics of sexuate difference would depend on a contiguous logic of relation so as to represent the co-existence of irreducibly different beings. Moreover, insofar as the Platonic privileging of the one and the same is linked to the father's form-giving force, it can be read as an idealization of the phallus as a single, unified organ. Similarly, the logic of contiguity that makes possible a non-reductive rendering of sexual difference echoes the morphology of the female body, insofar as this is re-presented as neither cave-like receptacle nor reflecting screen, but via the figure of the passage which permits one to co-exist with/in an other, without subsuming either.

The internal relation between the logic of contiguity and the morphology of the female body is taken up again in Irigaray's figure of the two lips, to which we will return in Chapter 6. In the section of *Speculum* on Plato's *hystera*, however, this relation is taken up in the figure of the *corps à corps*. This phrase appears at the end of Irigaray's analysis (*SF*, 457) and serves as a final example of the subversive doublespeak that characterizes her approach. The *corps à corps* refers to the one-on-one combat that was a typical part of the training of an Athenian citizen (who would of course have been male). However, it also represents the agonistic style of the polis, where citizens would wrestle with words so as to make their case heard. Irigaray's text foregrounds the way in which these rhetorical battles are constructed on the exclusion and silencing of women, and that this is as true of the dialectical struggles of metaphysics as it is of the space of political representation.

At the same time, however, within the context of sexual difference that *Speculum* provides, the *corps à corps* becomes a figure that recalls the original relation to the body of the mother, where two were able to co-exist without reference to a unifying truth and without either needing to dominate the other. It is this re-inscription of the phrase that Irigaray takes up in a later essay entitled '*Le corps à corps avec la mère*', where she writes that we need 'to find, rediscover, invent the words, the sentences, that speak of the most ancient and most current relationship we know – the relationship to the mother's body, to our body – sentences that translate the bond between our body, her body, the body of our daughter.'[24] As this passage indicates, the recollection of an originary relation to the mother's body is especially important for those who are born from her and share her sex. In reclaiming a relation to the mother, a daughter simultaneously takes up a direct relation to her own sex that does not depend on mediation through a male subject. However, in a representational economy that both appropriates and occludes the maternal body, a daughter has nowhere to turn if she wishes to articulate her own relation to the female sex. Hence the significance for the daughter of reclaiming the mother's body from an economy of metaphorical substitution and instead rendering her visible via figures that map contiguous relations. If the mother's body is figured as allowing one and another to coexist in a continuous and contiguous touching, it offers a model for mother-daughter relations in which the daughter's fate is not to become a mother-substitute in her turn. Instead, a daughter could stand alongside her mother, inseparable insofar as they are of a like sex, yet irreducibly different by virtue of the relation between them, in which one was born and one gave birth to the other. In this dissymmetrical generative relation, neither is wholly absorbed by the other and thus it can remain visible that they are alike – as well as uniquely singular.

As we have seen, the aim of Irigaray's project is to rearticulate female specificity and sexual difference in ways that release the female body from being reduced to the necessary 'other' on which an economy of the same depends. The Myth of the Cave is iconic for Irigaray insofar as it dramatizes the appropriation of the female form and hence the way in which the mother functions not just as an other, but a *necessary* other for Platonic metaphysics. By showing how the trace of the maternal body destabilizes the myth from within – in the 'wall face that works all too well', or the passage between that refuses a binary logic of oppositions – she shows how the figure of the mother refuses to be contained by the (father's) Forms. Despite the power of the metaphysical system, the mother remains resolutely other to the position of other that she has been assigned.

> Is comparing it [the soul] to the *others of the same* (*aux autres des mêmes*) the only thing to be done? But whom are we to call upon to arbitrate that specula(riza)tion except the 'father' once again? ... As for the relationship to *the others of the others* (*aux autres des autres*), *to the other of the other*, anyone who ventures near it will be threatened with loss of self (as same), for it does not exclude the possibility of there being a reversal. (*S*, 335; *Sf*, 419)

This last 'reversal' need not be one that swings about the axis of symmetry that governs the myth. That is, it need not necessarily threaten to return us to the darkness of the cave. The more radical and genuinely destabilizing reversal would be one allowing this maternal darkness to become 'other' to its position as the 'other' of the light of day. Such a reversal would require that the 'darkness' no longer be defined against the daylight realm, but in its own terms: terms that do justice to that which constitutes the maternal 'darkness' and makes it irreducible to a simple absence or lack of true and proper form.

That such a reversal can be articulated at all indicates that '[t]he outside, backside, other side cannot be ringed in once and for all': the maternal refuses to be completely subsumed within her multiple roles as 'other' of the Same, but remains stubbornly other to them too, an irreducible remainder. Thus the mother does not only supply a 'store of in(de)finite alterity' for the Platonic economy of the same, which appropriates her maternal-material resources for the reproduction of its 'proper' Forms (S, 335). She is rich enough to retain a genuine (improper) alterity, one that is not appropriable within a logic of sameness and that demands other terms to articulate its specificity. It is this demand, the call to figure woman as other to 'the other' on which metaphysics depends, to which Irigaray's work responds.

Reclaiming Diotima: The Wisdom of Love

Irigaray's re-telling of the Myth of the Cave works to re-evaluate its foundational role within western metaphysics. From the perspective she opens up, this myth's significance lies not only in the way that it orients metaphysical thinking, but more importantly, in the way that it reveals this thinking to be premised on the foreclosure of the relation to the maternal that orients each of us – male or female – in the world. Her subversive re-reading shows that along with the maternal, metaphysics has also foreclosed sexual difference as a horizon for human beings, who are always born of woman, and as sexuate beings themselves.

Her project is not simply destructive, however, for she seeks another wisdom, one that Platonic metaphysics largely obscures. As shown above, this metaphysics orients human beings in relation to a single origin of Being and a truth that is one and the same for all. Such a model forecloses the thought of beings who come into being via a singular and unrepeatable relation to a mother, and who exist as two different sexes that cannot be reduced to two versions or copies of the same. It is towards these relational beings, who exist as irreducibly two, that Irigaray seeks to reorient us, in both our thinking and our lives.

Perhaps surprisingly, given her thoroughgoing critique of Platonic metaphysics, Irigaray finds some of the resources for doing so within another of Plato's texts, namely, *Symposium*. Towards the end of this dialogue, Socrates tells how a wise woman from Mantinea, Diotima, once taught him about love (*eros*). Diotima's teaching culminates in her delineation of the so-called ladder of love: a properly educated soul will pass from love of a particular body, to a love of beauty in appearances in general, to the higher beauty of souls, and then of laws and knowledge, until finally it is drawn towards the ultimate encounter with Beauty itself.[25] In this way, the lover's journey repeats the passage from the world of the senses to the realm of the Forms that is dramatized in the Myth of the Cave. However, in her essay 'Sorcerer Love' (originally published a decade after *Speculum*), Irigaray suggests that in an earlier section of Diotima's speech there is another – forgotten – passage, which her reading seeks to reclaim.

Diotima begins by teaching Socrates of the intermediary nature of love: if love desires what it lacks, and love loves the beautiful and the good, then it cannot itself be beautiful and good. Rather, love is *between* the good and the bad, the beautiful and the ugly. Likewise, love is neither merely mortal, nor fully divine, but passes between mortals and immortals, conveying messages between gods and men. Love is thus an intermediary that allows for 'the encounter and the transmutation or transvaluation between the two' (*ESD*, 21).

Irigaray goes on to discuss what is for her the key passage in Diotima's speech. When asked what kind of activity receives the name of love, Diotima replies that it is a 'begetting in beauty, in respect to both the body and the soul'.[26] The Greek word for begetting here (*tiktein, tokos*) can be used not only of men but also of women, where it is usually translated as bearing or giving birth.[27] The emphasis on birth is justified by what follows, for Diotima expands on her cryptic statement by explaining that:

> All men [human beings] are pregnant in respect to both the body and the soul, Socrates, [...] and when they reach a certain age, our nature desires to beget. It cannot beget in ugliness, but only in beauty. The intercourse [*sunousia*, lit.: being with or together] of man and woman is a begetting [or giving birth]. This is a divine thing, and pregnancy and procreation are an immortal element in the mortal living creature.[28]

For Irigaray, this passage reinforces love's role as intermediary: *eros* brings lovers together in such a way that their being with one another allows them to release what they bear in a joyful engendering. Irigaray draws attention to Diotima's description of the intercourse or being-with one another of a man and woman as itself a bearing or begetting. Later in the speech, Diotima will emphasize the desire for immortality through one's offspring. However, in this earlier passage, the erotic encounter simply *is* a bearing or begetting: intercourse, or more literally, being with another in love, is generative and creative in and of itself. As Irigaray puts it: 'Love is fecund prior to any procreation' (*ESD*, 25–6). Whether or not a child is born, love engenders a being-together which is a rebirth of the lovers themselves, a regeneration of one with and by the other.

In keeping with love's intermediary nature, this mutual re-engendering permits a passage to immortality, not because it turns mortals into immortal *beings*, but because it constitutes immortality as a perpetual becoming, and thus a perpetual becoming-immortal that takes place within mortal life. Here there is no metaphysical turning away from the life of the body to find immortality through the soul alone; rather, immortality is realized *within* the movement of the lovers' coupled becomings.

Nonetheless, according to Irigaray, the overall direction of Diotima's speech miscarries. As her teaching progresses, the aim of love becomes its offspring: the child who replaces love as an intermediary between lovers, and turns love itself into a means to an end. Love is captured and frozen in something *outside* the lovers that confers immortality on them, rather than being realized in a perpetual becoming-immortal within their mortal lives (*ESD*, 27–30). Worst of all, love loses its intermediary character and becomes split between mortal and immortal, for Diotima goes on to distinguish between two kinds of offspring: the merely physical children of those who are lovers in body and the more enduring, spiritual offspring of those who are lovers in soul.[29]

If the soul is properly nurtured, it may ultimately be led towards a vision of Beauty itself, and inspired to give birth to true virtue, the most valuable offspring of all. Irigaray notes that the presentation of a rapturous *vision* of beauty inscribes a trace of the sensible even in this most metaphysical of encounters. As in the Myth of the Cave, where the Form of the Good is represented by the blazing light of the sun, here too the non-material eternal realm is represented by visual images borrowed from the sensible world. This appropriation is most violently enacted in the division between physical and spiritual procreation, which metaphorically appropriates the generative powers of the mother while simultaneously reducing actual procreation to a poor copy of 'proper' spiritual birth.

Tellingly, Irigaray's reading of *Symposium* does not focus on this metaphorical appropriation of birth, even though as we have seen, her analysis of the Myth of the Cave shows this to be the foundational act of western metaphysics. However, in the Myth of the Cave, this originary metaphorical appropriation is itself repressed, such that the significance of the mother's generational powers is precisely that which is occluded. By the end of Diotima's speech, by contrast, physical birth has been explicitly inscribed in contrast with the purely spiritual birth of ideas, and hence the significance – or rather, the *in*-significance – of actual birth has already been decided.

In this context, to insist on the difference between 'real' and metaphorical birth would only tend to reinforce the very split between body and soul that divorces physical birth from spiritual significance. Merely reversing the hierarchy and privileging physical over spiritual births would not allow the revaluation of the physical *as* spiritual which Irigaray seeks. Such a reading would still not be attentive to the lesson of the earlier part of Diotima's speech, which teaches that love moves *between* the physical and spiritual as well as between mortality and immortality, not in a hierarchical ascent, but in ways that entwine each ceaselessly in the other.

Hence Irigaray's emphasis on the passage which, for her, is the interpretative key to Diotima's lost teaching, and in which Diotima suggests that the 'being together' of lovers, each pregnant with possibilities, is a giving birth in and of itself, prior to procreation. This image suggests that the generative powers of the mother should be valued without being reduced to a reproductive function. Moreover, as we have seen, at this point in her speech, Diotima presents the lovers as pregnant in both body *and* soul. Thus, the birth that takes place between them is not merely a metaphorical appropriation in which spiritual growth is modelled on physical birth. Instead, their transformative encounter can be understood as constituting a *repetition* of birth in which the carnal and the spiritual are always already entwined.

By deliberately privileging the earlier passages of Diotima's speech against its overall trajectory, Irigaray recovers an alternative to the metaphysical framework that opposes bodily becomings to eternal Being, and devalues the maternal body while privileging spiritual birth. In contrast, Diotima teaches of an erotic encounter in which the generative powers aligned with pregnancy are valued without being reduced to a reproductive function, and mortality and immortality remain entwined rather than split between body and soul. Whereas the Platonic idealization of a single origin of Being obscures the way in which birth begins not with one but two, Diotima teaches of an encounter between two who are irreducibly different and mutually transformed.

In this chapter, we have seen how Irigaray's critical analysis of Plato passes into a creative engendering of philosophical resources. Through her intimate engagement with his texts, she recovers some of the figures through which we might begin to rethink human being in terms of an originary relation to both the mother and the generative interval of sexuate difference.[30] In turn, Irigaray shows how this rethinking would necessarily transform philosophy, re-orienting our approach to fundamental philosophical questions about the origin of being, and the relation of form and matter. If we are to cease repeating the logic which feeds off the mother's body while disavowing her significance, we need to rethink matter as not only receptive, but active and generative. By re-approaching the mother's body in ways that acknowledge her capacity to *engender* form, Irigaray reminds us that she was never fully contained by the walls of the cave, but always remained elsewhere, sustaining the generation of difference in fluid and contiguous relations. As we will see in later chapters, the figures of contiguity and touch that Irigaray recovers by recalling our maternal origins might help us rethink the relation between self and other from the perspective of a distinctively female subject. Whereas Platonic metaphysics both appropriates maternal matter as a resource and disavows that appropriation, Irigaray places our dependence on the mother at the centre of her account of being, while also acknowledging her own dependence on the body of Plato's work, wrestling *corps à corps* with Plato's texts to transform the contours of his thought.

One of the ironies Irigaray reveals is the inability of the Platonic logic of the One to recognize the value of the singular. By recognizing our beginnings in birth, we can reaffirm the singularity of each human being who begins in a unique relation with the body of the mother. This relation reminds us that birth never begins with one, but always (at least) two, embodied in the relations between mother and child as well as in the generative encounter between the sexes. It is this generative encounter which Irigaray recovers through

Diotima's speech, along with an affirmation of Being as two and an image of birth as the active transformation of spiritualized matter that depends on openness to the other, rather than the replication of the same. By reclaiming Diotima's voice from Plato's text, Irigaray thus furthers her project of transforming western philosophy, countering the Platonic love of wisdom with Diotima's wisdom of love.[31]

4

Woman as Other: Variations on an Old Theme

According to Plato, those who rule in the shadowy world of the cave live as if in a dream. In the previous chapters, we saw how Irigaray shows that the Platonic staging of western metaphysics is itself organized so as to sustain an 'old dream of symmetry', governed by a logic of sameness and replication.[1] Once analysed, this dream speaks of the repression of sexual difference and a foundational blindspot concerning maternal origins. In this chapter, we will see how both the dream and the blindspot continue to inform western philosophy, by examining Irigaray's analysis of the development of ancient Greek thought before turning to her engagement with two thinkers whose work frames philosophical modernity: Descartes and Kant.

Broadly speaking, the shift from Platonic metaphysics to modern – that is, post-Cartesian – philosophy involves the increasing centrality of the individual (male) subject. Whereas Plato locates the origin of Being in a transcendent realm of Ideas that orient the philosopher's search for wisdom, modern thinkers will re-ground both being and knowledge within the subject. In so doing, they will also find new ways of negotiating the relation between the finite and the infinite, the sensible and the transcendent, form and matter. Irigaray identifies a familiar pattern running through these transformations in two closely intertwined threads: the denial and/or appropriation of maternal generative power, and the rational (male) subject's dependence on a material (female) other. However, before examining the sections of *Speculum* in which Irigaray engages with the key figures of philosophical modernity, it is worth pausing to note the chapters on Aristotle and Plotinus, both of whom play a crucial role in the transition from ancient to modern philosophy.

Irigaray on Aristotle: Woman as a 'Mutilated Male'

Aristotle's works are incredibly wide-ranging, particularly from a modern perspective in which scholars tend to specialize in particular disciplines. He produced extensive studies of biology and zoology, as well as influential works on ethics, politics, tragedy, and 'first philosophy' – Aristotle's name for the branch of philosophy which investigates first principles or causes and which will later come to be known as metaphysics.[2] His work establishes logic as a formal discipline, while his study of *psychē* (soul or animating force, as the Latin translation of the title, *De Anima*, suggests) can be read as the founding text for what will later become psychology and philosophy of mind. However, for our purposes, what is most important about Aristotle is the way that he rejects Plato's theory of the Forms as transcendent entities. Instead, Aristotle argues that form (for which he uses both *eidos* and *morphē*) is immanent to matter. For this reason, one might think that Aristotle's metaphysics would be more amenable to feminists such as Irigaray, who wish to escape the Platonic dualism that opposes (transcendent) form and (sensible) matter, and privileges the former. However, as Irigaray shows, things are not so simple.

First and foremost, this is because of the way that Aristotle preserves the link between form and originary power, insofar as it is form that causes something to be what it is. Matter remains the substrate which by receiving form becomes a particular kind of being. Hence, he remains firmly within the hylomorphic tradition: 'According to Aristotle, a generated thing – natural or artificial – is material on which form has been imposed.'[3] In a manner somewhat peculiar to modern ears, the substance of a being – that which preserves its identity across time – is thus aligned with its form (or what Aristotle calls its formal cause), not its matter (the 'stuff' of which it is made). The formal cause is presented as an archetype or pattern, as well as in a phrase that is usually translated in terms of 'essence', for example, as an essential formula or statement of an essence.[4] As Vasilis Politis sums up, for Aristotle, 'the essence of a changing, material thing is its form (as opposed to its matter or to a combination of its form and its matter). By the form of a changing, material thing, such as, for instance, a particular human being, he means that which explains why the matter (e.g. the flesh and bones) of this particular thing, the human being, constitutes the thing that it constitutes.'[5] The form (formal cause) or essence of a changing material thing necessarily remains the same as long as that thing exists. Aristotle thereby founds a tradition of thinking about essence as that which remains the same through change which constitutes the backdrop to debates about Irigaray's own supposed 'essentialism' (discussed in Chapter 6).

By contrast with matter shaped into determinate beings by their essence or formal cause, unformed or 'prime matter' would be wholly indeterminate and amorphous. It thus remains analogous to the receptacle in Plato's *Timaeus*, and just as difficult to theorize. Indeed, strictly speaking, that which is utterly devoid of form has no 'being' and so cannot be said to exist. 'Prime matter' remains purely speculative, a theoretical projection. Nonetheless, because the beings we encounter in the world are always a combination of matter and form, a complete account of their nature makes such a speculation necessary.

Irigaray's reading emphasizes that, although it provides the necessary housing for forms, this speculative projection of matter is denied any autonomous existence and, crucially, any power to actively articulate forms of being for itself. In this way, 'matter has been sealed over again' (S, 162). If anything, the privilege accorded to form is more insidious in Aristotle's metaphysics: whereas Plato explicitly dramatizes the hierarchy between the sensible world and the realm of the Forms, Aristotle makes the form/matter distinction internal to nature. The fact that the specifically material aspect of nature is still deprived of any active powers to articulate forms for itself is thus less obvious.

Worse still, Aristotle's metaphysics repeats the appropriation of the generative powers of the mother and their re-ascription to a transcendent power which is itself eternal and unchanging, 'alien to all genesis'. This is a reference to Aristotle's God, who as 'primary substance' stands at the opposite end of the scale to 'prime matter'. The universe must have a beginning in something which does not itself begin: God is 'this Unbegotten being, this Origin beyond origins' (S, 161). Indeed, God is necessary, Irigaray suggests, to prevent the beginning of all beings being traced back to an originary matter: 'If the prime mover didn't install a brake on the wheel of *infinite regression*, for instance, might not all substance risk hurtling into some formlessness of prime matter? It might be seduced into returning to the womb of the mother-earth' (S, 164). As pure Being – that is, pure substance or form – God is wholly other to material nature; his activity consists in a purely intellectual intuition. Nonetheless, he is the reason why material nature comes into being and why it has the being that it has, for everything in nature strives to become more like its divine origin. Therefore, matter need play no active role in the world's coming into being, because nature is always already ordered in its entirety by, and in relation to, God. Hence Aristotle's 'onto-theology ... reduces the potential for generation, growth, change and expansion for all beings' (S, 164).[6]

If God is the intellectual source of the natural order, then by theorizing nature – that is, articulating its order according to the appropriate categories – man becomes more like God. Just as the Forms orient the gaze of the Platonic philosopher, so God orients the good life for Aristotelian man, who can nurture the divine part in himself by living a life of contemplation. The affinity between God and man is carried further in Aristotle's account of reproduction. If God is the origin of the world, then it is male beings who most closely imitate him, as it is the male of the species that has the power to generate living offspring. According to Aristotle, the sperm is the active element in generation, providing the form, the life-principle which brings a new creature into existence by animating matter. The mother passively provides this matter – but that is all she provides: dead matter that is brought to life, and given a specific kind of life, by the movement communicated to it by the sperm. Indeed, woman herself is only female because she *lacks* the animating and form-giving capacities of the male. For Aristotle, 'it is through a certain incapacity that the female is female'. She is 'as it were an impotent male', or even 'a mutilated male' that lacks 'only [!] one thing': 'the principle of soul'.[7] Hence the problem signalled by the title of Irigaray's chapter: 'how to conceive (of) a girl'. Woman is neither a well-formed man, nor does she have a different form or essence of her own. Thus, 'not only is she secondary to man but she may just as well not be as be. ... Theoretically there would be no such thing as woman' (S, 165–6).

For Irigaray, Aristotle's account of the form/matter relation, of reproduction, and of God all testify to a profound denial of human beings' beginnings in the body of the mother. As with Plato, Aristotle both signals such beginnings, at one point noting that 'the menstrual blood has in its nature an affinity to the primitive matter',[8] and refuses them, by denying such matter any active form-giving force. Irigaray reclaims the link between 'first matter'

and the female to ask if the former might be found in 'this bodili-
ness shared with the mother, which as yet has no movement of its
own, has yet to divide up time or space . ... Fusion, confusion,
transfusion of matter, of body-matter, in which even the elementary
would escape any static characterization. In which same and other
would have yet to find their meaning' (S, 161). This passage once
again speaks in more than one voice, suggesting the traditional
Aristotelian account of prime matter as formless and undetermined, yet simultaneously registering a different principle of
movement characterizing the pregnant female body that bears otherness within. A different account of space and time, as well as self
and other, would be required to articulate this body's capacity to
share its 'body-matter' without becoming simply indistinct.

Plotinus: Freezing over the Mother-Matter

In raising these possibilities, Irigaray takes advantage of woman's
anomalous place within Aristotle's philosophy. Whereas man's
form and function secure his place in nature and his relation to the
divine: 'She alone is in a position – perhaps? – to question her function in this all-powerful "machine" we know as metaphysics' (S,
166). Irigaray's own questioning continues via Plotinus. Between
the chapters on Aristotle and Descartes, *Speculum* includes a section
composed wholly of quotations from Plotinus' *Enneads*, a set of
treatises whose themes 'move from the earthly to the heavenly, from
the more concrete to the more abstract.'[9] Plotinus was a follower of
Plato (who died around 550 years before Plotinus was born) and
is commonly acknowledged as the founder of what has come to be
known as 'Neoplatonism'. Plotinus' version of Platonism is shaped
in part by his attempt to respond to Plato's critics, and in particular,
to the challenges posed by Aristotle. In contrast to Aristotle,
Plotinus seeks to recuperate a Platonic theory of Forms as eternal
and transcendent truths about an eternal and transcendent reality
founded ultimately on 'the One', which occupies the same kind of
priority as Plato's Form of the Good: 'The One is that on which all
else depends, what constitutes all else, present as such in, and part
of all else, yet also different from, and independent of, all else, thus
"beyond" all else'.[10] In keeping with this, 'Plotinus shares with Plato
the principle that eternal truths and the reality which grounds them
have a paradigmatic status for the sensible world such that the
latter represents or imitates or shares in the former.'[11] Irigaray's

selections suggest that Plotinus pushes the logic of Platonism to a certain extreme as regards the status of the sensible, material world, and that he does so by combining Platonism with certain strands of Aristotle's thought. In this way, Plotinus functions in *Speculum* as the culmination of a particular trajectory in Greek philosophy concerning the theorization of Matter.

If prime matter is a speculative projection for Aristotle, Plotinus takes seriously the implication that such matter does not exist: 'Matter has no reality and is not capable of being affected. ... It lives on the farther side of all these categories and so has no title to the name of Being' (S, 168).[12] Matter is thus that which 'we know only as the Void' (S, 169). In ways that recall Plato's *Timaeus*, Plotinus claims that matter can neither change nor be changed by the Ideal-Forms for which it acts as a temporary support. Matter merely reflects the appearance of the Forms which are 'visible against it by its very formlessness'. In all these 'mimicries of the Authentic Existents', matter remains empty. It is thus only 'like a mirror': a mirror has its own reality and gives back a 'faithful' image, whereas Matter reflects unreal semblances of the real (S, 169). Such faithlessness leads Plotinus to characterize matter as 'evil' because utterly lacking in the form of the Good, a view that will be taken up and reinforced in the Christian denigration of the flesh.

Unsurprisingly, Plotinus also likens Matter to a mother. However, he makes it explicit that this is only a metaphor. Matter is sterile and lacks the generative capacities of the mother. It is thus 'not female to full effect, female in receptivity only, not in pregnancy'. Matter is more appropriately represented by the eunuch: 'by what is neither female nor effectively male but castrated of that impregnating power which belongs only to the unchangeably masculine' (S, 179). Plotinus here repeats the appropriative gesture which attributes generative power wholly to the male, while laying bare the fact that the 'other' against which the masculine principle is defined is not properly speaking 'female' but a castrated or mutilated male. Thus his insistence that Matter is not completely 'like' a mother does not constitute a positive recognition of women's generative powers. Rather, it seals woman's occlusion: inadequate even as metaphor, woman is redundant in a metaphysics where the male principle is sufficient to explain both Being and non-Being, generation and lack.

In this chapter, Irigaray presents a series of passages which seem to require no additional voice: as direct quotations, they speak for themselves. Yet Plotinus' words only resonate with such

apparently 'immediate' significance because they have been torn
out of their original context and set against the backdrop of
Irigaray's own project. Like the back wall of the cave which works
'all too well', this textual backdrop transforms the significance of
the words projected onto it. *Speculum* is after all a concave mirror:
it concentrates the light on Plotinus so as to reveal the contours of
a metaphysical tradition that deprives maternal-matter of both its
generative power and a life of its own. Hence the chapter's punning
title, 'une mère de glace': *la mère*, meaning mother, is also homophonic with *la mer*, the sea, while *glace* means both mirror and ice.
Plotinus represents the mother-matter as a mirror devoid of any
active powers of her own. Instead she is frozen into a sea of ice, a
glittering surface of dead matter.

Nonetheless, by ending the chapter with the passage in which
Plotinus claims matter is 'female in receptivity only, not in pregnancy', Irigaray manages to suggest that even here, there is an
obscure opening, a trace of a remainder. If pregnancy indicates a
fertility that exceeds merely passive receptivity, this implies a generative activity on the part of women that does not belong to the
'unchangeably masculine', and that remains unaccounted for
within Plotinus' apparently complete account of Being and non-
Being. Ice, after all, can melt and flow into new forms.

Irigaray Reading Descartes

On Irigaray's reading, what is remarkable about Cartesian modernity is how firmly even this tenuous remainder of active materiality
is covered over. For Aristotle and Plotinus, the form-giving capacities aligned with the male are still dependent on Matter, and this
necessary 'other' is still aligned – however problematically – with
woman and in particular the mother. In Descartes' philosophy, by
contrast, Irigaray suggests that the subject has become its own
'other' in ways that allow it to give symbolic birth to itself. Any
reliance on a mother, on a foundational relation to a corporeal
female other, is severed.

If Plato is regarded as the father of western metaphysics,
Descartes is equally often seen as the father of modern philosophy.
In part, this is because of the way he overturns the scholasticism
of medieval philosophy; in part it is because of the way he is seen
to reverse the relation between faith and reason, so that rather than
faith securing understanding, reason secures faith by proving the

existence of God; and in part it is because of the way that, as indicated above, he positions the self at the heart of the philosophical enterprise. This is particularly the case in the text with which Irigaray's reading is most closely intertwined, Descartes' *Meditations on First Philosophy*. As the rather Aristotelian title suggests, Descartes is here engaged in a quest for first principles; however, his distinctive (non-Aristotelian) approach privileges a meditative process which needs to be undertaken by the reader as co-participant. By passing through a method of doubt which leads him to bracket out anything of which he cannot be certain, the meditator is led to the surprising discovery that the one thing he cannot doubt is his own existence as doubting, that is, as thinking. The intuitive certainty of the existence of the thinking self (what is usually referred to as the *cogito*) becomes Descartes' 'Archimidean point', the first principle of first philosophy.

As with the sketch of Platonism in Chapter 2, the above account of Descartes' significance is a somewhat reductive if characteristic image of his thought – as others have shown, his thinking continues to be informed by Aristotelian substance metaphysics in ways that complicate the notion that he makes a clean break with his philosophical past.[13] But again, it is the Cartesian heritage of Descartes' thought – not only the privilege of mind over body, but the image of the thinking subject as self-founding – which is the main focus of Irigaray's critique. And as with Plato, one of the reasons she works so closely with Descartes' texts is not to reveal their 'true' and hitherto unrecognized meaning, but to displace them as the unproblematic source and support for ideas that have come to dominate the tradition – such as the idea that the essence of human beings is found solely in the (ungendered) act of thinking.

Irigaray's chapter on Descartes loosely follows the structure of *Meditations*. She tracks through the key stages of the meditator's journey, passing from doubt to the certainty of the *cogito* and the existence of God, and from there back to the world of the body and senses. This metaphysical journey remains recognizably that of Descartes' meditator, while being critically transformed in ways that reveal the lengths to which this meditating self will go to sever its links to a maternal-material origin.

Along the way, Irigaray weaves in references to other texts by Descartes, including the *Discourse on Method* and *Principles of Philosophy*, as well as a number of other texts that (from a post-Cartesian perspective) would more readily be classified as 'scientific', such as his treatises on *The World* and *Optics*. The latter provides the chapter's intriguing title: 'And if, Taking the Eye of a Man Recently Dead, ...' is borrowed from Descartes' description of an experiment designed to show how images are formed on the back of the eye.[14] This selection provides several clues to Irigaray's approach. First, her reading will suggest that the 'natural light' of reason that guides the meditator's journey has been unnaturally severed from the living world that he inhabits. It is thus akin to 'the eye of a man recently dead'. Second, she will show how the mimetic function of Plato's Cave is incorporated within the Cartesian subject: the reflective powers of the back wall of the cave are transposed onto the back of the eye. Philosophy's dependence on a material other becomes even more obscured, as this 'other' is incorporated within the self. Nonetheless, as Irigaray will show, the reversing capacities of concave mirrors are also internalized, destabilizing the Cartesian subject from within.

In addition to the title, the chapter is also framed by a quotation from the *Optics*. Here Descartes describes how visual images formed in the brain may be passed 'along the arteries of a pregnant woman into some determined member of the child in her womb and form there those birthmarks which are a cause of such wonderment to all Learned Men'.[15] In contrast to this epigraph, the main text of Irigaray's chapter does not explicitly mention women or mothers, miming the way that *Meditations* seems to involve a purely rational, reflective process which is apparently gender-free. Indeed, Descartes is often seen as offering a philosophical approach that is less problematic for women than many others, precisely because his thinking subject does not appear to be gendered. There is no reason, it seems, why the meditating self may not be a woman, at least in principle.[16]

Just as optics is dealt with separately, so Descartes' approach seems to exclude questions of gender from metaphysics:

> Such optical considerations are examined in specific treatises. *Already outside ontology.*

> The same thing applies to the discussions of woman and women. Gynecology, dioptrics, are no longer by right a part of metaphysics – *that supposedly unsexed anthropos-logos whose actual sex is admitted only by its omission and exclusion from consciousness*, and by what is said in its margins. (S, 183)

For Irigaray, it is this denial of the metaphysical significance of gender that is itself the problem. Moreover, the 'supposedly unsexed' neutrality of metaphysics is a disingenuous illusion which

the epigraph from the *Optics* helps her to expose. Descartes' meditating self depends on an ability to withdraw from the world and
thus on a division between reason and the senses, mind and body,
that seems to make sexual difference irrelevant to subjectivity. Yet,
while *Meditations* counsels 'Learned Men' to doubt the evidence of
their senses and ground knowledge in rational judgement alone,
the passage from the *Optics* associates the female body with a
passive and entirely *unknowing* reproduction of images.[17] Descartes
thereby reinforces a deeply entrenched conceptual framework in
which woman is aligned with the body in ways that mean the
rational meditating subject is implicitly male.[18] Irigaray's choice of
epigraph thus helps her show how Descartes' thought continues
to be gendered, even if this is revealed by what is said in the scientific 'margins' of his explicitly philosophical project. Indeed, the
fact that the Cartesian subject does not seem to have a sex not only
makes the gendering of Descartes' metaphysics more difficult to
challenge; it is a further sign of the way the male subject position
is here taken as the implicit norm.

By framing her chapter with references to the *Optics*, Irigaray
performs another reversal of perspective. The treatise on optics,
along with writings on meteors and geometry, was originally
intended to be prefaced by the more philosophical *Discourse on
Method*. By reversing the order and beginning with passages from
the *Optics*, Irigaray suggests that Descartes' apparently gender-
neutral metaphysics is framed and informed by the gendering of
the material world inhabited by 'Learned Men'. More specifically,
as we will see, her reading aims to show that his philosophical
project is silently informed by its negative relation to the pregnant
woman, insofar as it seeks to deny the meditating subject's dependence on birth from a mother. This matricidal desire, she suggests,
is the silent foundation of 'first philosophy'.

The Self-Sufficient Meditator

Nowhere is the meditator's desire for self-sufficiency more forcefully apparent than in the *cogito*. Having subjected all of his previous beliefs to doubt, the meditator is relieved to find that simply
by being aware that he thinks, he can be certain of one thing: that
he exists (as a thinking being). Irigaray emphasizes how this
moment of introspective certainty is presented as an act of pure
self-reflection:

Once the primary identification has been achieved, – at least within the argument developed here – the possibility arises not only that the subject exists as such but that its condition of being results from self-reflection. ... what is now founding the subject's existence and reflection works like the backing of a mirror that has been intro-jected, 'incorporated', and is thus beyond perception; ... If the 'I' can desist from specific cerebration ... then, *for a moment*, it perceives itself as the *matrix* of everything that is thought (within it). (*S*, 180–1)

The thinking 'I' requires no one and nothing else to assure it of its own existence. Like someone gazing at their own reflection, all 'I' need do is reflect on my own activity as I think to be assured that 'I' am. Yet as others have noted, the self-certainty sought by the meditator in this moment of self-consciousness is forever out of his grasp: in the very moment where he is certain of his own existence, he splits in two, becoming the one who is thinking and the one who is aware of himself thinking.[19] As Irigaray puts it, 'when the "I" thinks about something, the object of its thought is in fact itself' (*S*, 182). The *cogito* doubles the self which becomes subject and object at once.

Thus the real threat to the meditator does not lie in the doubts that arise at the start of the meditative process. Rather, the project is destabilized from within because of the internal doubling of the I that reflects on itself, leading Irigaray to ask: '*What if illusion were constitutive of thinking?*' (*S*, 182). The issue here is not so much that the content of the meditator's thoughts might fail to match reality (though this will be a concern later), but that the success of the *cogito* depends on an illusory identity between the self that thinks, and the self that thinks *about* itself thinking. By accentuating the difference between them, Irigaray suggests that the *cogito* is based on a mere 'fiction of proof', and that the supposed 'unity and sim-plicity of the subject' on which it relies is 'a sham' (*S*, 182–3). On this reading, the self-identity of the Cartesian subject is irreparably fissured: the self is forever other to itself. This is a key insight for those like Lacan and Derrida who are concerned with destabilizing the modern subject and showing its supposed unity to be an illu-sion. Irigaray reinforces this critique, but also goes beyond it by showing that the internalized 'other' produced in the *cogito* is not a genuine other at all, but merely a projection or reflection of the self:

in my thought I am subject – the 'I' is 'subject' – to/of reversal itself. I shall remain in ignorance of the fact that, in this embrace of truth that I covet above all else, I am seeking, in simplest terms, to be

united with *an image in a mirror*. This is how I am. At last alone,
copula. I-me, coupled together in an embrace that begins over and
over again. And fails equally often, because of the glass that separates us. (*S*, 189–90)

As this passage suggests, for the *cogito* to function as a moment of
immediate self-certainty, the subject must remain unaware of its
own doubling. Nonetheless, this doubling allows the subject to
secure its own (non-)identity while displacing its dependence on
anything other than itself.

By making this displacement of dependency the guiding thread,
Irigaray's approach generates a re-interpretation of the method of
doubt that leads the meditating 'I' to certainty of the *cogito* in the
first place. According to this method, the meditator must set aside
everything which it is possible to doubt, in order to find something
indubitable, a firm foundation on which knowledge can be re-
established. This leads to a (temporary) rejection of the evidence of
the senses, whose testimony is found to be unreliable. Thus the
meditative journey depends on 'closing my eyes, blocking my ears,
turning away from all my senses, even ridding my thoughts of all
images of bodily things' (*S*, 189). On Irigaray's reading, this process
is driven less by the quest for certainty than the meditator's desire
to free himself of dependency on anything that originates outside
himself. This in turn is seen as symptomatic of the meditator's
refusal to acknowledge his own origin in others. In other words,
the epistemological project of *Meditations* is underpinned by a more
profound ontological desire to establish the self-sufficiency of the
meditator's very being.

Hence Irigaray draws attention to Descartes' desire to free
himself from any beliefs inherited from his philosophical ancestors
or dependent on what he was taught in childhood: '*The basis for
representation* must be purged of all *childish* phantoms or fantasies
or belief or approximations' (*S*, 181).[20] For Irigaray, this too constitutes a refusal of the ways in which each singular self is necessarily
dependent on others – on the previous generations whose wisdom
one inherits, as well as on one's parents, those by whom one was
conceived and raised: 'Once *the chain of relationships, the cord*, has
been *severed*, together with ancestry and the mysteries of conception, then there is nothing left but the subject who can go
back and sever them all over again whenever he likes. In a speculative act of denial and negation that serves to affect his autonomy'
(*S*, 182). At root, this denial springs from the meditator's refusal

to recognize his dependence on the maternal other who first brought him into the world. So powerful is the repression of this originary dependency that it drives the Cartesian subject to seek to give birth to itself all over again in the *cogito*, which, on this reading, becomes a symbolic act of self-generation.

> The 'I' thinks, therefore it is. A verb, a verbal process/trial serve as premises for existence, recreate 'being' just as it was about to succumb, drowning in deep water, with nothing and no one to hold on to. ... the first such [clear and distinct] idea to present itself is – at this moment – that 'I think'. Building on this seed, this germ cell of truth, and on the development of a 'natural' light – though you really must not ask me right now where it comes from and how it came into being, in case I lose hold of it, and so on indefinitely – the 'I' will confer existence upon itself. (S, 184)

In the midst of the deep whirlpool of doubt, the clear and distinct idea that he is thinking seems to provide the meditator with solid ground. By grounding his own existence on nothing but self-reflection, the meditator appears to have found *'one fixed point* from which to begin all over again' (S, 189). However, as we have seen, Irigaray's reading suggests that 'the self-sufficiency of the (self) thinking subject' can never quite be secured (S, 183). Despite – or rather, because – of the repression of its origins in a mother, the Cartesian self remains haunted by its need for an other. At the very moment where the meditating 'I' seems to establish its own existence, a necessary other re-appears, whether through the doubling of the self in its own reflection, or as a non-deceiving God.

The Need For An Other: God

The meditator's need for an other is most obvious in his arguments for the existence of God. By proving his own existence through nothing but an introspective act, the meditator seems to lock himself into an empty solipsism. He can think, know that he thinks, and know that he is, but no more. The content of his thoughts might still be entirely deceptive; the world about which he thinks could be an ingenious illusion; his own body could be a dream. As Irigaray puts it:

> 'I think' therefore. But at the price of clearing away all thought, razing to the ground all objective reality for my ideas. 'I' think, but about whom? About what? And, in some manner, what for? And

who will give me something to think about, and think about rightly, in this existence in which I am at present confirmed. And *confined*. Leaving me hungry for something other than my single certainty of being. When it comes down to it, who will replace or substitute for everything and everybody I have given up in order to be? (*S*, 186)

Just as the child cannot remain forever in the womb, so the self cannot remain forever '*in suspension*', but needs a way (back) into the world (*S*, 186). Above all, it needs some certainty that its ideas are not necessarily misleading, but correspond to the objective reality of the world 'outside' the self. Hence the need to prove the existence of God. If God exists, and deception is an imperfection, then God in his perfection would not have arranged things so that 'I' would be constantly deceived. As long as I do not misuse my God-given capacities, my ideas will match the world and their objective reality will be secured. God 'confers upon my words the truth of the objective realities that they aim for in ideas' (*S*, 186).

Irigaray's reading here takes up the common criticism that Descartes' position results in solipsism and gives it a new twist. On her interpretation, the need for a third term to bridge the gap between self and world is no longer simply a result of the solipsism engendered by the *cogito*. Rather, both this solipsism and the need for a third term result from the way the meditating self has severed his links to his origins and ancestors, and above all, to the mother's body through which he was first brought into the world. On this reading, God is a necessary supplement for the absent mother, who has been excluded from metaphysics and confined to scientific treatises on nature.

Irigaray draws out the complex manoeuvres the meditator has to perform to posit this divine other without re-implicating the self in relations of dependence. On the one hand, Irigaray suggests that the idea of God is 'guaranteed by its total innocuousness as far as I am concerned. By this I mean both that the infinitely perfect does not need me in order to exist in its full autonomy and that it can no longer deceive me or itself on pain of losing its absolute value' (*S*, 186). As a perfect and perfectly self-sufficient being, God fulfils the meditator's needs without threatening either his judgements or his autonomy. On the other hand, even though Descartes denies that we can generate the idea of God's perfection by extrapolation from our own imperfect being,[21] Irigaray suggests that this idea is nonetheless a projection of the self: not a rational extrapolation, but an image of perfect self-sufficiency that is an unconscious expression of the self's desire to escape dependency and that simultaneously fills the lack created by the mother's absence. Thus, the divine 'other' who reconnects self and world also turns out not to be a genuine other. The repression of maternal origins makes space for the self to project an other carefully conceived to serve its own needs: 'God is, but it is the "I" that by thinking has granted him that essence and existence that the "I" expects from God ... *The son*, after busying himself with his own genesis, *reproduces (for) himself*, "on the third day", a "father-mother" to his own specifications. Or *in his own image?*' (*S*, 187). Although the meditating 'I' grants God existence by conceiving his essence, this does not make God dependent on the rational subject. Rather, because God is made in the self's (idealized) image, he is represented as a perfectly autonomous being, despite being 'made' by man.

On Irigaray's reading, then, both the need for a divine other and the doubling of the self in the *cogito* are positioned as signs of the inescapability of the self's existential and ontological dependency. Try as he might, the meditator cannot prevent this dependency from re-surfacing. However, while God is interpreted as a kind of 'false other', a necessary projection of the self, Irigaray also identifies a genuine other which stubbornly persists and indeed motivates much of the meditator's journey. For as she notes, it is only because material things remain intransigently 'other' to the meditator that a third term is required to bridge the gap between self and world at all: God must exist because the meditator is unable to fully re-absorb matter's extension into thought (*S*, 187).

By conjoining *Optics* and *Meditations*, Irigaray uncovers a familiar pattern: a materiality aligned with woman (and with the pregnant woman in particular) remains resistant to metaphysical thinking which opposes mind to body, reason to the senses, and intellectual form (ideas) to matter. This suggests that a different way of thinking about matter is required if we are to make space for a subject who is not artificially divorced from their bodily ancestry of birth. However, rather than acknowledge this, Cartesian metaphysics seeks ways to explain and contain the resistant 'otherness' of matter. Irigaray thus pays close attention to what happens to materiality once the self is returned to the sensible world via God.

Nature without Gaps

Many feminists criticize the mind–body dualism that emerges from Cartesian metaphysics because of the ways in which it makes embodied specificity, and hence sexual difference, inessential to human being, thereby perpetuating the illusion that the self is 'gender neutral'.[22] Irigaray's reading reinforces this critique while focusing more on the thinking subject's relation to nature as a whole than the mind–body relation per se. In this way, she reminds us that challenging mind–body dualism necessitates challenging the more general Cartesian representation of the material world.

In 'Meditation Six', Descartes famously insists that the mind does not inhabit the body like a pilot in a ship but that they are 'very closely joined and, as it were, intermingled'.[23] Much critical debate has arisen concerning how mind and body can be so closely connected, given Descartes' insistence that they are essentially distinct.[24] Rather than rehearse this debate, Irigaray borrows the metaphor and re-deploys it against Descartes to describe the self's relation not just to his own body, but the external world in general: 'the subject will observe the world like the pilot of a ship taking to the open sea' (S, 185). She draws out the way in which the splitting of the self in the *cogito* is echoed in the split between the self and material nature. Just as the self becomes the object of its own thoughts, so the material world of the senses can be admitted back into thought once it is turned into an object that is clearly distinct from the subject:

> The eye/'I' (of the spirit) is closed to the charms of seductively deceptive things and, once its mechanism has been analyzed, it will frame and reproduce only what is technically set up in front of it.
>
> For this new 'subject' that enters the world again greedy for scientific powers, any (other) fantasy, and (other) dream, disturbing the precision of his theoretical instruments, must be frozen – any 'passivity' of senses that are still natural and therefore uncontrollably open to impressions from silent, forbidden matter. (S, 184–5)

Irigaray foregrounds the ways in which, even when the evidence of the senses is re-admitted, Cartesian metaphysics continues to oppose the senses to theoretical reason. Whereas the former are understood in terms of passive and uncontrollable openness, reason's ideas allow the subject to properly regulate his own thinking and gain control of the world around him.

Such control is dependent on a particular model of matter: 'So this sea [*cette mer*] where he is, or at least seems to be, lost, that overwhelms him on every side and so puts his life in danger, what is she [*qu'est-elle*]? Considered coldly, she [*elle*] consists of an *extended corporeal thing'* (*S*, 185; *Sf*, 231). Irigaray is again implicitly combining two key texts: Descartes' *Meditations*, where the world of the senses threatens to drown him in a whirlpool of doubt, and his treatise on *The World*. Here too Descartes invokes the sea, noting that 'people on some vessel in the middle of it may stretch their view seemingly to infinity; and yet there is more water beyond what they see.'[25] Descartes uses this image as a reminder of the limits of the senses and imagination. Despite this, it occurs as part of a thought experiment in which he himself imagines another world, via which he hopes to give his readers an ideal model for thinking about the real world they actually inhabit.[26]

In particular, Descartes wishes to help 'the philosophers' to overcome 'the memory of their "prime matter"', which has been 'stripped so thoroughly of all its forms and qualities that nothing remains in it which can be clearly understood'.[27] As Irigaray suggests, Descartes is seeking to escape the puzzling otherness of matter that persists in Aristotelian and scholastic thought. By contrast, in Descartes' thought experiment, the whole of nature is reduced to a particular form: that of 'external extension', that is, 'the property it has of occupying space.'[28] The essence of matter becomes not its singular qualities but its quantity, which is always calculable in terms of spatial dimensions.

While *The World's* account of space is presented as an imaginative exercise, it clearly fits with the account of matter as nonthinking, extended substance given in *Meditations*. By entwining the two, Irigaray foregrounds the ways in which Descartes' metaphysics is informed by a vision of nature as an object of knowledge fully masterable by the thinking 'I': 'From this place where he is now assured of existing, he can cut the sea into any number of pieces, subject her to any number of visual angles, inscribe her in an even vaster space in order to draw a line around her: a map of the world. The "I" can subject the sea to a whole range of techniques that will transform her into an *object of use'* (*S*, 185). Even the most fluid part of nature, the sea, is now understood as operating on the model of solid bodies. Like the rest of nature – and like Plotinus' *mère de glace* – it is deadened and fixed so as to be made measurable, manipulable, and useful to man.

Irigaray goes on to recast the laws of motion that govern Descartes' imaginary world – and that are supposed to provide the ideal model for thinking about our own. She draws attention to the fact that when bodies collide, they are said to impart movement to each other without merging; at the same time, they will never separate in such a way as to produce a vacuum. Once again, by translating Descartes' concerns into the context of sexual difference, Irigaray gives them a particular valence. The anxiety that bodies might interpenetrate becomes a further symptom of the repression of the maternal, of the pregnant body that becomes more than one in ways that are not fully open to the subject's gaze. In Descartes' writings, the problematic status of maternal materiality is not even signalled as an unthinkable absence, as in Plotinus' image of 'the Void'. Instead, Irigaray's reading suggests that the numerous occasions where Descartes insists that nature does not permit a vacuum are symptomatic of a fear of the female body with its 'holes' and 'voids'.

In a typically subversive mimicry of Descartes' voice, Irigaray thus writes that: 'if there were really a vacuum, "nature" of her own volition would close over, sealing the two lips of that slit.' Drawing on one of Descartes' own examples, she goes on to consider the objection that God could nonetheless choose to create such a vacuum by emptying a vase of its contents, 'leaving it devoid of anything that would justify *opening its neck*'. To this, Irigaray (still miming Descartes) retorts that: '*my conception finds that distasteful*, and that anyway God cannot possibly fail to satisfy *the principle of non-contradiction*' (*S*, 188). As Irigaray will develop more extensively elsewhere, the images of two lips and the opening evoke the morphology of the female body, whose sex is reduced to no more than 'a slit' by the male subject's gaze. Her textual mimicry of Descartes thereby simultaneously hints at the alternative images of space and self that would be required to do justice to a female subject who belongs to the sex that gives birth: in defiance of the principle of non-contradiction (which asserts that something cannot be both 'p' and 'not-p'), such a space would have to permit two to co-exist in the same place at the same time without simply becoming one.

In response to Descartes, Irigaray asks how metaphysics might be transformed if the mother were incorporated into thought rather than silently appropriated or repressed: 'And what if the "I" only thought the thought of woman? The thought (as it were) of femaleness? And could send back this thought in its reflection only because the mother had been incorporated?' (*S*, 183). At the very least, such a mode of thinking would involve acknowledging our maternal origins and hence demand a metaphysics capable of granting generative power to sexuate matter.

Thus Was I Reborn in Wonder

At the end of Irigaray's reading, she puns on Descartes' name to highlight the way the self is reborn through the meditative process: 'Thus was I reborn [*ainsi suis-je rené*: lit. thus was I reborn/René], cleansed of those fables and material impressions that darken the understanding of children' (*S*, 189). As in the Myth of the Cave, so in *Meditations*, birth can be seen as the model for a philosophical journey that simultaneously represses the significance of our maternal origins. Moreover, whereas the ancient Greek philosophers sought an origin of being beyond the self, the Cartesian mediator first secures his own being and then seeks to re-establish the world (and even the existence of God) on that firm foundation: 'by a stroke of almost incredible boldness, it is the singular subject who is charged with giving birth to the universe all over again, after he has brought himself back into the world in a way that avoids the precariousness of existence as it is usually understood' (*S*, 182). By denying his dependence on anyone other than himself, the meditator cuts the link to the mother, and seeks instead to re-birth both himself and the world through an act of pure self-reflection.

Irigaray returns to Descartes in one of the essays included in *An Ethics of Sexual Difference* (*ESD*, 72–82). Perhaps surprisingly, here she finds positive resources in Descartes' *Passions of the Soul*, specifically, in his account of the way that wonder (*l'admiration*) arises '[w]hen the first encounter with some object surprises us, and we judge it to be new or very different from what we formerly knew, or from what we supposed that it ought to be'.[29] Crucially, wonder occurs before we know whether an object is 'agreeable' to us, that is, whether it suits our dispositions or is otherwise useful to us. It arises when we encounter something or someone we have not yet 'made ours' by judging it on our own terms and assimilating it to ourselves (*ESD*, 75). Irigaray suggests that wonder therefore precedes the appropriation of the other; instead, this first passion manifests an openness to the unfamiliarity of that which is encountered. She thus argues that wonder is indispensable 'not only to life', but also to the creation of an ethics, and above all, to the creation of an ethics of sexual difference (*ESD*, 74). Such an ethics would not only involve an ethical relation *to* sexual difference. As we will see in Chapter 7, an ethical mode of being and relating to others would also be inaugurated *through* the cultivation of sexual difference, that is, by remaining open and attentive to the way that the sexuate other, whether male or female, 'should *surprise* us again and again, appear to us as *new, very different* from what we knew or what we thought he or she should be. ... Wonder must be the advent or the event of the other' (*ESD*, 74–5). Wonder is thus an *'opening'* or 'interval' through which the sexes may relate in their irreducible difference, without assimilating one another: 'Before and after appropriation, there is wonder' (*ESD*, 81, 73, 74). Insofar as this first passion constitutes a 'bridge' or 'point of passage between two closed worlds, two definite universes, two space-times or two others' (*ESD*, 75), it can also be read as an affective version of the passage that Irigaray sought to recover from Plato.

Irigaray proceeds to question whether this passion which allows for openness to the other, and thus for a positive relation to sexual difference, might not also be the place of man's second birth: a birth that would transform the nature of human being by opening the male subject to sexuate difference and allowing woman to come to be (*ESD*, 82). As wonder arises whenever we encounter something new, unknown, or different, such a rebirth will not occur once and for all in the foundational manner of the *cogito*. Rather, wonder testifies to a 'perpetual rebirth' in ongoing encounters with the irreducibly other, and thus to a 'perpetual newness of the self, the other, the world' (*ESD*, 82).

For Descartes, the passions in general arise because of the conjunction of body and soul. Wonder in particular involves an openness to the world we encounter. Thus Irigaray suggests that instead of fostering the separation of self and world, wonder permits a transcendence that remains *within* the sensible world. It is there that one encounters those surprising others whose difference opens one up beyond oneself. Wonder undoes or precedes the opposition of body and soul, mind and matter. It is allied not with the thinking substance of the *cogito* that 'turns back upon itself and fastens up the circle of (its) subjectivity' (*S*, 180), but with: 'A birth into a transcendence, that of the other, still in the world of the senses ("sensible"), still physical and carnal, and already spiritual' (*ESD*, 82).

Whether it arises in the encounter between one sex and another, or between the material and the metaphysical, wonder testifies to 'their possible conception and fecundation one by the other' (*ESD*, 82). Instead of replacing maternal power with an act of autonomous self-generation, wonder confirms the creative movement of birth that is repeated in encounters between two who are irreducibly different. In wonder, then, Irigaray finds resources within Descartes' thought that would allow two different subjects to co-exist in ways that escape the solipsism engendered by the *cogito*.

When lost in this first passion, rather than the pure self-reflection of first philosophy, '[t]he beginning of the position of the subject as such still welcomes as desirable that which it does not know, that which it ignores or which remains foreign to it. *Sexual difference* could be situated there' (*ESD*, 79).

Kantian Reversals

Despite the undoubted significance of Descartes for Irigaray, it is another philosophical figure who looms over the central chapters of *Speculum*: Immanuel Kant. Adding to our long line of philosophical father-figures, Kant's work is often seen as the culmination of Enlightenment thought and the beginning of a new approach in which philosophy becomes characterized by the dual notions of critique and the transcendental. Critique for Kant involves using reason to investigate its own limits: while Kant is often caricatured as a straightforward champion of reason, in fact, his approach is based on the necessity not only of establishing its proper limits, but on making reason self-disciplined enough to establish and adhere to these limits for itself. Transcendental philosophy is the search for the a priori (universal and necessary) conditions of a given phenomenon – whether knowledge of objects (dealt with in the *Critique of Pure Reason*), moral action (*Critique of Practical Reason* and *The Groundwork of the Metaphysics of Morals*), or aesthetic and teleological judgements about nature (*Critique of Judgement*). The notions of critique and the transcendental are intrinsically linked: it is because human beings are not purely rational beings but finite and limited that they can only have knowledge under certain conditions; establishing these conditions helps prevent reason from going astray by overstepping its limits.

Later thinkers have pursued Kant's critical and transcendental approach but radicalized it by suggesting that what conditions us is historical and material (Marx, Nietzsche, Foucault) and not always available to consciousness (Nietzsche, Freud). Irigaray radicalizes it in a different way by resituating our understanding of human limits in the conjoined contexts of sexual difference and our dependency on birth from a mother: we are finite because we have a beginning, and our beginning both depends on sexual difference and brings us into being as sexuate beings ourselves. Thus, rather than focusing on the notoriously problematic and sometimes simply sexist claims that Kant makes about women, Irigaray shows

how the question of sexual difference impinges on the central terms
of his philosophy in ways that necessitate their thoroughgoing
transformation. In so doing, she can be seen as fulfilling the motto
Kant proposes for enlightenment: *Sapere Aude!* – dare to think for
yourself.

Irigaray's engagement with Kant is foregrounded in the opening
chapter of the middle section of *Speculum*, 'Any Theory of the
"Subject" Has Always Been Appropriated by the "Masculine"'.
This chapter sets up the dependence of the philosophical subject
on a female other or object in terms that are explicitly Kantian. The
object is:

> a bench mark that is ultimately more crucial than the subject, for he
> can sustain himself only by bouncing back off some objectiveness,
> some objective. If there is no more 'earth' to press down/repress, to
> work, to represent, but also and always to desire (for one's own), no
> opaque matter which in theory does not know herself, then what
> pedestal remains for the ex-istence of the 'subject'? If the earth
> turned and more especially turned upon herself, the erection of the
> subject might thereby be disconcerted and risk losing its elevation
> and penetration. For what would there be to rise up from and exer-
> cise his power over? And in? The Copernican revolution has yet to
> have its final effects in the male imaginary. (*S*, 133)

The 'Copernican revolution' was an image Kant adopted to describe
the transformation brought about by his philosophy. Just as
Copernicus revolutionized the western understanding of the universe by showing that the earth moved around the sun, so Kant
sought to revolutionize the approach to knowledge itself, by showing
that it is centred not in the object but the subject. Thus, whereas
Copernicus displaces the earth – and its human inhabitants – from
the centre of the universe, Kant moves in the opposite direction,
anchoring objective knowledge in the subject and its faculties.

More specifically, Kant suggests that rather than seeking to make
our knowledge conform to the way objects really are, objects have
to conform to our modes of knowing (that is, our faculties).[30] The
problem with the former approach is the one that confronts the
solipsistic Cartesian meditator: how can one be sure that one's
ideas match the way the world really is? Rather than appeal to God
to bridge the gap, Kant reverses the relation: it is human subjects
who form inchoate sensations into coherent objects. There are no
objects 'out there' to which we must seek access. Rather, our understanding of the world is able to 'match' the way objects are because

it is we human subjects who constitute unified objects in the first place, by providing an undetermined flow of sensory intuitions with spatio-temporal and conceptual form.

Irigaray's rendering draws attention to the ways in which, despite his active role in constituting objects of knowledge, the Kantian subject remains doubly dependent on the objective material world: first, because this subject situates itself in relation to the objects it constitutes (the 'bench mark that is ultimately more crucial than the subject'); and second, because the subject must be given the matter of sensation (the 'earth') if it is to have anything it can work up into objective representations in the first place. Yet at the same time, the subject necessarily opposes his own form-giving activities to the chaos of disorganized matter. The subject is therefore dependent on a material 'otherness' from which he must nonetheless carefully distance himself, cutting himself off from direct contact with a sensible matter that he is only prepared to encounter when it is contained within a representational frame. As Irigaray emphasizes, the philosophical speculations of such a subject are sustained by a thoroughly *specularized* nature. In response, Irigaray will seek to show that, far from straightfor-wardly securing the subject of knowledge, the Copernican turn simultaneously destabilizes him by making him dependent on the very materiality he seeks to submit to his orderly forms, thereby centering man 'outside himself' (*S*, 133).

Irigaray's reading draws attention to both parallels and differences between Descartes and Kant. Just as Descartes splits the thinking 'I' from extended matter, so the Kantian subject is constructed against the unformed materiality that it orders into a world of objects. However, Kant explicitly positions himself against Descartes when he argues that awareness of ourselves depends on awareness of something permanent outside ourselves against which the temporal order of our changing inner states can be determined.[31] According to Kant, there can be no foundational moment of purely introspective self-certainty: self-awareness is not possible without a correlative awareness of an external world. As Irigaray notes, Kant's transcendental subject, 'was, of course, obliged to draw on reserves still in the realm of nature; a detour through the outer world was of course indispensable; the "I" had to relate to "things" before it could be conscious of itself' (*S*, 204). Thus, one of the advantages which leads Irigaray to foreground Kant is the explicitness with which he thematizes the interdependency of self and other, subject and object. This constitutive inter-dependence is a commonly noted feature of Kant's philosophy. What makes Irigaray's approach distinctive is the way in which she shows how the position of the object maps onto the position accorded to woman in western philosophy, while the materiality which the Kantian subject seeks both to order and to distance itself from is aligned with the maternal body.

Before examining Irigaray's reading of Kant in more detail, it is worth reinforcing the point made above about the ways in which she seeks to transform the fundamental terms of Kant's project. Indeed, the foregrounding of Kant at certain key points in *Speculum* is all the more appropriate because of the ways in which Irigaray's own project can be described as 'post-Kantian': both in the sense that her project follows on from Kant's in important ways, and because she nonetheless disrupts and displaces Kant by seeking a philosophical position that moves beyond his. At the heart of Kant's 'Copernican turn' lies an investigation into the conditions of possibility of knowledge and experience. In response, Kant identifies a framework which makes knowledge possible precisely because it allows human subjects to form objects of experience out of the flux of sensations.[32] This framework is a priori, that is, necessary and universal. As it is not *beyond* experience, but constitutes the immanent conditions making experience possible, Kant refers to it not as transcendent, but transcendental. Irigaray's project can also be described as transcendental, to the extent that her central question concerns the 'conditions of possibility' for a female subject – that is, the conditions which would allow a woman to relate to herself *as* female without being defined as the 'other' of a male subject.

However, by even raising this question, Irigaray breaks open the Kantian project: if it is possible for woman to be a subject in her own right, that is, for there to be a subject who is also specifically and irreducibly female, then there can no longer be a single set of universal conditions making experience possible for all human beings. If her challenge to Plato is to think Being as two, her challenge to Kant is to think more than one transcendental, allowing the question of sexual difference to transform the critical project.

Earthquakes and the Anxiety of Inversion

It sometimes happens that the sun causes the earth to shake underfoot, and people fear being knocked over [*l'angoisse d'un renversement*], or thrown sickeningly down into the pit [the abyss], or even flying off into the void. To reestablish the balance that has been so dangerously disturbed, the philosopher decides that from now on nature overall will be put under the control of the human spirit and her origins will be based on her necessary obedience to the law. So the ground will now rest upon a transcendental ceiling that is propped up by the forms and rules of representation and is thus unshakable. (*S*, 203–4)

This dramatic opening to the chapter on Kant invokes three early essays Kant wrote in response to the Lisbon earthquake of 1755,[33] as well as his later account of the sublime (an aesthetic experience provoked by the destructive power of nature, to which we will return below).[34] On Irigaray's reading, the Lisbon earthquake stands not as an exceptional event, but an extreme example of one of the ways in which nature is regarded within the Kantian frame: as a chaotic and threatening materiality which it is the subject's responsibility to order to the best of his abilities.

Indeed, on Kant's account, nature is not just brought under the conceptual control of the subject; rather, the material basis of experience ('the ground') is made dependent on the a priori frame ('the transcendental ceiling') which allows the subject to transform the chaotic materiality of sensible intuition into coherent objects. By organizing these objects into a systematic whole, a second nature is produced whose laws necessarily reflect the conceptual rules according to which the subject constitutes the objective world. Irigaray thus presents the terrifying power of nature to overwhelm man and throw him off course in terms of *l'angoisse d'un renversement*: anxiety of reversal, inversion, or over-turning. What is most feared is that the material world might prove so chaotically uncontrollable that it resists being ordered by the subject at all, and hence reverses the axis of the Copernican turn, displacing the subject from the centre of knowledge.

The image of *renversement* recalls the capacities of mirrors to reverse and invert what they reflect. This association is strengthened by Irigaray's choice of epigraphs. The first passage she cites, from Kant's *Prolegomena*, concerns the problem of incongruent counterparts, that is, the way that a left hand and its mirror image are identical yet non-substitutable, because of the reversal that takes place in reflection.[35] For Kant this paradox supports his claim that space is not a property of things in themselves but the a priori form of intuition that frames human perception of external objects. This is because the two hands are identical in terms of any internal features that can be conceptually identified:[36] if space were a property of things in themselves, it would be possible to pick out the objective inner differences between a hand and its mirror image. Instead, Kant tells us, these inner differences can only be felt via the senses, in ways that depend on the status of space as a form of intuition.

The second passage Irigaray cites also emphasizes that space is a form of intuition, this time via the example of a person in a dark room with which they are familiar, but in which the positions of the objects have been reversed from left to right. Although Kant does not say so, it is of course as if the room had been reversed in a mirror. Again, Kant emphasizes that in such a situation, he would make sense of the effects of this reversal and re-orient himself by 'the mere feeling of a difference between my left and right sides'.[37] Re-situated in the context of Irigaray's project, the fact that there is a sensible difference which orients us in the dark is suggestive of the primary (but obscured) status of sexual difference. Just as a 'mere feeling of difference' guides us when we are unable to visually identify individual objects, sexual difference operates as a ground of differentiation that orients human beings in the world prior to the oppositional distinctions that situate subject against object, self against 'other'.

As in the chapter on Descartes, these epigraphs have complex effects that resonate through Irigaray's interpretation. The close conjunction of the epigraphs with the image of 'renversement' in the opening paragraph allows her to position the Copernican turn itself as a kind of mirroring: her reading suggests that the shift from object to subject is akin to a reversal in a mirror. Moreover, this is no ordinary mirror. Like the wall at the back of the cave, the reflecting glass in which the Kantian subject gazes must be a concave one, for it stands the world on its head: the original material ground of experience is replaced with the transcendental 'ceiling'. The Copernican turn implicitly depends on a mirror which allows the subject to distance himself from the threatening powers of material nature by re-grounding experience within himself.

By reading the Copernican turn as a kind of mirroring, Irigaray suggests that the subject–object relation is set up in such a way that the object is a projection and reflection of the subject:

> For if, already, we know which time was needed to produce the window through which we see the universe, to frame the space whereby the infinite is determined a priori, always already defined

in/by the subjectivity of man, we have still to learn that the *space-time of specularization* is implicit in the intuition of space. And even if, conceptually, my right hand and my left hand, or my hand and its image in the mirror, are rigorously the same, or the same thing, this would not be true for the intuitive character of space in which *the paradox of symmetry* was taken into account. Thus already a mirror turns out to support the apprehension of objects. (*S*, 205)

Irigaray's reading implies that Kant is not rigorous enough in his search for the 'necessary and universal' conditions of human experience. Both the subject–object relation and the a priori forms of space and time are themselves conditioned by the oppositional relations implicit in a specular logic: 'the *space-time of specularization* is implicit in the intuition of space'. As Kant himself shows in his discussion of incongruent counterparts, one of the features of such relations is that a mirror image is, paradoxically, both identical with and yet different from its original. Similarly, objects in the world must be both outside and other to the subject, while simultaneously reflecting the terms that allow that subject to constitute itself as the subject of experience, that is, to secure its own identity. Read in this way, like the earthquake, the paradox generated by mirror images is not exceptional but indicative of the fundamental structure of the Kantian world. The object is set up to reflect the subject's terms: it is constituted via the spatio-temporal and conceptual frame that allows the subject to distance itself from threatening nature while simultaneously orienting itself in the world by providing itself with objects of knowledge.

Irigaray draws particular attention to the role of the imagination in the constitution of coherent objects against which the subject can situate itself. For Kant, the imagination mediates between sensible intuitions and the conceptual framework provided by the understanding by generating what he calls a 'schema'. It is the 'schema' which translates the (a-temporal) conceptual categories into a form that can be applied to the temporal flow of appearances, and thus allows us to synthesize intuitions into objects. Irigaray emphasizes that this always involves filtering out those aspects of our sensory experiences which do not lend themselves to being synthesized in accordance with the form of a unified object:

> Thus, the function of the transcendental schema will be to negate an intrinsic quality of the sensible world, and this irremediably. Nature is foreclosed in her primary empirical naivete. Diversity of feeling is set aside in order to build up the concept of the object, and the

immediacy of *the relationship to the mother* is sacrificed. The intuition of the transcendental aims, under some vague and undetermined generality, to unify all the various sensations that take place or have taken place. In this way the multiplicity of unlabeled sensations is blacked out, reduced to a single entity that can be used to legislate – in the cruelty of understanding – the bond to the empirical matrix. (*S*, 204)

One of the effects of the framework required to produce unified objects is that the subject has to separate itself to a great extent from the complex fecundity of the sensible world, screening out those aspects that do not fit within its conceptual frame. As we might expect, Irigaray reads this as a process whereby the subject cuts himself off from his original bond to the maternal materiality that brought him into the world. Indeed, the project of re-framing – and thereby taming – nature reflects the ways in which, within Kant's critical project, material nature has always already been positioned as 'outside' and 'other' to the subject, such that it is always a potential threat.

On Irigaray's reading, Kant distances the subject from the objective world of material nature as surely as if he had inserted a silvered pane of glass between them. This distancing is reflected in the way that the transcendental subject itself, as a mere reference point for sensible intuitions, is no more than a bare unity of consciousness that can never be an *object* of knowledge. Such a conflation of subject and object would destabilize the whole system. Thus, as Irigaray notes, the subject is in effect positioned as the back of the mirror which makes objective appearances possible yet does not itself appear:

> Are we to assume that a mirror has always already been inserted, and speculates every perception and conception of the world, *with the exception of itself*, whose reflection would only be a factor of time? Thus extension would always already be re-staged and re-projected by the subject who, alone, would not be situated there. Does the subject derive his power from the appropriation of this non-place of the mirror? (*S*, 205)

The Kantian subject can of course become aware of itself via introspection. However, this is an awareness of the *contents* of its consciousness (the empirical self), rather than that mere unity of consciousness that forms a reference point for thoughts and intuitions (the transcendental subject, whose unity is expressed in the grammatical subject, 'I'). Moreover, as Irigaray reminds us, Kant argues that empirical self-awareness is only possible in relation to an external world of objects against which the temporal flow of the subject's internal states can be measured. Nonetheless, as the transcendental subject is positioned as the necessary reference point for all intuitions, and hence as the condition of the appearance of objects, ultimately, it is the subject which is the condition of self-awareness: if the 'I' has to relate to an external world of objects before it can be conscious of itself, 'this initial period of cooperative creation [con-naissance] is forgotten in an arrogant claim to sovereign discretion over everything' (S, 204). The initial promise of Kant's emphasis on the subject–object relation is undone. The ways in which subjects and objects of knowledge (connaissance) are constituted or birthed together (co-naissance) are covered over by the ways in which the subject sets up the object on its own terms so as to position itself at a safe – and legislative – distance from material nature. Instead of a subject born together with an other, the other is turned into a projection/reflection of a subject who is therefore, strictly speaking, self-grounding. On Irigaray's reading, Kant is not in the end so very different from Descartes after all; instead, under the guise of acknowledging a constitutive inter-dependency with an other, the Kantian subject in fact more fully realizes the self-constitution desired by the Cartesian meditator.

An Unanalysed Remainder

The reduction of the object to a reflection/projection of the subject is both reflected and reinforced in Kant's comments on women. Irigaray foregrounds the ways in which Kant's aesthetic examples and anthropological texts consistently position woman as the beautiful object for a male gaze, while her procreative powers are used to align her with material nature. Her analysis traces the different kinds of pleasure the Kantian subject takes in this 'woman-object' (S, 207), moving from the immediate sensual pleasure he finds in feminine charms to the more cultivated and supposedly disinterested pleasure afforded by a woman's beauty. While the former is useful, insofar as it encourages procreation, the latter is more valuable, as an appreciation of beauty increases man's sense of the world as a place that harmoniously reflects his own ordering powers. As the object of aesthetic appreciation, however, the ideal woman will harmoniously fit the subject's faculties while being unable to take up the position of subject herself. She is like the hand in the mirror which is the same as the hand it reflects, yet unable to take its place.

Irigaray's analysis foregrounds the importance of what Kant calls 'reflective judgement'.[38] As Kant elaborates in his account of aesthetic judgement, because the world of experience is produced by the subject (not materially, but insofar as it is the subject who gives the manifold of intuition spatio-temporal and conceptual form), this world, perhaps unsurprisingly, appears to reflect and harmonize pleasingly with the subject's faculties.[39] Nonetheless, by using Kant's own examples to draw attention to the way in which a mirror image is irreducible to its counterpart, Irigaray also suggests that the reflective operations that secure the Kantian subject always produce 'a *remainder*'. The fact that there is a difference that can only be felt by the senses holds open the possibility that our sensible intuitions contain something yet to be thought, something that cannot be wholly captured within the subject's space-time and that resists his conceptual frame: '*One kind of difference, inverted in the mirror, will never be analyzed. Is this because that difference could not be mirrored as object?*' (S, 210) Irigaray does not say here that the difference which is not analyzed is sexual difference. Rather, the text presents the reader with a puzzle (*what kind of difference is this?*). The solution (*sexual difference*) depends on piecing together Irigaray's intricate analysis of the ways in which the transcendental frame both produces the 'woman-object' the subject requires as his counterpart, and distances him from his material-maternal origins.

Irigaray's suggestion that the unanalysed remainder 'could not be mirrored as object' implies that sexual difference is not only unconceptualized within the Kantian frame, but unconceptualizable. Her question suggests that this is partly because woman's sexed specificity cannot be identified with a single visible organ, and so cannot be adequately represented as an *object*; and partly because sexual difference cannot be thought in terms of a relation of *mirroring*. Such a relation will only repeat and re-double the terms of one subject, rather than making it possible to think two who are irreducible to one another: 'The forms of arrangement may vary, but they will all bear the paradox of forcing into the same representation – the representation of the self/same – that which insists upon its *heterogeneity*, its *otherness*' (S, 137). Even in Kant's system then, there is a sensible excess which testifies to a difference that cannot be captured in the framework which constitutes material objects for a knowing subject. Nonetheless, Irigaray does not simply celebrate the possibility of such sensible excess. On the contrary, her analysis reminds us that the subject also positions nature as an unconceptualizable excess, in order to provide himself with a potentially infinite resource for further conceptual speculation: it is only *because* material nature resists being grasped through concepts in her entirety that there will always be more sensible intuitions to be worked up into objects. Sensible excess is required to sustain the subject's desire for producing objective order.

Thus, as Irigaray shows, in Kant's self-professed desire for systematic completeness, even the apparently unconceptualizable is reclaimed as a resource for the thinking subject. Her analysis explores the multiple ways in which, whenever it exceeds containment in a concept, nature in fact *extends* the subject's powers, as well as his awareness of his own higher purpose (S, 208). This is revealed most clearly in Kant's sublime, where the imagination is initially overwhelmed by nature's apparent infinity or its destructive might.[40] Yet when 'faced with the non-specularizable' – with 'nature that remains unformed or deformed' – the imagination is forced to operate at a higher level (S, 209): its failure to represent nature's apparent infinity becomes a way of reaching towards reason's unrepresentable ideas of the absolute. Similarly, by overcoming his fear of nature's insurmountable physical might (what Kant calls 'nature without'), the subject gains a heightened awareness of his ability to overcome his own sensible limits ('nature within').[41] In this way, he becomes more aware of his capacity to strive towards freedom by determining his will through reason alone, and thus, more attuned to his moral vocation.

On Irigaray's reading, the Kantian subject's conceptual frame 'alleviates the horror of the inchoate and unpossessable as well as the disgust for the misshapen refuse that will be excreted under the form of matter' (S, 205). Nonetheless, where this frame fails, the resulting excess does not pose a real threat. Nature's empirical excesses provoke the subject to resist in ways that reaffirm his own capacity to reach beyond nature. As Irigaray notes: 'Nature has also proved useful, we are told, in elaborating a spiritual plus that will not surrender to the sensible for all that' (S, 208).

Thus, Irigaray does not simply valorize those aspects of the sensible which might make themselves felt, but which resist containment in concepts. Given that, as her own analysis shows, sensible excess is built into the Kantian system as a necessary resource,

merely reversing the hierarchy to privilege this excess over conceptual thought would not really change anything. It would simply
spin the Copernican mirror on its axis once more. Instead, we need
to pay attention to *how* the sensible has been sacrificed within the
Kantian frame. This is why Irigaray repeatedly emphasizes the
way that sensibility is split from understanding.

The problem with Kant's account of the paradox of symmetry is
that it depends upon a clear cut distinction between conceptual
forms (according to which the hand and its mirror image are the
same) and sensible intuition (via which their difference is felt).
Thus what is most important about the example of incongruent
counterparts is not that it presents us with a material excess we
should seek to reclaim, but that it reveals the way in which the
world of the Kantian subject is fundamentally divided between the
conceptual and the sensible. Likewise, in Kant's account of space
and time as a priori forms of intuition, the problem (on Irigaray's
reading) lies in the division *between* spatio-temporal forms and the
matter of sensation, which reduces the latter to the *un*formed and
inchoate.

It is this fundamental cut between spatio-temporal and conceptual forms on the one hand, and sensible matter on the other,
which underpins the specular economy that opposes subject to
object. It also repeats, albeit in a new way, the hylomorphic model
that Irigaray has traced across the work of Plato, Aristotle and
Plotinius, according to which active form is imposed on passive
and unformed matter. It is therefore this divide, the original inser-
tion of the frame, that needs to be resisted.

Re-Framing the World

Irigaray's reading shows that displacing the oppositional subject–
object relation that characterizes Kant's philosophy will necessitate
re-working the transcendental frame: not by privileging sensible
matter over form, but by changing the relation between them so
that experience is no longer constituted by imposing form on inherently form-less matter. In this regard, it is telling that when Irigaray
describes the schema as a 'screen or obstacle', what it is said to
screen out is 'contiguity [*contiguïté*]' (*S*, 209, *Sf*, 260; translation
modified). This reference also helps to explain a number of passages where Irigaray might sound as if she is (too simply) privileging an unconceptualizable sensible excess, for example, when she

writes of nature being 'foreclosed in her primary empirical naivete' or of the 'immediacy of *the relationship to the mother* [being] sacrificed' (*S*, 204).

If the 'immediate' relation to maternal matter is understood in terms of contiguity, then this relation is not simply lacking in form in ways that collapse the differences between one and another. Rather, as explored in the previous chapter, contiguity involves an intimate proximity between two who stand alongside one another. Such contiguous relations thus suggest a relationship between human beings and nature which is no longer specular or oppositional: instead of being cut off from nature, subject and maternal-materiality would remain in touch without either being subsumed by the other.

While Irigaray does not use the phrase in the chapter on Kant, it is in her critical engagement with him that her notion of a 'sensible transcendental' is situated.[42] A 'sensible transcendental' would not be one that privileged the sensible over the transcendental. Rather, it would involve rethinking the conditions of experience in ways that no longer depended on opposing concepts and intuitions, subject and object, form and matter. Such a frame would make it possible to recognize the ways in which the sexuate, material aspects of our being give pattern and meaning to the world by actively shaping and taking shape within our bodily encounters – our contiguous relations with others. The finitude of human beings that Kant so significantly recognizes would thereby be re-situated and thought not so much in terms of the limits of the faculties, as rooted in the originary relation to the mother as well as the ways in which sexuate difference conditions and limits human being (as two).

In this regard, it is telling that Kant says that the incongruence between the left hand and its mirror image is due to 'inner differences'. For Irigaray, this signals that the difference which remains to be thought (sexual difference) concerns the inside of the body and in particular, the way the female body allows an other to co-exist within.[43] Such a body is fundamentally at odds with the specular economy of the Kantian system in which the 'other' is projected outside the self, whether as bounded object or chaotic excess. Indeed, Irigaray suggests that just as a fear of maternal dependency drives the Cartesian desire for self-conception, so an anxiety about the originary relation to the mother underpins the Kantian subject's quest for autonomy: 'by wishing to reverse the anguish of being imprisoned within the other, of being placed inside the other, by making the very place and space of being his own, he becomes a prisoner of effects of symmetry that know no limit' (S, 137). The Copernican turn is here presented as dependent on another, prior and unseen reversal. The Kantian subject seeks to invert the original condition of his existence – being placed within another – by projecting the other outside of himself and ensuring that 'everything *outside* remains forever a condition making possible the image and the reproduction of the self' (S, 136).

By making himself dependent on his relation to an external 'other' or 'outside', this subject becomes susceptible to a new vulnerability. Every time the 'other' refuses to behave as it should – for example, when the earth shakes underfoot and threatens to engulf the subject – he will have to find new ways of re-presenting and re-containing it. Just as the Cartesian meditator remains haunted by his need for an other, so the Kantian subject remains haunted by the possibility that restless and unstable matter might not always cohere with the objective forms by which he is secured.

Thus we might speculate with Irigaray that the reason the subject's relation to the sensible world must be so carefully managed is not, in the end, because he might be overwhelmed by chaotic matter, terrifying though that might be. The greater threat is that there might be an entirely different way of relating the sensible material realm to transcendental forms: that it might be possible to imagine a spatio-temporal frame that would not just bring *different* objects into view, but re-work the very concept of an object, such that sharing in its materiality would no longer preclude one from being a subject. Such a framework would permit a different kind of embodied (and thus sexed) subject, as well as a world of (sexuate) experience shared between subjects whose differences could be sustained, rather than reduced to unthinkable excess.

Just as the wall face in Plato's cave works all too well, once the Kantian subject sets his specular projections in motion, the multiple 'effects of symmetry' threaten to spin out of control. Irigaray thus wonders what would happen 'if the earth turned and more especially turned upon herself' (S, 133). Such a revolution would prevent the material-maternal realm from being reduced to 'object' or 'other' for a male subject. Instead, the figure of the earth turning upon herself suggests the possibility of both an active matter that gives (itself) shape and form, and a female subject defined in relation to her own sex.

To further this radical shift in perspective, in some of her more recent work Irigaray has taken up the Kantian model of the autonomous subject as one who *thinks* for themselves, and re-cast autonomy as *breathing* for oneself.[44] Breath is *of* the body without being material substance: it animates our carnate being, allowing the body to become spiritualized in living movement. Irigaray's re-casting of autonomy is thus in keeping with her search for a 'sensible transcendental' in which matter and spirit are no longer opposed. This model of autonomy is not only more appropriate for a subject who is always bodily (and hence sexuate), but for a relational self born from a mother who breathes for us while we are in the womb. Learning to breathe for oneself means learning to take up a relation to the mother as a distinct being: such a spacing allows our former dependence to be acknowledged, along with the gift of breath and birth, while nonetheless allowing us to remain in touch with the mother through the air that flows between us. On this model, there is no need to cut oneself off from the mother as a threat to one's autonomy; instead, breathing for oneself also gives one's mother space to breathe as a female subject in her own right.

By taking up the figure of breath, Irigaray can be read as reclaiming one of the Greek terms for soul or spirit, *psychē*, which also meant breath. As mentioned at the beginning of this chapter, *psychē* ‾‾ is the subject of one of Aristotle's treatises; in the western tradition which follows, *psychē* will be inscribed into a framework where the subject of psychology – the mind and the capacity for thinking – is seen as essentially independent of the bodily rhythms of breathing. For Irigaray, by contrast, the fluid passage of air, between inside and outside of a body as well as between one body and another, is a reminder both of our own bodily being and of the maternal body within which we all began. As a way of recalling this body to philosophical thought, Irigaray journeys through the works of her philosophical fathers (Plato, Aristotle, Plotinus, Descartes, Kant) to construct a genealogy of maternal matter. As we have seen in this chapter, this genealogy takes us from the puzzles of prime matter, which has no being of its own yet must be thought to exist; to the Void that matter 'beyond Being' becomes; to the carefully reframed and externalized nature that forms a necessary counterpart to the modern subject. Irigaray's perspective suggests that, if the roots of western metaphysics lie in a disavowed appropriation of maternal generative power, the philosophical frameworks of Descartes and Kant make it even harder to recover the trace of an active maternal matter. Instead material nature is positioned as 'outside' and 'other' in ways that foreclose the possibility of subjects who are constitutively sexuate.

By revealing how this possibility is foreclosed, Irigaray begins to suggest the terms in which it might be recovered: by allowing that the world will not end if bodies interpenetrate, but that this is in fact a condition of our coming into the world; by rethinking matter as self-regulating and generative, and thus, as neither inert nor merely chaotic excess; and by re-grounding the self not in pure introspection but a bodily self-relation that is always inflected by sexual difference. As we have seen, such difference might be affirmed through the non-appropriative passion of wonder: as with Diotima, so in her reading of Descartes, Irigaray shows how, despite its disavowal of (sexuate) difference, the tradition harbours difference within. However, before examining how Irigaray develops these openings towards the kind of 'sensible transcendental' required for sexuate subjects, we need to turn to *psychē* once more, this time not as breath, but as it reappears in the form of psychoanalysis. Thus, in the next chapter, we will return to the beginning of *Speculum*, to see how Irigaray's analysis of Freud informs her journey through western thought.

5

Freud, Lacan, and Speaking
(as a) Woman

If Kant was shaken by the Lisbon earthquake of 1755, Lacan and Freud theorize in response to the earthquakes that shake us from within: 'The reasons for the quakes must be sought out, these seismic convulsions in the self must be interpreted' (*S*, 137). Irigaray suggests that despite, or perhaps because of, this reversal of perspective, the Kantian and psychoanalytic projects continue to mirror one another: both are sustained by the appropriation of maternal-matter and the reduction of woman to the 'other' of a male subject.

Nonetheless, psychoanalysis remains one of the key frameworks informing Irigaray's approach to both philosophy and the question of sexual difference. The first section of *Speculum* offers a critical re-telling of Freud on femininity, forming a counterpart to the final section on Plato. Several key essays and interviews in the accompanying volume, *This Sex Which Is Not One*, also focus on Irigaray's critique of psychoanalysis as well as the challenge she poses for it by seeking to think woman as a subject: to *parler femme*, speak (as a) woman. As others have examined Irigaray's engagement with Freud and Lacan in depth, this chapter will focus on how that engagement helps her to expose the dreams, desires and blindspots that sustain traditional metaphysics.[1] It will conclude by examining how Irigaray's own mode of writing (as a) woman subverts both philosophy and psychoanalysis from within.

Irigaray's engagement with psychoanalysis goes beyond negative critique. As she shows, psychoanalysis is valuable to feminism both because it takes seriously the role of sexuality in the development of identity, and because of the descriptive force with which it exposes the alignment of woman with the 'other' of a male subject. Psychoanalysis helpfully reveals the sexual *in*-difference of the structures of subjectivity, insofar as these take only *one* sex as norm and ideal: 'in the process of elaborating a theory of sexuality, Freud brought to light something that had been operative all along though it remained implicit, hidden, unknown: *the sexual indifference that underlies the truth of any science, the logic of every discourse*' (*TS*, 69). For this reason, psychoanalysis is a powerful tool with which to re-approach philosophy, whose privileging of a disembodied and universal reason works to conceal the gendering of its conceptual structures.

Irigaray's doubled relation to psychoanalysis is particularly clear with regard to Freud's notion of the unconscious. For Freud, the unconscious is a necessary presupposition, a condition of possibility for making sense of conscious life.[2] Irigaray appropriates this model to show how the maternal operates as the unconscious grounding of philosophical accounts of origin, subjectivity, and truth, as we have seen in her analyses of Plato, Descartes and Kant. At the same time, she folds her critique back onto psychoanalysis, insofar as it continues to theorize the unconscious in relation to a male subject who remains dependent on the repression of the maternal. Thus, 'if Freudian theory indeed contributes what is needed to upset the philosophic order of discourse, the theory remains paradoxically subject to that discourse where the definition of sexual difference is concerned' (*TS*, 72). Psychoanalysis perpetuates a 'logic of the same' by taking one sex – the male – as the model for its account of both sexes. By giving '*a priori* value to Sameness' in this way, 'Freud's contribution remains, in part – and precisely where the difference between the sexes is concerned – caught up in metaphysical presuppositions' (*TS*, 73). It is this repetition of sexual indifference that leads Irigaray to critically distance herself from psychoanalysis, despite its importance for her approach.

Whereas for Plato and Kant, human beings are oriented by a relation to an 'other' projected outside of themselves (the Forms, the object), for psychoanalysis, the unconscious functions as 'the Other, lapsed within' (*S*, 135). To this extent, psychoanalysis can be positioned as a continuation of Cartesianism, albeit one which makes the internal doubling of the self critically explicit. However, Irigaray will argue that this 'other within' continues to be an 'other of the Same', in ways that re-entrench the fundamental structures of western metaphysics. If Plato orients us towards the transcendent, psychoanalysis plunges us back down into the cave of the psyche: 'When the Other falls out of the starry sky into the chasms of the psyche, the "subject" is obviously obliged to stake out new boundaries for his field of implantation and to re-ensure – otherwise, elsewhere – his dominance. Where he was once on the heights, he is now entreated to go down into the depths' (S, 136).[3] This time, the darkness is not so much to be escaped, as mastered through exploration and analysis.

Freud on Femininity

Speculum opens with a lengthy close reading of Freud's 1933 essay 'Femininity'. Along the way, Irigaray incorporates a wide range of references to other key texts by Freud on sexuality and psychic development. Just as she offers a densely woven re-telling of the Myth of the Cave, so here Irigaray quotes extensively from 'Femininity', weaving her analysis out of Freud's text. Via interpretative commentary and ironic repetition, she lays bare the values and assumptions that govern his account, offering alternative perspectives on infantile sexuality that call into question the supposed necessity or 'obviousness' of Freud's own conclusions.

Often these alternative perspectives are opened up by sustained lines of questioning which invite her readers to rethink female sexuality for themselves, rather than simply telling them what to think. Why, she asks, must we assume a phallic stage not only in the development of the boy's sexuality but also the little girl's, yet never raise the possibility of 'a vulvar stage, a vaginal stage, a uterine stage, in a discussion of female sexuality?' (S, 29) Why privilege penis envy in the little girl's development, but never raise the possibility of envy of the vagina, or uterus, or vulva on the little boy's part? Her analysis continually draws attention to the strain put on Freud's account by the way he tries to explain how the little girl becomes a woman while taking the male subject as the developmental norm. At times, her engagement is marked by a barely suppressed laughter at the conceptual somersaults Freud is forced to perform as he tries to map femininity onto the same Oedipal and phallic model as male sexuality. 'Becoming a woman', she notes, 'really does not seem to be an easy business' (S, 39).

Irigaray repeatedly turns Freud against himself by exploiting his suggestion that gaps in conscious thought and speech are signs of repression that can only be explained via an appeal to the unconscious. She is especially attentive to the tensions, omissions and aporia that mark the essay on femininity, a text that Freud himself describes as incomplete and fragmentary.[4] One such tension concerns the role of anatomy. Freud himself cautions against treating the anatomical distinction between the sexes as a sufficient basis for explaining the psychological differences between masculinity and femininity. Yet as Irigaray shows, he nonetheless treats what he takes to be 'natural' male and female roles in sexual relations, in which the male is assumed to be active and the female passive, as a model for these psychological differences. Thus the alignment of femininity and passivity seems to be 'naturally' inscribed 'according to a *mimetic order*, with anatomical science imposing the truth of its model upon "psychological behaviour"' (S, 15).

Irigaray suggests that Freud is unconsciously drawn to such appeals to anatomy because they seem to put an end to uncertainty on the mysterious subject of woman. Thus, despite his own warning that 'what constitutes masculinity or femininity is an unknown characteristic which anatomy cannot lay hold of',[5] Freud proceeds to suggest that a woman who develops 'normally' will take up a femininity to which she is 'biologically destined'.[6] As he famously writes elsewhere, 'Anatomy is destiny' – though as Irigaray shows, the 'normal' destiny of a woman is very strange indeed.[7]

If Freud treats woman as an object of the scientific investigations of men (S, 13), Irigaray turns the tables by putting Freud – or at least his text – on the couch and subjecting it to analysis. As the title of this part of *Speculum* suggests ('The Blind Spot of An Old Dream of Symmetry'), she treats his essay as a dream governed by a logic of the Same that depends on the repression of sexual difference, that is, on blocking out the very possibility that woman might exist as a sexuate subject in her own right. If Freud's essay begins by positioning woman as a riddle, Irigaray suggests that he is blind to the solution implicit in his own text, which repeatedly shows how taking the male subject as the norm makes woman's sexuate specificity a puzzling impossibility.

In what Irigaray calls 'a sort of blind reversal of repressions', Freud posits the little girl's desire to be 'the same' as a man, while remaining blind to the way it is his own discourse which is governed by 'the desire for the same, for the self-identical, the self (as) same' (S, 26). Thus, he positions the little girl as taking *the same* phallic pleasure in her clitoris as the boy takes in his penis, a pleasure that is lost only when the girl comes to see her own body as lacking and develops 'penis envy'. As Irigaray observes, as far as

sexual differentiation goes, 'one term will be constituted as "origin",
as that by whose differentiation the other may be engendered and
brought to light. *The same re-marking itself* – more or less – would
thus produce the other, whose function in the differentiation would
be neglected, forgotten' (S, 21). On this model, insofar as the little
girl is permitted to recognize her difference at all, it is only in comparison to the male subject and in terms that position her as lacking
in relation to him (he is 'more', she has 'less'). Moreover, until this
painful moment of dispossession, the little girl's sexual development is mapped entirely onto that of the boy. The problem is thus
not just that 'THE LITTLE GIRL IS THEREFORE A LITTLE MAN' (S, 26),
but that even more damagingly: 'In the beginning ... the little girl
was (only) a little boy. In other words, THERE NEVER IS (OR WILL BE)
A LITTLE GIRL' (S, 48).

On Freud's account, in order to become a woman and hence
'unlike' the little boy, the little girl must pass through the most
traumatic stage of her development: that in which she comes to see
her own sex, as represented by the mother, as castrated. As Irigaray
notes, 'the little girl is, must become a man minus certain attributes
... A man minus the possibility of (re)presenting oneself as a man
= a normal woman' (S, 27). For Irigaray, making castration and
penis envy the basis of female sexuality constitutes the most
obvious instantiation of a culture that defines both woman and
desire in relation to the male subject: 'to castrate woman is to
inscribe her in the law of the *same* desire, of *the desire for the same*'
(S, 55). Woman is once again reduced to a poor copy: 'a sort of
inverted or negative alter ego ... Inverse, contrary, contradictory
even' (S, 22).

Irigaray calls Freud's account into question by asking why the
little girl should be assumed to feel the same way about the mother
not having a penis as the little boy. For the little boy, it at least
makes sense to think that the absence of a penis could potentially
represent the threat of losing something (though Irigaray still asks
why the *mother's* having 'nothing to be seen' would necessarily
threaten *the little boy's* libidinal economy; S, 49). But given that her
body is *like* the mother's, it is not at all clear why the little girl
should find it strange or horrifying that the mother does not have
a penis, nor why she should regard this as the loss of something
that was once there, as Freud suggests.[8] As Irigaray shows, such
analyses only make sense if the female sex has already been mapped
onto the male body such that the clitoris is seen as a penis equivalent, and the little girl is assumed to regard possession of a penis

as the bodily 'norm'. Instead of taking her 'likeness' to the mother as primary, Freud's account of the little girl's reactions assumes she is just like a little boy.

On this account, the hatred the little girl feels when she comes to see the mother as lacking, and thus as the cause of her own lack, leads her to transfer her affections to the father.[9] This permits her both to become a 'normal' adult woman and to reclaim the phallus, above all, by bearing the father's child (preferably, of course, a son). Thus, as Irigaray observes, at every stage 'normal' femininity reaffirms the value of the phallus: 'If *she* envies what *he* has, then it must be valuable. The only thing valuable enough to be envied? The very standard of all value' (*S*, 53).

By contrast, this standard reduces woman to nothing. By positioning the mother's body as castrated, woman comes to be defined by a hole, a lack, a horrifying void: 'the little girl, the woman, supposedly has *nothing* you can see. She exposes, exhibits the possibility of *a nothing to see*. Or at any rate she shows nothing that is penis-shaped or could substitute for a penis' (*S*, 47).[10] Elaborating on this view to draw out the seriousness of its consequences, Irigaray notes that:

> Woman's castration is defined as her having nothing you can see, as her *having* nothing. In her having nothing penile, in seeing that she has No Thing. Nothing *like* man. That is to say, *no sex/organ* that can be seen in a *form* capable of founding its reality, reproducing its truth. *Nothing to be seen is equivalent to having no thing. No being* and *no truth*. (*S*, 48)

Freud's account makes the visibility of the male sex organ paradigmatic in ways that obliterate the sexed specificity of woman. On this model, if there is no 'thing' to be seen, no clearly defined object available to the gaze, there is nothing there at all. This precludes the possibility that women's sexuate bodies might need to be articulated in different terms, that their sexual being might be distributed across multiple sites, folds and surfaces, not all of which are open to the gaze. Irigaray thus reminds us that where there is 'nothing to be seen', there may still be 'something not subject to the rule of visibility or of specula(riza)tion', 'something' which 'might yet have some reality' (*S*, 50). After all, the tradition has repeatedly grounded reality in that which cannot be seen – the Forms, the *cogito*, the unconscious – so why not allow the status of reality to the female sex? As Irigaray says, woman's sex may be 'nothing the same, identical, identifiable': but is not nothing (*S*, 50). However, within the economy of selfhood and desire which psychoanalysis delineates, the horrifying 'nothingness' of the mother's sex is required for the little boy to become a man. It is this 'horror' which prompts him to relinquish his Oedipal attachments, enabling him to transfer his desire to a series of other women who will function as mother-substitutes. Nonetheless, as Irigaray notes, while the little boy may fear castration, the burden of representing 'the *nothing* of sex, the *not* of sex, will be borne by woman' (*S*, 52). It is *her* sexual organ, after all, that 'represents *the horror of nothing to see*' (*TS*, 26).

Irigaray shows that psychoanalytic theory is valuable for feminism if it is read as revealing this representational burden, that is, if it is read as a *description* of the ways in which the 'logic of the Same' results in the negation of woman. The problem, however, lies in the extent to which psychoanalysis continues to *reinscribe* this homogenizing logic as the basis for so-called 'normal' female sexuality, and hence to *prescribe* it as a regulatory norm (*TS*, 70). As Irigaray puts it: 'The interpreters of dreams themselves had no desire but to rediscover the same. Everywhere. And, indeed, it was not hard to find. But was not *interpretation* itself, by that fact, caught up in the dream of identity, equivalence, analogy, of homology, symmetry, comparison, imitation ... ?' (*S*, 27) In this way, psychoanalysis continues to perpetuate a sexual indifference driven by an underlying desire for the same. By mapping all aspects of women's sexuality onto a male norm, reducing all possibilities of pleasure to their masculine equivalents, psychoanalysis continues to leave women's own desires unarticulated and her sexuate specificity unacknowledged: 'Off-stage, off-side, beyond representation, beyond selfhood' (*S*, 22).

Mirroring Plato

Irigaray's reading of Freud provides additional clues for rereading metaphysics from a feminist perspective. In particular, she draws attention to the ways in which Freud and Plato cast critical light on one other: reading Freud into Plato helps make explicit the sexual imaginary built into the foundations of metaphysics; reading Plato back through Freud exposes the deep metaphysical roots of the patterns of thought that position woman as 'other'. Insofar as Plato and Freud can be seen as the beginning and culmination of the western theoretical tradition, woman remains trapped between them as a necessary absence, like the space between opposing mirrors that allows them to reflect the same image to infinity.

Like the Myth of the Cave, Freud's analysis of femininity is marked throughout by a confusion of cause and effect, beginning and end. The reproductive female sexuality which is supposedly the *effect* of normal sexual development is projected back into the analysis of the pre-pubescent girl: it is because of her reproductive 'destiny' that the little girl 'must' come to hate the mother, 'must' feel penis-envy, and 'must' transfer her desire to the father. As Irigaray puts it, the game is played out and its rules agreed upon long before reproduction is a physical possibility (S, 25). Irigaray questions why this reproductive role should necessarily be the determining factor in woman's sexuate identity, especially when Freud himself warns against treating anatomy in this way.

Further confusions arise when Freud foregrounds the difficulties involved in determining the relative influence of infantile impulses and later conflicts in the development of sexual pathologies. As Irigaray notes, despite recognizing these difficulties, in the case of women's supposed penis envy, Freud is surprisingly clear that it is infantile development which is the key. At one point he even insists on the significance of 'the first instalment of penis-envy in the phallic phase' in ways that conflict with his own account, in which penis-envy ought not to arise prior to the castration complex.[11] This rules out the possibility that penis envy is a retroactive formation, an expression of the social injustices a woman faces as a result of not being a man which is subsequently projected back onto childhood.

Unlike the Myth of the Cave, in the psychoanalytic account of the subject's journey into adulthood, the significance of the mother is explicitly acknowledged. However, as we have seen, woman is normatively identified with her reproductive function such that being female is equated with being a mother. In this way, psychoanalysis continues to cover over each human being's origin in a mother who is also a *woman*. As Irigaray puts it, 'theory will always already have excluded her appearance as a sexuate female subject' (S, 64).

Once again, the question of origin is crucial here: as for Plato, so for Freud. Insofar as both male and female sexuality are explained with reference to the phallus, the male subject is positioned as the origin of all desire. In turn, insofar as subjectivity is explained with reference to sexuality, being a subject is modelled on being male.

138 Freud, Lacan, and Speaking (as a) Woman

If woman's reproductive end governs the way the story of her sexual beginnings is told, this is because this story is already guilty of 'putting the Phallus at the beginning, and at the end.' In ways that are never explicitly stated, Freud posits the phallus 'as *terminus, origin*, and *cause of desire*' (S, 60). Thus, despite its apparent emphasis on the mother, psychoanalysis once again reflects man's desire to determine his own origin by positioning himself as the origin of desire. The phallus 'would not be the privileged signifier of the penis or even of power and sexual pleasure were it not to be interpreted as *an appropriation of the relation to origin and of the desire for and as origin*' (S, 33). Hence Irigaray's conclusion that the (phallic) tropes that govern Freud's theorizing reflect an implicit rivalry between man and his mother.

Later thinkers such as Lacan will insist on the status of the phallus as symbolic construction, not to be confused with the physical penis. But Irigaray's analysis suggests that this very process of symbolic idealization both reinforces and conceals the ways in which desire is modelled on a specifically male body: 'The penis – or better still the phallus! *Emblem of man's appropriative relation to the origin*' (S, 42). The phallus may be a symbolic idealization of the penis, but this itself suggests that the penis is in some way 'like' the ideal. The slippage between 'phallus' and 'penis' that characterizes Irigaray's analysis is not due to a lack of rigour, but a deliberate exposure of the way it is the *male* sex organ that is taken up as the governing symbol (what Lacan calls the 'transcendental signifier') of the structures of subjectivity, sexuality and desire. As she reminds us, 'the phallus ... (even in its hold over the signifier) is the sign of the male sex organ' (S, 28). Thus, by making the phallus 'necessarily the archetype for sex', the penis is rendered 'the best representational equivalent of the Idea of sex' (S, 58).

By contrast, woman is given no valid signifiers with which to represent either her own sex or her own desires. Instead, her relations to her own sexuate being, as well as to her mother, are mediated through a phallic economy of the same. Thus 'there will be no possibility of interplay between two different modes of relationship to the origin, the primary, the desire for origin' (S, 60). In Freud's essay, the little girl's relation to the mother is characterized either in terms of the phallic desire to give the mother a child, or in terms of phallic lack, as the female child resentfully breaks from the 'castrated' mother. Once this break is made, the little girl will have no way of relating to her own maternal origin *except* in terms of lack:

[S]he [the little girl] will have nothing ... to make up for, substitute for, or defer this final break in physical contact with her mother: she cannot turn back toward her mother, or lay claim to seeing or knowing what is to be seen and known of that place of origin; she will not represent 'her' relation to 'her' origin; ... She is left with a *void*, a *lack* of all representation, re-presentation, and even strictly speaking of all mimesis of her desire for origin. (*S*, 42)

On Irigaray's account, it is not the phallus that the little girl is lacking, but ways of representing the specificity of *her* relationship to maternal origins, especially insofar as – *unlike* the little boy – she shares the sex of her mother. But if she has no way of relating to the mother as a *woman*, rather than as an inadequate man, then the possibility of taking pleasure in her own sex is foreclosed. Hence the need to find ways of articulating woman's relation to her beginnings in birth which are not mediated through the male subject, as well as a different, non-phallic model with which to represent female desire in its own terms.

For this reason, Irigaray pauses at Freud's suggestion that, as well as wishing to give the mother a child (to make the mother pregnant), the little girl typically wishes to bear her one too. 'One might advance the hypothesis', Irigaray suggests, 'that the child who is desired in the relationship with the mother must be a girl if the little girl herself is in any degree valued for her femaleness' – or, indeed, if the little girl is in any degree to value her *own* femaleness. What if, then, the little girl desired to bear the mother another daughter? 'Engendering a girl's body, bringing a third woman's body into play, would allow her to identify both herself and her mother as sexuate women's bodies. As *two* women, defining each other as both like and unlike, thanks to a third "body" that both by common consent wish to be "female"' (*S*, 35). By taking her place between them, such a daughter would mediate the relation between the mother and the little girl, preventing them from being simply elided with one another. By enabling the little girl to relate to her mother via a female figure, this might help her to recognize her mother as a woman and herself as 'a woman in the making': 'In other words, this fantasy of the woman-daughter conceived between mother and daughter would mean that the little girl, and her mother also, perhaps, want to be able to represent themselves as woman's bodies that are both desired and desiring – though not necessarily "phallic"' (*S*, 36). This distinctively female fantasy opens up a space for imagining a little girl who desires to *be* a woman and to relate to her origins *in* a woman, without seeking either to take her mother's place or to be 'just like' a little boy.

The Mute and the Melancholic

On Freud's account, the little girl is a 'little man who will suffer a more painful and complicated evolution than the little boy in order to become a normal woman!' (*S*, 26). Thus, as Irigaray notes, it is hardly surprising if the sexuality of adult women tends to take pathological forms, of which the archetype in Freud's account is hysteria. As shown by Plato's *Timaeus*, both the word and concept of hysteria derive from the Greek word for womb, together with the ancient view that an unfulfilled womb had the capacity to roam around the female body, causing no end of disorder.[12] The Freudian hysteric was typically a woman whose disordered sexuality was expressed in a variety of symptoms with no discernable physical cause, such as inexplicable mutism.

Irigaray sometimes suggests that such symptoms can be one – desperate – way in which women seek to re-exert their autonomy by refusing to play their allotted role in a culture that reduces them to desirable objects of exchange among men. By excessively mimicking the ways in which woman's own desires are silenced, the 'hysterical' mute can be read as taking woman's 'normal' role too far in an unconscious act of resistance. However, Irigaray is clear about the limits of such disruptive acts: insofar as they play out the fears and fantasies of male desire, they are too easily recouped as further signs of feminine 'instability' and 'excess'. Thus, when we turn to Irigaray's own strategy of disruptive mimicry later in this chapter, it will be crucial that this differs from the hysteric's role as 'delirious double' (*S*, 141).

Freud himself controversially suggests that the origins of hysteria are often found in fantasy rather than actual sexual trauma. This claim has been criticized for down-playing the real extent of sexual abuse. Irigaray would not necessarily disagree, but adopts a different critical approach. Part of what makes women's relation to sexuality traumatic within a phallocentric culture, she suggests, is the way in which they are deprived of the imaginative resources with which to represent their own desires, and thus to construct non-traumatic fantasies of sexual inter-relation. Thus the 'vicious circle' which Freud's analysis describes, but also reinscribes: *because* women lack positive representations of their sex, it is difficult for them to be 'anything but suggestible and hysterical' (S, 59), in ways that reinforce their perceived status as neurotic or 'abnormal'. In sum, the little girl is consigned to a condition of dereliction with regard to her own sex. Using Freud against himself again, Irigaray suggests that his own account of melancholia provides unrealized resources with which to theorize this condition and explain why women are so often trapped within 'a "mental constellation of revolt"'.[13]

Whereas mourning is a process through which it is possible to come to terms with loss, melancholia arises when someone is not fully conscious of what it is that has been lost; mourning is thus impossible and the loss remains irresolvable. As Irigaray puts it, borrowing from Freud: 'in melancholia ... "the patient cannot consciously perceive what he has lost"' so even if he knows '"whom he has lost"' he does not know '"what he has lost in him"'.[14] The little girl finds herself in a similar situation with regard to the loss of a relation to her mother as a woman:

> The little girl, obviously, does not know *what* she is losing in discovering her 'castration' or in the 'catastrophe' of her relationship first with her mother and subsequently other woman. She has then no *consciousness* of her sexual impulses, of her libidinal economy and, more particularly, of her original desire and her desire for origin. In more ways than one, it is really a question for her of a 'loss' that radically escapes any representation. Whence the impossibility of 'mourning' it. (S, 68)

In a culture which defines femininity in relation to male desire, and identifies women with their maternal function, the little girl lacks the terms with which to identify the mother (or herself) as a woman. Thus she is unable even to articulate 'what has been lost' when her primary relation to her mother is broken.

In the end, Freud poses two decisive, critical challenges to the tradition. The first lies in the way 'he destroys a certain conception of the present, or of presence' through 'the impact of so-called unconscious mechanisms on the discourse of the "subject"' (S, 28). Thus, Freud undoes the Cartesian dream of introspective self-presence: instead, the unconscious means that the subject is to some extent always 'other' to himself. Nonetheless, this subject remains in a better position than woman, who lacks any means of representing her sexuate subjectivity except in his terms. Just like the unconscious, she is 'his' other, defined in relation to him. Thus, the second, 'blinder and less direct' challenge Freud poses 'occurs when – himself a prisoner of a certain economy of the logos, of a certain logic, notably of "desire", whose link to classical philosophy he fails to see – he defines sexual differences as a function of the a priori of the same, having recourse, to support this demonstration, to the age-old processes: analogy, comparison, symmetry, dichot-omic oppositions, and so on' (S, 28). By seeking to explain feminin-ity in terms which so clearly map the little girl onto the little boy, Freud exposes the logic of the same that maps woman onto man's 'other'. This he does despite himself, but in ways that show how the apparently neutral and universal structures of subjectivity are in fact those of a male subject. In this way, he makes explicit the gendering of western thought:

> In order to remain effective, all this certainly needed at the very least to remain hidden! By exhibiting this 'symptom', this crisis point in metaphysics where we find exposed that sexual 'indifference' that had assured metaphysical coherence and 'closure', Freud offers it up for our analysis. With his text offering itself to be understood, to be read, as doubtless the most relevant re-mark of an ancient dream of self ... one that had never been interpreted. (S, 28)

Just as the imagery of Plato's Myth of the Cave speaks of the mater-nal origins it appropriates and disavows, so Freud's account of femininity exposes the logic of the same which erases the feminine. By making this erasure visible, he makes it available for analysis, in ways that help Irigaray address the absence of a female subject in western thought and culture.

Freud himself gestures towards this absence in his 1931 paper on 'Female Sexuality', where he notes that the little girl's pre-Oedipal relation to the mother has an importance yet to be fully recognized. In ways that uncannily foreshadow Irigaray's critique of the gendered limits of psychoanalysis, Freud suggests that the little girl's 'first attachment to the mother' is 'so difficult to grasp in analysis' that 'it was as if it had succumbed to an especially inexorable repression'.[15] He even goes as far as suggesting that the significance of this period for the little girl is so great that 'it would seem as though we must retract the universality of the thesis that the Oedipus complex is the nucleus of all neuroses'.[16] As Irigaray emphasizes, this implies the little girl's relationship with her mother might require an analysis in non-Oedipal terms to do it justice.

For Irigaray, it is in these comments that Freud comes closest to seeing what the pathology of the female hysteric might owe to the foreclosure of a relation between mother and daughter defined in terms of their shared female sex: 'And there, in what he recognizes as outside the range of his systematic prospecting (beyond the self?), Freud is in fact indicating a way off the historico-transcendental stage, at the very moment when his theory and his practice are perpetuating ... that very same stage, which we may now call the *hysterico*-transcendental' (*S*, 139). To Irigaray's disappointment, Freud does not pursue this glimpse of an opening beyond his own historically conditioned approach and towards a non-Oedipal account of the journey towards becoming a female subject. If the Freudian account of the little girl forces her to mimic the little boy, Irigaray suggests that Freud is a mimic too, unconsciously repeating, even as he exposes, the 'a priorism of the same' which has sustained 'every figure of ontology' in the western tradition since Plato (*S*, 27; translation modified).

Mothers and Others: Lacan and the Non-Existence of 'Woman'

Alongside Freud, the work of Lacan is crucial to Irigaray's project, as it is for many of the post-structuralist thinkers with whom she is often allied, including Derrida and Kristeva. If Lacan is the key inheritor of Freud's theories, it is an inheritance he first had to reclaim, by displacing what he saw as the damaging brand of ego psychology which had come to be particularly dominant in the United States. By contrast, Lacan himself foregrounds the constitutive role of language in the formation of the subject, to the extent that, for Lacan, the unconscious is 'structured like a language.'[17] Lacan's approach is deeply informed by the philosophical tradition on which Irigaray also draws. Moreover, by undermining the supposedly unified identity of the phallic subject, Lacan gives a certain kind of privilege to the feminine. Despite this, Lacanian theory – Irigaray suggests – does not result in much of an improvement so far as *women* are concerned. Thus, while it is from Lacan that she appropriates the language to re-position woman as 'other' to the 'other' of the male subject, as we will see, she is thereby using him against himself. And it is Lacan, rather than Freud, who is the target of her most biting criticisms. This is particularly evident in her close analysis of Lacan's lectures on woman in her essay 'Così

Fan Tutti' (TS, 86–105). In *Speculum*, however, there is no single section focused explicitly on Lacan. Instead, Irigaray remains in tacit dialogue with him throughout: Lacan's is one of the dominant voices woven into the concluding chapter of *Speculum*'s central section, 'Volume-Fluidity', although (tellingly) Irigaray's critical engagement with him is at its most intense in '*La mystérique*', the chapter which is structurally positioned at the focal point of the book.

The fact that Lacan is not a named interlocutor and instead functions more like an ever-present absence is a knowing rhetorical strategy on Irigaray's part. As we will see, for Lacan, 'woman' as such does not exist, while the 'feminine' is privileged as an excess which overflows and eludes the bounds of identity. By making Lacan a nameless presence who nonetheless pervades the text, Irigaray ironically takes him at his word: she gives him the feminine position he desires, while demonstrating the way in which this positioning results in erasure and silencing.[18]

Among the many threads that compose *Speculum*'s textual fabric, several are devoted to the multiple ways in which Lacan's framework aligns woman and the mother with the 'Other'. This tripartite framework consists of what Lacan terms 'the imaginary', the 'symbolic' and the 'Real'. The 'Real' should not be confused with 'reality': the world we inhabit as subjects is constituted through the symbolic, understood not only as language but the entire network of signs that create meaningful socio-cultural order. The 'Real' is that which erupts into this world with an immediacy that defies representation; thus, it is typically experienced as traumatic. In the face of the Real we are always at a loss. The imaginary is a crucial liminal field which in some ways can be thought of as 'between' the symbolic and the Real, and which is constituted in relation to both.

It is in the imaginary that the subject-to-be begins to be formed. More particularly, this takes place in what Lacan calls the 'mirror stage' where the ego is first constituted. He describes how in a crucial developmental stage, the young infant (Lacan specifies between six and eighteen months) will be fascinated by his image in a mirror, with which he will come to identify.[19] This identification is necessary for the child to come to have some sense of itself as a unified being, yet is based on an illusion: the coherent bounded image covers over the polymorphous and fragmentary nature of the child's lived bodily experience. The primary identification is thus a *mis*-identification. As in Irigaray's analysis of Descartes, the mirror stage exposes the split that occurs in the moment of self-reflection that constitutes the Cartesian ego.[20] Lacan thereby lays bare the ways in which the (male) subject of the western philosophical tradition is neither as unified nor as self-sufficient as he projects himself to be. However, Irigaray also highlights the ways in which the mirror stage simultaneously perpetuates that tradition – despite Lacan's claim that psychoanalysis is 'at odds with any philosophy directly stemming from the *cogito*.'[21]

A crucial feature of the image with which the infant identifies is that this image comes from *outside* the self;[22] it is thus not necessarily an image in a literal mirror but can be found in the way the child sees itself reflected in others' eyes. As Lacan notes that all this takes place while the infant is still 'trapped in his motor impotence and nursling dependence',[23] Irigaray emphasizes that the primary other in whom the infant will tend to see itself reflected will be the mother. In Lacan's mirror stage, then, we find the archetypal scene that is re-staged throughout *Speculum*, in which woman operates as the m/Other who supports and sustains the subject, '[i]n whose sight everything *outside* remains forever a condition making possible the image and the reproduction of the self' (*S*, 136). The Lacanian account may problematize the subject's identity insofar as this is shown to be based on mis-identification, but this does not change the fact that the mother supports the constitution of this fissured self, and not vice versa.

The reasons why there cannot, on the Lacanian account, be a female subject (unless 'she' takes up a masculine subject position) emerge more clearly when we turn to his account of the symbolic. Becoming an ego is not enough for becoming a subject. The child in the mirror stage remains locked in a dyadic relation with the mother. Lacan's account of how the specular unity of the ego becomes a fully fledged subject reworks Freud's account of the castration complex. To take up the position of an individuated subject, the child must accept what Lacan calls 'the Name of the Father'. In French, this phrase puns on the name of the father (*le nom du père*) and the father's prohibition, the 'no' (*le non du père*). The father's word *is* a prohibition, forbidding the incestuous desire for the mother. By accepting this prohibition and separating itself from the mother, the child can take up a position like the father in language (can accede to the father's name) by referring to itself as 'I'.

Becoming a subject requires entry into the symbolic order and thus necessarily means becoming a 'speaking subject'. Nonetheless,

the split engendered in the mirror stage is deepened and exacerbated on accession into language. The symbolic order which allows
the subject to refer to itself as such not only pre-exists this subject,
but is independent of it.[24] The very sign with which the subject
seeks to mark its singularity – 'I' – can be used to refer to any and
all subjects, quite anonymously. It circulates within a system of
signs that does not depend on any particular subject at all: on the
contrary, language speaks – and thereby constitutes – the subject.[25]
Thus the symbolic is radically 'Other' to the subject it makes possible, and who is therefore alienated from himself in the very
moment that he comes to be. As Yannis Stavrakakis puts it, 'The
subject is petrified and alienated exactly in the place where it seeks
the birth of itself'.[26]

Irigaray draws attention to the way that this birth of the subject,
and indeed the 'Otherness' of the symbolic which makes it possible, is dependent on the role of the mother as Other. As we have
seen, the condition of acceding to the position of the subject is the
act of symbolic castration in which the infant sacrifices its bond
with the mother so as to separate itself out as an individuated 'I'.
Once again, for Irigaray, this is paradigmatic of the process through
which the subject has constituted itself throughout western thought:
'The ban upon returning, regressing to the womb, as well as to the
language and dreams shared with the mother, this is indeed the
point, the line, the surface upon which the "subject" will continue
to stand, to advance, to unfold his discourse, even to make it whirl'
(S, 140). Though the need to separate himself from the mother as
Other means the subject comes to be lacking in the very moment
he comes to be, and though this subject is forever alienated in the
very language that makes him an 'I', it is nonetheless *his* fissured
subjectivity which is at stake, while the mother must be sacrificed
as the very condition of this (quite normal) drama. She is the lack
which makes signification possible: if a sign is to signify something,
there must be a difference, a gap or break, between signifier and
signified. To enter into language, the child must give up a world
of replete immediacy and accept this gap which makes symbolic
mediation possible. The break with the mother is the forging of this
necessary gap or lack. But if the mother must be sacrificed to constitute the lack on which the symbolic depends, she herself will
always be absented from language. She is – necessarily – condemned to a mute silence. Thus, while the subject may speak in
endlessly whirling sentences of his own alienation, '"she" comes
to be unable to say what her body is suffering' (S, 140).

Speculum does not contend that this silencing results solely from the Lacanian system. Rather, Lacan functions like the focal point in a concave mirror, condensing a tradition in which the mother is both appropriated as a resource and excised from the system she silently sustains. Thus, *Speculum's* analyses of the philosophers are also permeated by references to the 'cut' from the mother through which the subject secures his own identity. At the same time, Irigaray's analysis of symbolic matricide in the philosophies of Plato, Descartes, and Kant is simultaneously an implicit critique of Lacan for repeating and re-entrenching this foundational sacrifice.

The similarities between Lacan and Plato are particularly telling. Thus, Irigaray parallels Lacan's privileging of the symbolic as the origin of the speaking subject with Plato's ascription of originary power to the Forms.[27] Just as Plato privileges the Forms' radiant Otherness and aligns this with the father's generative power, so Lacan foregrounds the Otherness of language and privileges the phallus as the governing signifier of the symbolic order. Irigaray also parallels the role of the receptacle in Plato's thought with that of woman in Lacan's: both operate as the female Other, making the reproduction of the father's form possible, without having access to symbolic forms of her own. The Lacanian m/Other is like the receptacle in *Timaeus* insofar as each 'receives the marks of everything, understands and includes everything – except itself – but its relation to the intelligible is never actually established. ... And it would not have access to its own function with regard to language or to the signifier in general, since it would have to be the (still perceptible) support of that function' (*TS*, 101). The Platonic division between the world of the senses and the Forms is repeated in the Lacanian split between the perceptible (the image) and the intelligible (the symbolic order). Within this structure, woman continues to operate as the sensible–perceptible support. Just as *Speculum* circles back round to the beginning of the philosophical tradition by ending with Plato, so where woman is concerned, Lacan brings us full circle, back to the originary scene of metaphysics. For better and for worse: for while Lacan does at least make the Othering of woman explicit, he does not call her exile from the symbolic into question. Thus, like Freud's account of femininity, Lacanian analysis does not merely describe but reinscribes the cultural and symbolic dereliction of woman.

As Irigaray shows, this dereliction is confirmed in Lacan's account of woman's position in relation to the symbolic order. On the one hand, the mother from whom the child tears himself away to enter the symbolic is herself necessarily lost to representation. In her inassimilable excess, she becomes a constant threat to the symbolic order, and is thus allied with the Real. On the other, the maternal bond that is sacrificed is retrospectively projected as a lost union, generating a fantasmatic 'phallic mother' who is both desired and feared: to be re-absorbed into her plenitude would mean losing oneself as an individual subject. The mother is thus allied with either a fantasy of wholeness modelled on phallic completion, or a radical lack which is traumatic in its disruptive force. She is never a woman, or a female subject able to take up her own relation to others.

That such a possibility is foreclosed within the logic of his system is recognized by Lacan when he famously writes that 'There's no such thing as Woman'.[28] If the symbolic order is governed by the Name of the Father, if the phallus stands for the completeness that the subject desires, then insofar as 'woman' signifies one who lacks the phallus, by definition, it signifies one who cannot be a subject. But if she cannot exist as a speaking subject, she cannot exist at all, except as lacking: 'There's no such thing as Woman because, in her essence ... she is not-whole [elle n'est pas toute].'[29] Thus 'Woman cannot be said. Nothing can be said of woman.'[30] As Lacan adds: 'when any speaking being whatsoever situates itself under the banner 'women', it is on the basis of the following: that it grounds itself as being not-whole [de n'être pas-tout] in situating itself in the phallic function.'[31] By defining woman as the pas tout(e), Lacan perpetuates Freud's alignment of woman with nothingness. In contrast to the ideal wholeness symbolized by the phallus, she is that which is not whole, which is lacking, and – therefore – that which is not, which does not exist: 'Woman certainly does not know (herself to be) everything/whole (ne (se) sait pas tout), even knows (herself to be) nothing (ne (se) sait même rien)' (S, 231; Sf, 287; translation modified).[32]

Of course this only makes sense within a symbolic order governed by the Name of the Father in which the phallus is the ideal form that defines and regulates all relations and representations. Within such an order, it is completely logical for Lacan to insist that there can be no sexual relation: strictly speaking, there are not two sexes, but one sexed subject and his other.[33] This signals precisely what Irigaray is concerned about: not only does woman have no existence as a sexed subject in her own right, but no relation between two different sexes is possible. The world inaugurated by the Lacanian symbolic is a world bereft of sexuate difference.

The Other of the Other

Insofar as woman does enter into the symbolic order, it is in one of two ways. First, she can become the object of man's desire. She is thus identified with what Lacan calls the 'object *a*'. As Jane Gallop neatly explains: 'The object is designated by a lower case "a" to place it in a relation of inferiority to the capital *A* in Lacan's writing which stands for the *Autre*, the radical Other that is other than any objectifiable other. The object *a* is a domestication of the Other.'[34] Such objects of desire are stop-gaps in the economy of lack that underlies the subject. Thus, just as women bear the symbolic weight of nothingness in Freud's account, so here women 'bear the fault of the unsayable': they become an endless supply of fetish objects that cover over a lost and irretrievable plenitude (*TS*, 98). Women are thus not only exiled from language, but mask their own absence. As objects of desire, they become mirrors of the male subject once more: mimics caught up in the '*masquerade of femininity*' that allows them to reflect man's desires, at the price of giving up their own (*TS*, 133–4). Alternatively, woman can seek recompense for her absence as a subject by stopping up her lack with her own 'object *a*': a child. Hence the second way that woman can appear within language: by allowing herself to be symbolically identified with her maternal function.

Irigaray suggests that in the end Lacan (no less than Plato) appropriates maternal generative power and attributes it to a phallocentric symbolic order which sustains only one (male) subject. Woman is non-existent, except in her socially recognized maternal role; as the object of man's desire; or as his necessary but necessarily sacrificed m/Other. He may be a split subject, but she is no subject at all. Instead, she takes up the supplementary roles required to sustain the drama of his formation and self-alienation:

> The 'subject' henceforth will be multiple, plural, sometimes di-formed, but it will still postulate itself as the cause of all the mirages that can be enumerated endlessly and therefore put back together again as one. A fantastic, phantasmatic fragmentation. A destruct(tura)tion in which the 'subject' is shattered, scuttled, while still claiming surreptitiously that he is the reason for it all. (*S*, 135)

Lacan may show that the subject is founded on misrecognition and alienation in ways that undo it from within, but the Other remains defined in relation to this subject in ways that make an other (female) subject impossible.

Language, rather than anatomy, now consigns woman to her role as object and Other, but she is no less trapped: indeed in some ways, Irigaray suggests, the situation is worse. Freud's appeals to anatomy, problematic though they are, nonetheless allow Irigaray to foreground the ways in which the female body does not map onto a phallic model. This in turn allows her to call for a different language, one more able to do justice to women in their bodily specificity. By contrast, Lacan insists that woman's position as *pas toute* or non-existent is a necessary feature of language, inscribed by the structure of lack on which the symbolic is founded. It is thus, as Irigaray notes, 'the effect of a logical requirement' (*TS*, 89). This makes it impossible to appeal to *another* language in which woman is not defined in terms of lack but might instead participate as a speaking subject herself (*TS*, 87–9).

Moreover, as noted above, for Lacan, the unconscious is also 'structured like a language'.[35] As that which cannot be directly represented *in* language, the unconscious is like the white space on a page, a necessary absence shaped by the gaps left between words. If language is organized around the phallic signifier, so too is its inverse, the unconscious as the Other of the symbolic order.[36] However, insofar as woman also functions *as* an absent 'Other', she cannot have her own relation *to* the Other. Without such a relation to the unconscious which forms the necessary counterpart of language, she cannot become a speaking subject – unless, of course, she mimics the male subject position.

The possibility of women having their own relation to the unconscious *as* women is one of the things ruled out by Lacan's repeated comment that 'there is no Other of the Other'.[37] If one becomes a subject only in relation to the Other, if the Other is the Other *of* the subject, there can be no 'Other of the Other', for this would in effect turn the Other into a subject itself. Thus, as Irigaray draws out, if woman is positioned as the Other of the subject, then there can be no Other of woman (indeed, how could there be an Other to that which does not exist?), and thus woman cannot herself take up the position of a subject. More specifically, if the mother is the Other whose sacrifice – whose 'othering' – is required for entry into the symbolic order, allowing that there could be an 'Other of the m/ Other' would imply that the *mother* might become a subject: that is, that she might speak as a woman, as a sexuate subject irreducible to her reproductive function.

Of course, if the mother is to become a subject in ways that do not simply duplicate the masculine subject position, then her relation to the 'Other' will have to be radically re-thought so that it is no longer constituted through lack and the logic of the sacrificial 'cut'. This is the challenge Irigaray faces, and it is why her work demands a thoroughgoing transformation of the underlying structures of both self and other. To this end, she appropriates and reworks Lacan's reference to the 'Other of the Other', turning his words against themselves by using them to suggest that there could be an 'other' way of positioning the m/other, one which does not reduce her to silenced exclusion.

Thus, in a key passage (already cited in Chapter 3), she entwines Lacan with her critical analysis of Plato:

> Is comparing it [the soul] to the *others of the same* (*aux autres des mêmes*) the only thing to be done? But whom are we to call upon to arbitrate that specula(riza)tion except the 'father' once again? ... As for the relationship to *the others of the others* (*aux autres des autres*), *to the other of the other*, anyone who ventures near it will be threatened with loss of self (as same), for it does not exclude the possibility of there being a reversal. (*S*, 335, *Sf* 419)

This entwining allows Irigaray to position Platonic philosophy as a metaphysics of 'the same' which is threatened not so much by the 'other' as by the possibility that this 'other' might escape definition in the same terms that are supposed to govern all speculation. At the same time, her appropriative (and non-capitalized) reference to the 'other(s) of the other(s)' deliberately blurs woman's Lacanian position as both the radical m/Other against which the subject is constituted, and the 'domesticated' other that functions as an object of desire. This helps her to suggest that there could be other ways of thinking woman than as either Other or object for a male subject, ways which might instead allow her to take up the position of a subject in relation to other (sexuate) subjects herself.

By pluralizing Lacan's phrase and rendering it as '*the others of the others*', Irigaray also gives it a more general resonance, signalling the multiple ways in which woman is positioned as 'other' across different theoretical systems, while simultaneously suggesting that there are many potential alternatives to this positioning. Thus, the notion of the 'other of the other' comes to stand for Irigaray's general project: the search for ways to re-figure woman in her sexuate specificity as 'other' than the other of a male subject.

As we will see in subsequent chapters, a key aspect of this project is how a sexuate female subject might relate to those who are irreducibly other to herself, if neither self nor other are constituted by structures of lack, opposition or negation.

Finally, as noted above, Lacan identifies the symbolic order itself as 'the field of the Other'.[38] Thus the phrase 'there is no Other to the Other' implies that there can be no other symbolic order, and no other process for becoming a subject than the logic of lack that demands the sacrifice of the mother. As her multiple reappropriations of the 'other of the other' show, Irigaray is challenging this prohibition on there being another symbolic order. She shows that this challenge cannot be met merely by finding alternative ways of representing woman within the Lacanian symbolic, because the 'Othering' of woman is one of its constitutive structures. Finding the terms with which to articulate woman in her specificity thus means challenging those constitutive structures: the division between self and other, intelligible and perceptible, language and body.

Irigaray seeks to do this through her own relation to language. As we have seen, *Speculum* is written in ways that destabilize traditional categories until language seems to work against itself and alternative ways of thinking begin to emerge. Here we are returned to the fundamentally performative nature of Irigaray's project, as highlighted in Chapter 1. However, Irigaray's relation to Lacan indicates another reason why this performative style is so risky: its playful subversiveness holds her in close proximity to Lacan at the very moment she seeks to move away from him.

Speaking in the Feminine/Speaking (as) Woman

Lacan's own writings and lectures are full of puns, jokes and sophisticated *double* (or even triple) *entendres*, which deliberately over-determine the text. This textual excess is a way of reminding his audience that he is seeking to speak of that which language cannot grasp – of the relation to the Other which makes his own position as a speaking subject possible even as it continually fissures him. The slippages of meaning he creates allow the unconscious to speak in the only way it can: indirectly, through gaps and stammers. In this excessive language, Lacan in effect aligns himself with the feminine. This is possible because the feminine is defined not anatomically but as a position of lack. Thus, there are some who are male, he notes, who can situate themselves 'on the side of the not-whole'.[39]

More specifically, Lacan can be read as positioning himself alongside the male mystics who he associates with what he calls feminine *jouissance*, a term referring to the pleasure or joy of orgasm understood not just as a moment of physical intensity but a kind of ecstatic release in which the subject loses him- or herself. Phallic *jouissance* for Lacan is characterized by its quest for lost plenitude or for the 'One'; it therefore erases the very possibility of a relation to the other sex – that relation between two which Irigaray seeks to recover. However, Lacan also posits an 'Other' – feminine – *jouissance*, about which, he says, women know nothing, except perhaps that they experience it.[40] This lack of knowledge makes sense when one remembers that for Lacan, 'Woman' does not exist. There is no female subject to recall the 'experience' of this 'Other' *jouissance*, in which she who is not, is carried beyond her own lack. Thus, it is not the subject's phallic fantasies but feminine *jouissance* which is privileged as most fully manifesting the radical and excessive lack at the heart of the subject's de-centred existence.

As Irigaray shows, the value of this ecstatic excess appears only from the side of the subject: it is the radical lack of the Other which is the truth of *his* existence that is stammered forth. Woman may be the possible site of this shuddering excess, but she remains unable to articulate her own relation to it. For the male subject, as Lacan's own playful style indicates, feminine excess offers 'new riches': if language speaks the subject, by allowing it to be permeated by the feminine, both language and the subject it speaks are to be found 'dancing, playing, writing [themselves] more than ever' (S, 140). For women, however, *jouissance* remains:

> Pleasure without pleasure: the shock of a remainder of 'silent' body-matter that shakes her at intervals, in the interstices, but of which she remains ignorant. 'Saying' nothing of this pleasure after all, thus not enjoying it. ... If there is such a thing – still – as feminine pleasure, then, it is because men need it in order to maintain themselves in their own existence. It is *useful* to them: it helps them bear what is intolerable in their world as speaking beings, to have a soul foreign to that world: a fantasmatic one. (TS, 96)

Woman's ecstatic excesses help sustain the speaking subject's relation to the Other, and thus, *his* relation to existence. As Irigaray notes, it is telling that for Lacan, the exemplary figure of feminine *jouissance* is a statue by Bernini: the frozen, silent figure of the mystic St Teresa, locked forever in ecstatic self-loss.

Irigaray takes up the figure of the female mystic in '*La mystéri-que*', a neologism that links the supposed 'mystery' of femininity to woman as mystic and hysteric.[41] At one level, this chapter seeks to articulate the 'unknowing silence' of feminine *jouissance*, which it inscribes in recognizably Lacanian terms:

> This is the place where consciousness is no longer master, where, to its extreme confusion, it sinks into a dark night that is also fire and flames. This is the place where 'she' – and in some cases he, if he follows 'her' lead – speaks about the dazzling glare which comes from the source of light that has been logically repressed, about 'subject' and 'Other' flowing out into an embrace of fire that mingles one term into another, about contempt for form as such, about mistrust for understanding as an obstacle along the path of jouissance and mistrust for the dry desolation of reason. (*S*, 191)

Woman's alignment with the 'Other' allows her to become the site of an excess that escapes the logical structures of identity within which the subject has secured but also trapped himself, in a 'prison of self-sufficiency'. By breaching 'the philosopher's closed chamber', she holds open a path beyond reason towards transcendence and the divine (*S*, 192). However, the very notion of an excess that *undoes* logical distinctions is itself only an inversion of the logic that sustains the supposedly rational subject. By emphasizing these patterns of opposition and inversion, Irigaray shows how feminine *jouissance* is only the most extreme version of the Other of the subject, a supplement that once again erases the specificity of women in favour of a projection of excess required by a masculine imaginary.

Despite this, a number of passages in '*La mystérique*' can be read as suggesting an excess that does not merely transgress the symbolic order of the masculine subject, but belongs to a different order altogether. To this extent, Irigaray's own text is marked by a kind of excessive but productive doubling. Thus, when she writes of 'this shimmering underground fabric that she had always been herself, though she did not know it' (*S*, 193), this can be read as referring either to the feminine as the subject's excessive and unconscious counterpart, or to the glimmers of a buried fabric of specifically female existence through whose recovery woman might come to know herself. What is at stake here is what it means to be '*Outside of all self-as-same*' (*S*, 200): whether this outside is a projection of the subject, his inverted illogical Other; or another other, one who does not conform to his logic at all. By exposing the mechanisms that produce the first of these 'outsides', Irigaray hopes to recover the second.

Attuning ourselves to the complexities of '*La mystérique*' is one of the keys to reading *Speculum* as a whole. In this chapter, and across the book, Irigaray writes not simply *of* the female mystic – the subject's unconscious Other – but *as* a mystic, making language twist and turn until it begins to stammer in a voice that defies the logic of the subject: '*one must know how to listen otherwise than in good form(s) to hear what it says*' (*TS*, 111). As existing systems of representation only repeat and reinforce the destitution of woman in language, Irigaray has to disrupt and disturb this syntax so as to allow woman to speak in other terms. Hence the unavoidable riskiness of her mode of writing: she can sound at times like she is mimicking the (Lacanian) master's voice all too well by celebrating that feminine mode of self-loss that the subject loves so much.

Thus, in passages such as the following, it is crucial that Irigaray is not simply advocating a rebellious but ultimately unproductive celebration of feminine 'irrationality'. Rather, she risks taking up the supposedly illogical voice of the female hysteric and mystic so as to disrupt the subject's discourse, not as an end in itself, but to try and make space for a different kind of language, a different logic, and different circuits of desire:

> But how is this to be done? Given that, once again, the 'reasonable' words – to which in any case she has access only through mimicry – are powerless to translate all that pulses, clamors, and hangs hazily in the cryptic passages of hysterical suffering-latency. Then. ... Turn everything upside down, inside out, back to front. *Rack it with radical convulsions*, carry back, reimport, those crises that her 'body' suffers in her impotence to say what disturbs her. Insist also and deliberately upon those *blanks* in discourse which recall the places of her exclusion and which, by their *silent plasticity*, ensure the cohesion, the articulation, the coherent expansion of established forms. Reinscribe them hither and thither *as divergencies*, otherwise and elsewhere than they are expected, in *ellipses* and *eclipses* that deconstruct the logical grid of the reader-writer, drive him out of his mind, trouble his vision to the point of incurable diplopia at least. *Overthrow syntax* by suspending its eternally teleological order, by snipping the wires, cutting the current, breaking the circuits, switching the connections, by modifying continuity, alternation, frequency, intensity. Make it impossible for a while to predict whence, whither,

> when, how, why ... something goes by or goes on: [...] Not by means
> of a growing complexity of the same, of course, but by the irruption
> of other circuits, [...] with no possibility of returning to one single
> origin. (S, 142)

Disrupting the ways we normally write and speak can allow the blanks and silences on which the speaking subject normally depends to become visible and audible. Only by making language work against itself, exposing the constitutive occlusions (of woman, of the feminine, of the mother) on which its coherence depends, might it be possible to begin to speak differently, to speak (as a) woman in a voice no longer defined as the 'other of the Same'. As Irigaray notes, such an operation 'though anarchic in its deeds of title, nonetheless demands patient exactitude' (S, 143). Thus, far from simply adopting the illogical language of the Lacanian mystic, *Speculum* sets this feminine excess alongside all the other figures of woman as 'other': woman as sacrificed m/Other or phallic plenitude; as horrifying lack or object of desire; as inert receptacle, chaotic matter, or flowing formlessness. In the passages between these figures, a different yet distinctive voice begins to emerge. By 'switching the connections', Irigaray's text composes an apparently contradictory female figure that is both fluid *and* frozen, lack *and* excess, in ways that defy a masculine logic that insists on opposing one to an other.

Like the wall face that works 'all too well', Irigaray's text ceases to be a well-behaved mirror reflecting the unity and identity of the male subject. Instead, it takes up his multiple projections of woman and illicitly conjoins them to reveal the illogical over-determination of masculine discourse. For the more the latter seeks to preserve the self-sufficiency of the subject, the more it remains dependent on an ever-proliferating set of female 'others', 'scattered into *x* number of places that are never gathered together into anything she knows of herself' (S, 227). Against this cacophonous multiplicity, the absence of a distinctively female voice becomes an ever more palpable silence.

Thus Irigaray's aim is not to celebrate feminine excess but to 'jam the theoretical machinery' (TS, 78), both by revealing these masculine dependencies and by allowing the repeated silencing of woman to be heard. This project is disruptive, but not merely negative. If masculine discourse is not entirely self-sufficient, that is, if it is not complete in itself and thus not *tout* (whole), woman can no longer be defined against it as *pas toute*. At the same time, recognizing that the masculine subject is itself *pas toute* (incomplete, not all) makes it possible to recognize that another (female) subject might also exist. The aim of Irigaray's subversive strategies is thus to suspend 'the production of a truth and of a meaning that are excessively univocal' (*TS*, 78) and instead to allow this 'other' woman to speak in her own voice: 'why not double the misprision to the limits of exasperation? Until the ear tunes into another music, the voice starts to sing again' (*S*, 143).

In response to the univocal logic of the same, Irigaray calls for 'a *double syntax*, without claiming to regulate the second by the standard of representation, of re-presentation, of the first' (*S*, 138). As we have seen, this call for another language, one capable of articulating woman in her specificity, is made as much by the doubled voice in which Irigaray writes as by what she says. This subversive doubling manifests itself not only in '*La mystérique*', but throughout the 'Volume-Fluidity' chapter of *Speculum*, where Irigaray plays with Lacan's formulation of ~~Woman~~ as '*pas tout(e)*' as well as with the title of his lectures on feminine sexuality, *Encore*.[42] As a call for more, '*encore*' suggests the radical excessiveness of feminine *jouissance*, which can never be completed or contained, in ways that reinforce woman's (non-)existence as not-whole. In 'Volume-Fluidity', Irigaray allows woman to respond to the male subject's desire to define and identify with feminine excess with the words 'pas ... encore' (*S*, 232, *Sf*, 288). This multivalent phrase captures the way woman is repeatedly condemned (not only by Lacan, but by western thought more generally) to not-being (she is not ... again), while at the same time constituting a rejection of Lacan's account of feminine sexuality (not *encore*). More importantly, the ellipsis makes visible both the logical gap between claiming that woman 'is not' and suggesting that she 'is not *yet*', and the temporal gap between her theoretical non-existence and the future in which she might yet come to be.

This subversive appropriation of Lacan's own terms is extended as Irigaray reworks the negating figure of woman as *pas tout(e)* into an affirmation of a different conception of female being: because she is not-whole, woman's form is not non-existent, but never completable as one. She is always becoming, without becoming one *or* the (Lacanian) Other; instead, she remains in touch with the other in ways that allow her to change form without becoming form-less. In ways we will examine in more depth in the next chapter, 'Volume-Fluidity' thus suggests that woman's being *pas tout(e)* does not have to be understood in terms of either lack or excess, but as signalling the need for a new logic or syntax with which to articulate female beings. It also reinforces Irigaray's point that, if there is to be a 'double syntax', it is crucial that neither is regulated by the other. This is a call for two who are no longer strictly speaking 'doubles': two who are no longer determined by a mimetic logic of the same, but whose irreducible voices resound alongside one another without becoming one.

As we might expect, another way in which Irigaray begins to forge this double syntax is through the figure of the mirror. Instead of the flat mirror which splits the subject from his opposing image and allows him to identify with it, she turns to the curved mirror, and in particular, the concave mirror of the speculum:

> But which 'subject' up till now has investigated the fact that a *concave mirror* concentrates the light and, specifically, that this is not wholly irrelevant to woman's sexuality? [...] Which 'subject' has taken an interest in the anamorphoses produced by the conjunction of such curvatures? What impossible reflected images, maddening reflections, parodic transformations took place at each of their articulations? (*S*, 144)

The concave mirrors that allow the inside of the female body to be reflected have the power to drive the subject mad, facing him with reflections he cannot comprehend. Such mirrors set his phallocentric logic ablaze, just as *Speculum* itself operates as a burning glass of theory, whose concentrated focus on the oppositions that sustain an economy of the same burns up their supposed coherence.[43] At the same time, the curved surfaces of the speculum also represent the possibility of woman reflecting (on) herself, defining herself in relation to her own sexuate being, rather than operating as a mirror for a male subject.

Finally, the disruptive capacities of the concave mirror help Irigaray to challenge the alignment of woman with a 'faithful, polished mirror, empty of altering reflections' (*S*, 136). Instead of a glassy surface with no life of its own, she asks us to imagine a living mirror whose silvering has become liquid and mobile:

> Mirror made of matter so fluid, so ethereal that it had already entered and mingled everywhere? What if matter had always, already, had a part but was yet invisible, beyond the senses, moving in ways alien to any fixed reflection. ... This silvering at the back of the mirror might, at least, retain *the being* (*l'être*) which we have been perhaps and which perhaps we will be again – though our mirage

has failed at present or has been covered over by alien speculations. A living mirror, thus, am I (to) your resemblance as you are to mine. (S, 196–7)

As this last phrase suggests, the evocation of a 'living mirror' is here interwoven with Irigaray's analysis of woman as the 'other' required for the subject's reflections: she is his 're-semblance' – even for the decentred, alienated Lacanian subject, whose 'absence of being' ~~Woman~~ reflects in her nothingness (S, 197). Likewise, the reference to 'alien speculations' recalls the mis-identification of the mirror stage just as effectively as it invokes the masculine projections of the feminine that have 'covered over' woman. Yet, even as she exposes the way feminine excess operates as an inexhaustible supplement to the subject, Irigaray simultaneously evokes a fluid mirror which would no longer allow self and other to be 'cut in two', divided and opposed as if separated by the frozen surface of a glass (S, 200). Neither would this living mirror reproduce immobile copies of unchanging originals. Instead, by 'moving in ways alien to any fixed reflection', such a mirror might allow likenesses to emerge between two whose flowing forms reflect one other's living being without need of being the same. In this fluid inter-relation, the distinction between self and other would not be lost. Rather, they would take shape together in a non-oppositional process in which 'the one is in the other, and the other in me' such that self and other 'spawn – and slit – each other in(de)finitely' (S, 200).

In passages such as these, a non-oppositional process of self-constitution begins to emerge which would allow woman to become a subject in her own right, without sacrificing the sexuate specificity of her being. For as Irigaray notes, and as we will see more fully in the next chapter, 'for her, *the one doesn't rule out the other*' (S, 202; my emphasis).

6

The Status of Sexuate Difference

In response to both Kant's 'Copernican' turn and Lacan's linguistic one, Irigaray calls for another, sexuate, revolution. Instead of producing yet another double of man, this revolution would generate figures that do justice to the sexuate specificity of woman and the radically dissymmetrical difference between the sexes.[1] Thus Irigaray seeks a language allowing woman to relate to herself in her own terms rather than those of the male subject. This chapter will begin by exploring some of the key figures Irigaray employs to re-imagine woman as a subject, paying particular attention to the image of two lips. In so doing, it will show why the charge of 'essentialism' that has sometimes been made against Irigaray's work is misplaced. While recognizing that there are risks involved in Irigaray's appeals to the female body, I argue that her aim is not simply to find alternative ways of representing the female sex. Rather, she is seeking to refigure the very relation between the body and language by escaping the hylomorphic model in which symbolic forms are imposed on inert and essentially form-less matter. Irigaray's claim is neither that our existence as women is determined by our anatomical sex, nor that we think differently because we have female bodies. Instead, she is arguing that we need to re-think the relation between our being and our bodies, as well as between form and matter, self and other, if we are to be able to think of woman as a sexuate subject.

Irigaray's explorations of female self-relation are designed to engender figures for a female autonomy that would permit us to affirm being (as) two. In the second half of this chapter, I examine the concern that the increasing emphasis on 'being two' in Iriga-ray's later work signals an inadvertent return to a kind of hetero-sexism that compromises her earlier project. Addressing this concern will help clarify the difference between the sexual and the sexuate, along with the ontological status of the latter and its rela-tion to Irigaray's notion of 'genre'.

When Our Lips Speak Together

In Chapter 3, we saw that Irigaray's reading of Plato's Myth of the Cave draws attention to what she calls 'the forgotten passage'. This phrase signals both the forgetting of the appropriation of the mater-nal body in the imagery of the myth (the forgetting of the passage of the mother's body into philosophical metaphor), and the forget-ting of the passage itself as a space between. As we also saw, by recalling the mother's body to the Platonic scene of representation, Irigaray refigures the passage as the birth canal while reminding the reader of the passage between mother and foetus sustained by the umbilical cord and placenta.

In a number of later texts and an interview with the embryolo-gist Hélène Rouch, Irigaray develops the notion of a placental economy. Rouch's account of the role of the placenta allows Irigaray to elaborate a model in which otherness is tolerated within the self, rather than assimilated, excluded, or negated:

> One of the distinctive features of the female body is its tolerance of the other's growth within itself without incurring illness or death for either one of the living organisms. Unfortunately, culture ... has given no interpretation to the model of tolerance of the other within and with a self that this relationship manifests. ... Whereas the female body engenders with respect for difference, the patriarchal social body contracts itself hierarchically, excluding difference.[2]

The placental economy is regulated by a space between one and another that belongs to both and to neither, and that is character-ized by intimate relations of contiguity and contact, rather than substitution or negation. It thus allows differences to remain pal-pable between two beings who are nonetheless not straightfor-wardly separable.

In the fluid darkness of the pregnant body, Irigaray finds a space and time that do not belong to the logic of the unified subject:

[D]eeper than the greatest depths your daylight could imagine ...
Neither permanently fixed, nor shifting and fickle. Nothing solid
survives, *yet that thickness responding to its own rhythms is not nothing.*
Quickening in movements both expected and unexpected. Your
space, your time are unable to grasp their regularity or contain their
foldings and unfoldings. (*EP*, 13; my emphasis)

Such passages confirm Irigaray's rejection of the assumption that
'what appears to the subject constitutes the totality of what *is*',[3] for
this living darkness is not nothing, even though there may be
nothing much to see with the subject's objectifying gaze. Instead,
it is replete with fluid movements which are rhythmic, not random:
this fluid quickening cannot be reduced to a permanently shifting
excess lacking any determinable form at all. Its rhythmic pulsions
generate dense patterns of folding and unfolding that are sufficiently strong and flexible to allow for the unexpected, and that
hold together a space-time that has no need to demarcate self and
other via fixed boundaries: 'I caress you, you caress me, without
unity – neither yours, nor mine, nor ours. The envelope, which
separates and divides us, fades away. Instead of a solid enclosure,
it becomes fluid: which is far from nothing. This does not mean
that we are merged' (*EP*, 59–60). Here the singular identities of 'I'
and 'you' no longer depend on self-enclosed unity. Instead each is
sustained with the other in fluid interrelation. While the space
between them is no longer solid, it is neither void nor vacuum, but
what Irigaray calls an 'almost palpable density' (*EP*, 105): a fluidity
that is not devoid of form, but a 'thickness' shaped by rhythmic
movements that articulate self and other together.

In re-figuring pregnancy via the passage and the placental
economy, Irigaray releases the materiality of the maternal body
from its traditional role as inert container for the male subject's
forms. The womb is no longer a cave with walls of petrified matter.
Instead, Irigaray begins to find the terms for a female subject
characterized by a fluid materiality capable of embodying a non-
oppositional relation between self and other. Thus she reminds us
that: '*The/a woman never closes up into a volume.* The dominant representation of the maternal figure as a volume may lead us to
forget that woman's ability to enclose is enhanced by her fluidity,
and vice versa' (*S*, 239). As always, in foregrounding female fluidity, Irigaray has to play a double game: she needs to find ways of
taking up this fluidity, which has traditionally been represented in
terms of a *lack* of form, and show how it can become the basis for

a different way of generating form, along with a different form of (female) subject.[4] Her refiguring of the pregnant body is part of this project, as are her writings on female (and male) sexuality.

For Irigaray, the question of sexuality is inseparable from the question of how a subject is formed. Male sexuality has typically been organized around the idealization of a single, visible sex organ, in ways that reflect and reinforce the model of self-identical unity. Irigaray contrasts this with the multiple sites of woman's sexual pleasure – 'breasts, pubis, clitoris, labia, vulva, vagina, neck of the uterus, womb ...' (S, 233) – which are suggestive of the way the female body does not conform to the bounds of male identity. Nonetheless, even if woman 'does not have *one* sex organ, or a unified sexuality', Irigaray's task is to show how this does not mean 'that she has no sex' (S, 233).

A key role is played in this project by Irigaray's discussion of female and male auto-affection: at one level, this term refers literally to masturbation as well as the different ways in which men and women touch (themselves) to give (themselves) pleasure. At another, it refers to the way a subject relates to itself, such as in the founding moment of self-reflection that grounds the Cartesian self. Irigaray suggests that, because he has been identified with a self-contained form (whether the penis, the phallus, or the bounded ego), the male subject needs an external instrument with which to touch himself: a hand, a woman, language, or a self-representation (S, 232). As a counter-measure, Irigaray turns the traditional alignment of the female body with both lack and excess into a positive resource for re-figuring female auto-affection:

> this excess is (not) nothing: the vacation of form, the faults in form, the return to another edge where she re-touches herself without anything/thanks to nothing. Lips of the same form – but of a form that is never simply defined – ripple outwards as they touch and send one another on a course that is never fixed into a single configuration. (S, 230 translation modified)

What can only be seen as a 'hole' or lack if the male body is taken as the standard becomes a spacing between lips which allows them to touch on each other, closing without becoming sealed into one, opening without losing all contact, continually taking up different forms without ever becoming form-less: 'She is indefinite, in-finite, *form is never complete in her*. She is not infinite but neither is she one unit(y) ... This incompleteness in her form, her morphology, allows her continually to become something else, which is not to say that she is ever univocally nothing' (*S*, 229, translation modified). By refiguring the female body together with women's capacities for auto-affection, Irigaray helps us imagine a female subject whose constitution does not depend on the unity of self-identity; instead, 'This self-touching gives woman a form that is in(de)finitely transformed' (*S*, 233).

The figure of the lips goes on to play a particularly important role in Irigaray's quest for a grammar with which to articulate a distinctively female subject, perhaps most famously in 'When Our Lips Speak Together', though she returns to this image throughout her work (including the poetic text *Elemental Passions*, published eight years after *Speculum*, on which I also draw here).[5] In these texts, the image of the lips is offered as a way of figuring a female morphology according to which – contra Freud and Lacan – woman is defined not as the lack or absence of the phallus, but in relation to herself. Irigaray works to recover the possibilities both for self-relation and for pleasure afforded by the '*nonsuture of her lips*', possibilities that are sacrificed when woman is reduced to the closed volume of a reproductive container (*TS*, 30). By invoking both the labia and the mouth, the image of the lips playfully suggests that by re-figuring the female sex, woman might begin to speak in a sexuate voice. In parallel with the concave mirror which allows woman to see herself, the lips also present woman as constantly touching (on) herself, as indicated in the passages cited above. This shift in emphasis from sight to touch helps Irigaray escape a specularizing economy in which woman is objectified by a male gaze.[6] Rather than fixing her against a male subject, the lips provide a figure of female auto-affection that allows woman to take shape in her own fluid movements.[7]

Thus, the lips are not simply deployed to refigure female sexuality in ways that no longer take the male body as paradigmatic. As 'strangers to dichotomy and oppositions', the lips offer an alternative model to that in which identity is secured via opposition to or a constitutive cut from an other (*ESD*, 18). While each lip is inseparable from the other with which it moves, the two are not simply indistinguishable:

> We – you/I – are neither open nor closed. We never separate simply ... Between our lips, yours and mine, several voices, several ways of speaking resound endlessly, back and forth. One is never separable from the other. You/I: we are always several at once. ... One cannot

be distinguished from the other; which does not mean that they are indistinct. (*TS*, 209)

The lips through which a woman touches herself as they touch on each other are neither one nor two, nor do they relate as (active) subject to (passive) object. In 'that contact of *at least two* (lips)' there is no possibility of distinguishing 'what is touching from what is touched' (*TS*, 26). Each moves and is moved by another such that they mutually define each other without need for division or rupture. Instead, they are held together by a spacing that allows each to touch on the other while remaining distinct. In the movements that flow between them, they remain in contact without being the same, shape one another while taking on their own form.

The male order of the subject covers over this fluid economy because its oppositional logic 'freezes the mobility of relations between. It produces discontinuity. Peaks, pikes, fissures' (*EP*, 90). By contrast, the lips gather and shape differences together. Between women's lips, different voices pass without being split in two. Yet this lack of definitive separation does not mean they are talking nonsense: rather, they belong to a different logic than that governed by the opposition of self and other and the desire for identity in sameness. The lips figure a self-shaping female corporeality whose fluid movements bring woman into definition without needing to exclude otherness and thus without needing to mirror the (phallic) unity of the male form. Instead, between lips and passage, '[t]he one and the other interpenetrate and transmute each other such that the dichotomy between them no longer exists'.[8]

Crucially, in their fluid interrelation, neither lip need mirror the other: while they move together and always affect each other, they need not move in the same way at the same time. As Irigaray puts it, the lips 'are re-doubled before the time of any mirror. They seem to mime each other. But the separation which permits that miming is still foreign to them. ... The wall between them is porous. It allows passage' (*EP*, 66). Or again:

> [Y]ou are neither my counterpart nor my copy. How can I say it differently? We exist only as two? We live by twos beyond all mirages, images, and mirrors. Between us, one is not the 'real' and the other her imitation; one is not the original and the other her copy. ... No need to fashion a mirror image to be 'doubled', to repeat ourselves – a second time. Prior to any representation, we are two. ... we are always one and the other, at the same time. (*TS*, 216–17)

Here Irigaray writes of two who relate to each other without being divisible into two ones, whose differences cannot be mapped in terms of the relation between an original and its inverted mirror-image, and whose similarities are irreducible to relations of doubling or copying. The lips are inseparable but not the same; are two without being sundered. Each is shaped by the other such that the other partially constitutes its unique form; indeed, each is itself *because* of the ways in which it is bound together with another which is not its mirror image. In this relational process of constitution, each is always one and the other at the same time, without becoming indistinct – on the contrary it is the relations between them that shape one and another into distinctness together.

Irigaray thus presents the lips as a figure for a relational female subject, 'Outside any possible symmetry or inversion' (*EP*, 63). In fact, the figure of the lips introduces a dissymmetry twice over: not only does each lip not simply mirror the other, but together they figure a process where self and other take shape in ways that neither reflect nor invert the oppositional process through which the male subject is formed. It is this double dissymmetry that releases woman from her role as the 'other of the Same' by making it possible for her to become other to 'the other'. Instead of a second sex made in the image of the first, instead of two who are really one, Irigaray finds the figures for an irreducible female subject who is neither one nor two, but located incalculably in-between.

Appealing to the Body: The Risk of Essentialism

The figures of the placental economy and the lips offer an alternative to the oppositional model in which a subject is constituted via a split from the m/Other. Instead, self and other take shape together in ways that would allow a woman – and more specifically, a daughter – to remain in touch with her mother. By relating to her own sex in the body of the mother, the daughter would be able to enter a horizon of sexuate belonging and relate to herself as a woman without being defined against a male subject. At the same time, the language of the placental economy allows the daughter's debt to birth to be acknowledged in terms of a dynamic *relational* bond that prevents the mother from disappearing into a fantasy of amorphous plenitude.[9]

Nonetheless, some readers have been troubled by Irigaray's appeal to figures that draw on a specifically female and maternal body. There are of course good reasons for feminists to worry about any framework that seems to reinforce the traditional alignment of woman with 'the body' or 'nature'. As Irigaray's own analysis shows, the rational subject has typically been constructed against the natural realm that has been aligned with women, and this in turn has been used to block women from laying claim to the powers of reason that legitimate claims to knowledge as well as full participation in ethical or political life. The identification of woman with her body has been central to her positioning as the 'other' of the subject: less rational, more emotional, less capable of transcending the realm of the senses, more tied to, and determined by, her bodily being.

Irigaray's own appeal to the female body has thus led to the charge of 'essentialism'.[10] On this view, she is guilty of making the female body 'the rock of feminism' in ways that reinscribe two fundamentally patriarchal claims:[11] first, that woman can be identified *with* her body, and second, that woman is determined *by* her body. A third related concern is that by celebrating the fluidity and multiplicity of female sexuality, Irigaray reinscribes a traditional (phallocentric) image of feminine excess. Finally, Irigaray is sometimes read as seeking to recover the feminine in ways that lead her to posit a universal essence of *woman* that cannot do justice to the multiple differences between *women*. As Schor notes, Irigaray is thereby seen as subscribing to 'the belief that woman has an essence, that woman can be specified by one or a number of inborn attributes that define across cultures and throughout history her unchanging being'.[12] She is thus charged with repeating another patriarchal fallacy, namely, that of treating a specific kind of subject (white, western women) as a universal norm in ways that exclude others.

The concern that Irigaray's own perspective reflects a western bias is a legitimate one which impacts on all those of us who theorize from a western context. Theorists such as bell hooks and Gayatri Spivak have taught white western feminists in particular a much needed attentiveness to the limits of our own perspectives, and helped us to listen for, and allow ourselves to be changed by, other feminist voices.[13] However, there is no intrinsic reason why Irigaray's project cannot be fully inflected by the ways in which sexual difference intersects with other differences, whether of race, class, ethnicity, age or sexuality. Irigaray foregrounds the importance of attending to such intersections when she states that: 'the most important thing to do is to expose the exploitation common to all women *and to find the struggles that are appropriate for each woman*, right where she is, depending upon her nationality, her job, her social class, her sexual experience, that is, *upon the form of oppression that is for her the most immediately unbearable*' (*TS*, 166–7; my emphasis). Combating the oppression women face *as* women does not mean seeing all women as 'the same'; on the contrary, it is crucial to address the form oppression takes in the singular situation of each woman.

Neither is it the case that Irigaray is blinded to differences between women by a search for some kind of (falsely) universalizing 'essence' of the feminine. As we have seen, she is explicit that her project is not to define woman. Rather, she seeks to establish a female subject position which different women can inhabit in different ways.[14] Irigaray thus distances herself from any group which undertakes 'to determine the "truth" of the feminine, to legislate as to what it means to "be a woman"' (*TS*, 166). As Tina Chanter suggests, such distancing testifies to 'the seriousness with which [Irigaray] takes differences at all levels' in ways that are in keeping with her thoroughgoing challenge 'to the tendency of Western thought to reduce everything to the same'.[15] This challenge means that, even if sexuate difference has ontological priority for Irigaray (as I think it does), her project does not negate the importance of other kinds of differences. I will return to this issue in subsequent discussions of Irigaray's perceived heterosexism (in this chapter) and the question of the relation of sexuate difference to race (in the next). For now however, it is worth emphasizing that for Irigaray, far from being indifferent to other kinds of difference, an ethics of sexual difference safeguards alterity in ways that make it possible to do justice to differences 'at all levels'.

Taking all of this into account, a generous reader might ask how it is possible to read Irigaray's appeals to the body such that they do not operate as attempts to define female identity in terms of a universal essence. Likewise, given her critique of the phallocentric 'othering' of woman, and her quest for a different logic and syntax for a woman other to this other, we might ask how it is possible to read her appeals to plurality and multiplicity in ways that do not simply reinscribe femininity in terms of disorder and excess.

Part of the answer to these questions has already been given: Irigaray makes it clear that she is not seeking to celebrate feminine excess, but to completely rethink the constitution of the self such that this no longer depends on a cut from the other. '*Never simply being one'* – being plural, fluid, more than one – does not mean 'lacking unity', if by this we mean being formless and indistinct. Rather, it means rethinking a notion of unity to allow for the ways in which distinct identities can be shaped by relations between two (or more) who are neither the same nor completely separable. As Irigaray puts it, 'Woman always remains several, but she is kept from dispersion because the other is already within her' (*TS*, 31).

Again, the pregnant body can offer us a starting point for thinking a subject who is more than one without being alienated from herself like the Lacanian ego or 'I'.[16] The pregnant subject is not constituted by (mis-)identification with external reflections/projections; instead, the other emerges within – without mother and foetus simply becoming one. However, by invoking the pregnant body, we come back to the central question: how can Irigaray's appeals to the female body operate without defining woman in terms of biological or anatomical essence? The next section will examine some possible answers to this question. As we will see, to answer it fully, we will need to return to the way Irigaray's project challenges the traditional conceptualization of matter.

From Strategic Essentialism to Symbolic Transformation

In response to claims that Irigaray succumbs to the temptation to define woman via a naïve and 'essentialist' appeal to anatomical sex, a number of feminists more sympathetic to her project have argued that this so-called 'essentialism' is a deliberate discursive strategy. This 'strategic essentialism' is seen both as a form of resistance and as a provisional stage which feminism must pass through so as to arrive at different ways of thinking sexual difference.[17] Many of these readings are subtle and generous towards Irigaray.[18] They position her appeals to the female body as a deliberate reappropriation designed to counter and displace phallocentric representations of woman while simultaneously insisting on that within the feminine which remains irreducible to patriarchal discourse. Thus, Diana Fuss argues that: 'To the extent that Irigaray reopens the question of essence and woman's access to it, essentialism represents not a trap she falls into but rather a key strategy she puts into play, not a dangerous oversight but rather a lever of displacement.'[19] Given that we are historically encased within the reductive essentialisms of patriarchal thought, finding alternative ways of representing the female body is a crucial stage in the project of thinking woman differently.

Nonetheless, reading Irigaray as a 'strategic essentialist' remains problematic in two related ways. First, there is a danger that Irigaray's position becomes wholly identified with such an approach in ways that obscure the extent of her positive project. Thus, it is important to separate the subversive mimicry of a hysterical/mysterical voice – which *is* a strategy for disinterring a distinctively female way of speaking otherwise – from the project of re-figuring woman as a sexuate subject – which is not itself merely a 'strategy', but the goal which demands such thoroughgoing cultural and philosophical transformations. Second, positioning Irigaray as a strategic essentialist can also obscure the ways in which the transformation she seeks would undo traditional models of essence, insofar as these rely on a constitutive opposition between form and matter.[20] As we have seen, for Irigaray, rethinking the form/matter relation is an inextricable part of rethinking woman as other to the 'other'. Thus, in the end, her project problematizes even 'strategic' appeals to biological or anatomical 'essence'.

The strongest interpretations of Irigaray deploy the notion of strategic essentialism in ways that are attentive to these risks. Thus, both Fuss and Whitford position Irigaray as mobilizing an *apparently* 'essentialist' language to help open the way towards alternative *non-essentialist* constructions of feminine subjectivity. On this approach, Irigaray speaks the language of essentialism so as to leave essentialism behind. Moreover, as Whitford argues, it is *because* of the essentialist definitions of woman within the tradition that '[o]ne cannot get "beyond" essentialism ... without passing through essentialism'.[21] Irigaray's 'so-called essentialism is primarily a strategy for bringing to light the concealed essentialism of philosophy'.[22] However, exposing the ways in which western thought has typically aligned woman with the body and excluded her from full recognition as a subject is not on its own enough to *shift* that pattern of thought. Strategic essentialism can also play a role in helping to prevent this pattern from repeating itself by providing alternative figures of woman – 'however provisional'.[23] Whitford's reading shows that such creative re-appropriations are necessary to open a (psychic and linguistic) space within which female specificity can be cultivated in positive terms; they are part of the work required to generate an alternative syntax that would allow women to speak without sacrificing their female specificity. When such creative language work is (mis-)taken as an attempt to simply identify women with their bodies, 'what has been lost sight of is the horizon. It is to fix a moment of becoming as if it were the goal.'[24] As Schor helpfully summarizes:

> for Whitford mimeticism is the strategy, essentialism is the stage, and that stage is obligatory if women are to become subjects in the symbolic. ... Whereas the male philosophers are free because of their founding exclusion of the maternal-feminine to deny their own essentialism, as a philosopher in the feminine Irigaray is obliged not only to pass through essentialism but also to speak its language. ... The major misreading of Irigaray according to Whitford consists then in taking her essentialism for the final stage, the last word, when it is only part of a process.[25]

Both Whitford and Fuss help us to see that what some have seen as 'essentialist' appeals to the female body in fact point in quite the opposite direction. For when Irigaray invokes women's bodies in images such as the two lips, the very fact that the lips are an *image* shows that the female body is never simply anatomically determined but always mediated via symbolic figures.

More specifically, for Whitford and Fuss, the figure of the lips embodies a shift from a logic of *metaphorical substitution* to a *metonymic logic of contiguity*.[26] Whereas metaphor uses one term in place of another to suggest a certain likeness (thus Irigaray reads Plato's cave as metaphor for the womb), metonymy uses the name of one object to call up another with which it is associated (one lip brings to mind the other). Thus, while metaphor substitutes one term for another in ways that foreground what they have in common, metonymy depends on the relations between different terms that allow them to be associated or placed alongside one another. The lips are thereby taken to figure a shift from a logic that privileges equivalence and sameness, to one which relies on perceiving likeness between non-identical terms, and which thus allows sameness to co-exist with difference. Whereas the former has sustained the identity of a masculine subject, the latter offers a way of figuring female specificity without reducing woman to the 'other *of* the Same'.

Thus, when Fuss suggests that the two lips operate as 'a metaphor *for* metonymy', she points to the way in which positioning woman as other to the 'other' of the male subject requires not simply alternative *images* of the feminine, but a different *process* of self-constitution.[27] This shift is explored in depth in Whitford's account of Irigaray's critical appropriation of Lacan, in which

Whitford can be seen as taking Fuss's insights further by showing how the two lips function as a symbolic figure for an alternative (non-phallic) imaginary that would allow a distinctively feminine process of self-formation. Like the lips which touch on one another without being the same, a little girl is *like* her mother without being identical to her: 'the two can be seen as together yet separate; both the girl and her mother can be separate beings, while remaining in relationship.'[28] Whitford suggests that the two lips help us represent the position of a female child who forms a sense of her own sexuate identity via contiguous relations with her mother, rather than a process of mirroring that relies on separation, opposition and substitution. As a figure for this alternative process of feminine self-formation, the image of the lips contributes to a symbolic order capable of representing relations between women without simply identifying them with one another or treating them as substitutable.[29]

Whitford's reading shows that psychoanalysis is crucial for Irigaray because it presents both the subject and sexuality as formed (via imaginary processes and symbolic structures) rather than naturally given. This holds open the possibility that these processes and structures could be transformed to allow for a feminine subject. Those who read the image of the two lips as an appeal to anatomical or biological essence thus miss the point. Irigaray deploys the two lips to show that 'biology (or nature) must receive a symbolic mediation which is more adequate for women', where 'more adequate' means not a more truthful description of the female body, but a representation which does not reduce women to their functions as m/Other for a male subject.[30]

This point is reinforced by other readers such as Elizabeth Grosz and Moira Gatens. They too insist that for Irigaray, 'we have no unmediated access to the "real" body, the "raw" or the "natural" body ... the human body and sexual difference are always *lived in culture*, mediated by its values, its oppositions and its discourses.'[31] Far from taking the biological body as given, Irigaray directs our attention to how the body is *represented*, and the complex ways in which those representations are internalized to shape the ways we live our bodies as well as our sense of self. Bodies as they are lived are always already full of meaning, always socially, historically and culturally informed. Thus, both Gatens and Grosz emphasize Irigaray's insistence that her concern is not with anatomy but morphology, understood as 'the way in which the shape or form of the female body is represented in culture. Morphology is not given, it is interpretation, which is not to say that it has nothing to do with our cultural understandings of biology.'[32] Thus Grosz concludes:

> Contrary to the objection that she is describing an essential, natural or innate femininity, unearthing it from under its patriarchal burial, Irigaray's project can be interpreted as a contestation of patriarchal representations *at the level of cultural representation itself*. The two lips is a manoeuvre to develop a *different* image or model of female sexuality, one which may inscribe female bodies according to interests outside or beyond phallocentrism, while at the same time contesting the representational terrain that phallocentrism has hitherto annexed.[33]

On this reading, the figure of the two lips is not an anatomical description but offers an alternative female morphology, that is, an alternative interpretation that constructs the female sex in terms of plenitude rather than lack:

> Freud's morphological description of the female sex as castrated, as lacking, receives no more nor less 'confirmation' from biology than does Irigaray's positing of the female sex as made up of (at least) two lips. The difference is that Freud's morphological description of the female sex amounts to the inverse of male morphology which is taken to be full, phallic; while Irigaray's description presents the female form as full, as lacking nothing.[34]

Refiguring the Female Body and the Form/Matter Distinction

The approaches outlined above offer a strong defence of Irigaray as a non-essentialist thinker. Each reflects Irigaray's emphasis on finding alternative ways of representing the female body as a key element in the project of thinking woman differently. Nonetheless, they also draw our attention to a significant tension between this emphasis on the symbolic representation of woman and Irigaray's challenge to the form/matter distinction. As shown by Whitford's account, this tension is particularly acute in relation to the psychoanalytic frame, even one that is radically re-appropriated and transformed for distinctively feminist ends.[35] On the one hand, as Whitford observes, the symbolic structures of subjectivity would remain empty formalisms without the imaginary processes of self-identification which 'flesh it out'. On the other, the imaginary depends on the symbolic to give it representational form: 'The symbolic is structure (form) which is given content by the imaginary, and the imaginary pours itself into the available structures to form representations. Subjectivity, then, belongs to the symbolic, but it is empty without the imaginary; identity is imaginary, but it takes a symbolic (representational) form.'[36] By contrasting the symbolic as structure or 'form' with the imaginary which provides such forms with representational matter or 'content', Whitford's account brings out very clearly the way in which the Lacanian frame repeats the form/matter distinction of which Irigaray is so deeply critical. As we have seen, this distinction has structured western metaphysical thought in ways that oppose a form-less maternal matter to a masculine form-giving activity that appropriates the material resources of its feminine Other.

Whitford's rendering of the relation between the imaginary and symbolic also brings out the Kantian resonances of these Lacanian concepts by echoing Kant's famous dictum: 'Thoughts without content are empty, intuitions without concepts are blind. It is, therefore, just as necessary to make our concepts sensible ... as to make our intuitions intelligible'.[37] As discussed in Chapter 4, for Kant as for Lacan, the subject and its experience are not empirical givens but constituted under certain universal and a priori conditions. Irigaray can thus be read as seeking the conditions – that is, both the conceptual categories and the forms of space and time – for a female subject. This is signalled in the opening essay of *An Ethics of Sexual Difference*, where, referring directly to Kant, she notes that the inauguration of such an ethics 'requires a change in our perception and conception of *space-time* ... an evolution or a transformation of forms, of the relations of *matter* and *form* and of the interval *between*' (*ESD*, 7). To put it in more Kantian terms, she is seeking to re-schematize reality.[38] Read in this way, the figure of the two lips allows Irigaray to explore the kinds of spatio-temporal relations required for the female object/other to be reconstituted as a subject. However, as we also saw in Chapter 4, the Kantian framework depends on the way that spatio-temporal and conceptual forms actively organize the sensible matter of intuition into unified and intelligible objects. Irigaray's mode of post-Kantianism thus requires a more fundamental transformation, displacing this underlying opposition between passive matter and form-giving activity and giving manifold matter an active role in the re-casting of spatio-temporal relations.

Thus, while emphasizing the psychoanalytic (or post-Kantian) dimensions of Irigaray's project helps show why the charge of essentialism is so misplaced, it also threatens to trap her attempts to articulate the terms for a female subject back within a hylomorphic tradition she seeks to escape. Likewise, by insisting that for Irigaray, there is no 'body' per se but only bodies as they are socially and culturally represented, the charge of essentialism can be firmly (and rightly) rebutted: 'Bodies are not conceived by Irigaray as biologically or anatomically given, inert, brute objects, fixed by nature once and for all. She sees them as the bearers of meanings and social values, the products of social inscriptions, always inherently social.'[39] Yet at the same time, foregrounding the search for alternative ways of representing or symbolically mediating the body's sexed specificity also risks implicitly reinforcing the view that the materiality of the body is in and of itself *form-less* until inscribed with meaning. Both Gatens and Grosz explicitly reject this view: the body is not a *tabula rasa* passively awaiting a socio-cultural overlay.[40] Instead, Irigaray's concept of the body is understood as referring to 'a body that *exists as such* only *through* its socio-linguistic construction'.[41] Such bodies are far from passive or inert: thus Grosz draws attention not only to a 'creative coding or inscription, a positive marking of women's bodies', but also to the ways in which, '[a]s sexually specific, the body codes the meanings projected onto it in sexually determinate ways.'[42]

This final comment leaves the question of how the body is constituted – as such, and hence, as sexually specific – rather more open. If this is indeed seen as *wholly* the result of cultural and symbolic processes, then – as Alison Stone argues – this still implies the existence of some kind of indeterminate matter which those processes shape into determinate bodily forms. Such a view entails that matter itself 'cannot shape the process whereby it is acculturated and made corporeal'.[43] It is thus profoundly at odds with Irigaray's critique of the form/matter distinction. Unless we attend to the materiality of the body as not only *bearing* meanings and values, but actively *participating* in their – and its own – constitution, we risk perpetuating the opposition between passive matter and active form-giving powers that Irigaray shows to be fundamental to the cultural devaluation of both mothers and women.

To some extent, the tensions that arise as a result of emphasizing Irigaray's view of bodies as culturally constructed are to be found within her own texts. In *This Sex Which Is Not One*, she suggests that it may be time to return to 'that repressed entity, the female imaginary' so as to foreground 'the possibility of a different language', of 'women's language', as well as the need for 'two different syntaxes' (Irigaray, *TS*, 28, 80, 33, 132–4). In keeping with this, *Speculum* critiques Freud's theories for their non-symbolization of female desire and for reducing woman to lack in ways that afford her 'too few figurations, images, or representations by which to represent herself'; as a result, 'access to a signifying economy ... is difficult or even impossible for her' (*S*, 71). While all these terms need to be treated with caution, especially when taken out of context, they do imply the need for a female symbolic in ways that continue to work with a broadly Lacanican framework even as they work against it. Likewise, taken on their own, Irigaray's appeals for different ways of *representing* both woman and the mother do not necessarily challenge an underlying division between the materiality of the body on the one hand and the linguistic and cultural forms (the representations) which give that matter meaning on the other.[44]

Nonetheless, as we have seen, for Irigaray, it will remain impossible to find adequate figurations of the female body unless we also refigure matter itself as capable of actively generating form. Thus, while Irigaray undoubtedly does call on us to recognize (and transform) the ways in which women's bodies are shaped by the social and linguistic significances they are given, crucially, her project also demands that we find social and symbolic forms in which matter's own form-giving powers are acknowledged, given value and even celebrated. This means that, alongside the quest for alternative cultural representations of woman, we also need to rework the way we represent the processes through which the body's cultural forms are produced, in order to take full account of the body's capacities to actively participate in such processes. The images of the lips and the placental economy contribute to this project, helping us conceive of an actively self-shaping matter that can bear otherness within and that is replete with form-giving powers. Such images do not just provide new representational figures for the female body; they represent the body itself as capable of generating both figure and form.

The so-called problem of Irigaray's essentialism is itself a problem of representation. On the one hand, the essentialist charge is often motivated by the concern that Irigaray's appeal to figures such as the two lips unhelpfully reinforces the (patriarchal) view that the anatomical form of women's bodies causally determines their existence and identity. The essentialist charge thereby reflects an underlying representation of the body as fixed and determined matter, so that any appeal to the specifically female body is in turn seen as 'fixing' and 'determining' women's existence. On the other hand, defending Irigaray from this charge by positioning bodies as (entirely) the product of socio-cultural forms implicitly reinscribes a representation of matter as inherently undetermined and formless. Thus, even as it foregrounds the political need for alternative representations of women, as Stone notes, such a defence 'paradoxically repeats the very devaluation of female matter which it aspires to expose and undermine at the symbolic level'.[45]

By contrast, the originality of Irigaray's approach lies in the way in which she calls for alternative representations of the female body while simultaneously calling into question how the body's form is itself determined. She challenges the dominant model in which form must be imposed on inert matter by an active ordering power, and instead asks us to rethink bodily forms as emerging through the movements of a mobile and fluid materiality. Thus, as Stone notes, Irigaray's project works towards an understanding of 'the *forms* of bodies, as well as their material composition, as fluid.'[46] This makes it hard to read her appeals to the female body as invoking any kind of fixed 'essence'.[47] On the contrary, the fluid movements of the lips, or the passage between mother and child, provide a model in which form emerges out of matter understood as an active patterning of relations. Matter is neither deadly inertia nor formless flux, neither passive receptacle nor chaotic excess. Instead, it becomes actively self-shaping in a fluid giving of forms.

Ethics and/as Poetics: Recalling Being (as) Two

Given Irigaray's rejection of the traditional (hylomorphic) form/ matter distinction, it is worth asking whether there are ways of thinking about her deployment of figures such as the two lips which position them neither as attempts to find true descriptions of the anatomical essence of the female sex, nor as alternative rep-representations or symbolic constructs that inscribe the materiality of the body with sexed significance. Irigaray's own emphasis on language as invention is helpful here. In keeping with her non-essentialist position, Irigaray is clear that there is no already present, 'essentially feminine' language of the body which women merely need to 'liberate' from masculine oppression: 'Why speak? you'll ask me. ... If we don't invent a language, if we don't find our body's

language, it will have too few gestures to accompany our story. ...
Let's hurry and invent our own phrases' (*TS*, 214–15). Thus, as
Gatens and Grosz indicate, it is not a matter of recovering the
'natural' (in the sense of biologically determined) language of the
female body which patriarchy has covered over. On the contrary,
Irigaray calls on women to *invent* the words and gestures that allow
their bodies to speak, that is, to express their distinctiveness in
ways that no longer take the male subject as norm, and that are
therefore no longer constrained by an oppositional framework that
pits self against other. What is required is not just a new way of
thinking, but 'the creation of a new *poetics*' (*ESD*, 5). The inventiveness required for such a poetics is not wholly unconstrained; rather,
given the constraints of the (phallocentric) language already in
place, we will have to be inventive if we are to find words allowing
the distinctiveness of the female body to speak.

In keeping with this, Irigaray's own writing is engaged in a
reciprocal relation with the body. Her texts draw on the sexuate
female body whose fluid movements *give* us figures for rethinking
woman as well as our representations of self and other; at the same
time, she gives meaning and significance *back* to that body, by
seeking linguistic forms that acknowledge its active and generative
powers. The relation to the body is thus primarily an ethical one:
just as we are given life by a female body that births, so that body
offers us figures for conceptualizing our existence. The question
then becomes how we take up that body and those figures in our
thought: do we return maternal generosity by giving the female
body significance, or do we appropriate these resources in ways
that do not acknowledge the mother's existence as a woman? To
put the point differently, borrowing from Irigaray's own model of
the placental economy: the female body is able to give birth because
it manifests tolerance of an other within, but western culture has
not yet returned this generosity by giving woman's bodily being
an interpretation that values its specificity. Irigaray, of course, is
seeking to be generous.

One way of thinking about the inventive generosity for which
Irigaray calls is what we might term, following Heidegger, a kind
of 'projective announcement'. While Irigaray does not, to my
knowledge, draw explicitly on this particular Heideggerian
thought,[48] this approach is in keeping with a distinctive (though
not uncritical) Heideggerian strand which runs through her work,
becoming more pronounced in some of her recent texts.[49] In the
course of his 1936 essay on the 'The Origin of the Work of Art',

Heidegger presents art as *'the becoming and happening of truth'*.[50] Truth here does not consist in describing or re-presenting some already existing thing; rather, truth establishes itself in the disclosure of a particular being, and thus takes place in 'the unconcealedness of beings' [*das Un-verborgene/Unverborgenheit*].[51] The work of art is one of the possible sites where truth can establish itself, insofar as the work allows a being to come into being *as* that being which it is. Thus, the work constitutes 'the bringing forth of a being such as never was before'.[52] At the same time, such a work also 'opens' or 'sets up' a world.[53] For Heidegger, the world is neither an object nor a set of objects, but that which allows a being to enter into relation with other beings (thus making relations between subjects, as well as between subjects and objects, possible). By 'hold[ing] open the Open of the world', the work sustains the very possibility of relationality.[54] World is that 'to which we are subject as long as the paths of birth and death, blessing and curse keep us transported into Being.'[55]

Irigaray's call for 'a new poetics' lends itself to being read on this model. In seeking to speak (as a) woman, she is seeking to open a world in which woman could appear as a sexuate subject. Such a poetics would sustain the possibility of relations between the sexes in which each would be open to the sexuate specificity of the other.[56] Approaching Irigaray through this Heideggerian lens helps show why the project of 'speaking woman' (*parler femme*) should not be positioned as an attempt to represent a pre-existing essence of woman. Instead, speaking woman is more appropriately paralleled with the Heideggerian notion of speaking Being, of letting Being speak in such a way that a being is 'brought forth' as the specific being that it is. I will return below to Heidegger's distinction between questions of Being (i.e., those that concern what it means to be) and beings (those concerning the existence of particular kinds of entities).[57] For now what is most important is that different beings come to be (or are brought forth) depending on the different ways in which Being expresses itself (or 'speaks') in and through them; and that both the artwork and language work are privileged sites of such generative speaking (what Heidegger, drawing on the Greek, calls *poiēsis*).[58] On this model, 'speaking woman' would mean finding the figures that allow woman's being to be articulated in its sexuate specificity, where 'articulation' means neither the communication of a pre-existing idea, nor the representation of a pre-existing bodily entity, but the configuration of a mode of being in a kind of 'projective announcement'. For Heidegger, 'projective announcement' is a kind of naming, where this is not a process of labelling but a creative act (i.e., *poiēsis*):

> Language, by naming beings for the first time, first brings beings to word and to appearance. Only this naming nominates beings *to* their being *from out of* their being. Such saying is a projecting of the clearing, in which announcement is made of what it is that beings come into the Open *as*. ... This projective announcement forthwith becomes a renunciation of all the dim confusion in which what is veils and withdraws itself. Projective saying is poetry.[59]

'Projective announcement' is thus a naming that allows a hitherto undetermined being to become what it is; or rather, it allows a being already over-determined with a 'dim confusion' of meanings (in the way that woman has been over-determined by patriarchy) to be 'cleared' or released from such overburdening, and to become what it (or she) is, to take up what becomes its/her own specific being. Irigaray's appeals to the female body can be understood on this model. Thus, when she writes, for example, that 'By our lips we are women' (*TS*, 209–10), this ought not to be read as a reductive reference to an anatomical essence. Nor should it be seen as a representation inscribing either already existing bodies or otherwise indeterminate matter with a significance previously lacking. A more productive approach is to read the image of two lips as a projective announcing that calls into being that which it names by calling forth a figure of woman who speaks and appears in her sexuate specificity, *as* other than the 'other' of man, and hence *as* distinctively female.[60] Such a (sexuate, female) being would be intrinsically bodily and material, rather than matter on which form has been imposed.

In ways that Irigaray takes up in her more recent work,[61] Heidegger's later texts align the generative speaking of *poiēsis* not only with the work of art but with language itself. Language allows beings to speak not insofar as it represents them as objects for a subject, but by allowing beings to show themselves in the saying of language. An example of such saying which 'shows' might be Irigaray's own trope, *parler femmes*, insofar as these words both say and show the kind of speaking – *par les femmes* – of which they speak. For Heidegger, the saying which shows is 'what brings all present and absent beings each into their own [*sein jeweilig Eigenes*], from where they show themselves in what they are, and where they abide according to their kind.'[62] Similarly, Irigaray is seeking a way of speaking which allows woman to come into her own, and to abide in a world where she belongs to a distinctively female kind or (to use Irigaray's word) *genre*.

The notion of being 'brought into one's own' in play here implies an active appropriation of one's own mode of being: 'Appropriation (*Das Ereignis*) grants to mortals their abode within their nature, so that they may be capable of being those who speak.'[63] As Heidegger's original German makes clear, 'appropriation' here involves neither taking up an already existing identity nor appropriating the other as one's own; rather, being brought into one's own (*sein Eigenes*) is a happening or event – *das Ereignis* – through which one comes into being as the being that one is. It is this sense of appropriation which Irigaray invokes when she writes of cultivating a 'proper' or 'appropriate' relation to one's own sexuate kind (or *genre*): in so doing, she does not mean finding adequate representations of a pre-given essence or identity, but actively generating the cultural forms which allow men and women to be brought into being – to be articulated – as sexuate subjects. Nonetheless, it is important to distinguish appropriation in this sense, as taking up a relation to one's own sexuate being, from the negative sense in which this term is more often encountered in Irigaray's work, where it denotes the appropriation of the other. Becoming the being that one is can all too easily become appropriative in this second, negative sense, if identity is premised on the exclusion of the other whose difference is denied and who is instead turned into another version of oneself.

In her extensive dialogue with Heidegger, Irigaray suggests that such appropriative relations to the other still haunt his own thinking despite the radical challenge he poses to western metaphysics.[64] By locating being in the 'house of language',[65] Heidegger forgets our more originary dwelling within the body of the mother.[66] Thus, despite his recuperation of both earth and world from representational and hylomorphic modes of thinking, Heidegger continues to forget the air which makes speaking possible, the air which the mother breathes for the foetus in the originary relation that brings us into being and allows us to speak.[67] If '[t]he way to speaking is present within language itself',[68] we need to find ways of allowing language to speak of our debt to the mother, to the specifically *female* body that brings us into the world, and hence, into language. Irigaray thus reminds us that the horizon of Being is not death (as it is not only for Heidegger, but for much of western philosophy), but birth.[69] If for Heidegger, 'Appropriation grants to mortals their abode within their nature, so that they may be capable of being those who speak',[70] for Irigaray, appropriation – understood as the active cultivation of a relation to both our maternal origins and our sexuate being – grants to *natals* an abode within our nature, and makes it possible for there to be beings capable of speaking *as women*.

Heidegger's thinking provides Irigaray with a set of openings towards a sexuate philosophy, as signalled by the parallel she draws between Heidegger's analysis of the forgetting of Being and her own concern with the forgetting of sexual difference: 'Sexual difference is one of the major philosophical issues, if not *the* issue, of our age. According to Heidegger, each age has one issue to think through, and one only. Sexual difference is probably the issue in our time which could be our "salvation" if we thought it through' (*ESD*, 5; my emphasis). Nonetheless, even as she draws on such productive resonances, Irigaray remains critical of Heidegger. For if, according to Heidegger, western metaphysics has forgotten its own forgetting of Being, Heidegger himself, according to Irigaray, perpetuates a more fundamental act of dereliction: the forgetting of Being as two, the forgetting of the originary and ontological status of sexual difference. This difference means that, rather than a particular instantiation of a neutral and univocal Being, each unique being, in its gendered embodiment, is a singular and *sexuate* incarnation of Being as two. Unless we recall Being as two, the possibilities for relating – to ourselves, to others, and to the world – which language shows or announces will remain appropriative in ways that never allow us to come into our own as the sexuate beings we are. Thus, in seeking to allow Being to speak, what Heidegger forgets is the ethical demand that Being makes on us to find ways of allowing 'being two' to be heard, that is, ways of speaking that are attentive to sexuate difference.[71] Irigaray's project is to reorient us towards this ethical demand and to recall us to a Being that is irreducibly two.

The Sexuate, the Sexual, and the Heterosexist

The 'two' of sexuate difference, alongside an increased emphasis on relations between the sexes, has led some critics to see Irigaray's later work as reinscribing a normative heterosexism. This concern is encapsulated in Judith Butler's comment that Irigaray's later writings display 'a kind of presumptive heterosexuality' which turns heterosexuality 'into the privileged locus of ethics, as if heterosexual relations, because they putatively crossed this alterity, which is the alterity of sexual difference, were somehow more ethical, more other-directed, less narcissistic than anything else.'[72] Butler is one of Irigaray's most important contemporary interlocutors.[73] Her comments reflect a more general concern that has arisen among queer theorists in particular that a focus on sexual difference inevitably 'privileges heterosexuality over other sexualities'.[74]

Butler's specific comments on Irigaray were made in the course of an important interview discussion with Pheng Cheah, Drucilla Cornell and Elizabeth Grosz. This discussion reveals both the significance of Irigaray's work for contemporary feminist thinkers and the contestation to which it gives rise around a number of key issues. As the interview shows, the charge of heterosexism is itself contested and is often made with a sense of disappointment: by turning increasingly to the need to rework the relation between the sexes as part of the project of cultivating being (as) two, Irigaray's later writings seem to pull back from the radicality of her earlier work. In particular, she seems to have betrayed her earlier call for a language allowing woman, 'the object', to speak – and above all to speak *as* a woman without being defined in relation to the male subject – and to have refocused the question of difference in terms that make women's relations to men central all over again.

Irigaray does sometimes make comments in her later writings which seem to give heterosexual relations a certain kind of privilege: these comments are problematic not only in themselves, but because they are out of keeping with the philosophy of sexuate difference that her work unfolds. Thus, in what follows, I will argue that we need to hold the notion of sexuate difference apart from both heterosexual relations and from sexual difference where this is understood as a question of sexual orientation. It is sexuate difference, not heterosexuality, which has ontological (and, as we will see in the next chapter, ethical) priority in Irigaray's thought. This priority raises questions of its own, particularly with regard to the relation between sexuate difference and race, to which I will also return in the next chapter. However, here I want to show why I think the charge of heterosexism is misplaced insofar as Irigaray's notion of sexuate difference is not necessarily or inherently heterosexist. I will do so partly by insisting on the continuity between her earlier and later texts and the importance of reading the latter firmly in light of the former. Broadly speaking, I agree with Gail

Schwab on this issue when she notes that 'what Irigaray is talking about is not *heterosexuality*, but *sexual difference*', and that this is 'not at all the same thing'.[75] Nonetheless, I think there are important lessons to be learned from this debate, partly because responding to it helps clarify some key aspects of Irigaray's thought; and partly because it serves as a humbling reminder of the risks we inevitably take – of generating new exclusions, or inadvertently reinforcing old blindspots – whenever we seek to address questions of difference.

In some ways, the attention which Irigaray pays to heterosexual relations throughout her work is completely understandable, and indeed, necessary. Precisely because heterosexual relations have operated as the most intense (and destructive) site for the reproduction of patriarchal norms, it is not only legitimate but imperative that we make every effort to reframe these relations in terms of an encounter between two (sexuate) subjects, instead of one (male) subject and his 'other'.[76] Thus, while criticizing what she sees as an (unnecessary) hardening of the sexuate into more fixed (heterosexual) relations in some of Irigaray's later writings, Penelope Deutscher observes that:

> Irigaray's ideal for the reconstruction of relations between the sexes should not be decontextualized. Because the feminine has been accorded the position of lack and atrophy in relation to the masculine, she considers that male–female relations must be reconceived as a cultural imperative. The imperative for this reshaping derives from this historical context, rather than from a global privileging of heterosexual and heterosocial interrelations in an Irigarayan politics.[77]

The claim that Irigaray goes beyond reframing male–female relations in non-oppressive ways, to become oppressively heterosexist herself, is not only troubling but surprising, given that, as Grosz notes, Irigaray's work repeatedly affirms 'the necessity of women exploring their sexualities, bodies, and desires through their corporeal and affective relations with other women.'[78] Such an affirmation is found in Irigaray's response to Freud on female homosexuality: 'what exhilarating pleasure it is to be partnered with someone like oneself. With a sister, in everyday terms. What need, attraction, passion, one feels for someone, for some woman, like oneself' (*S*, 103). This positive emphasis on relations between women continues throughout her later works, including those most associated with the heterosexist charge: in *I love to you*, for example, Irigaray foregrounds the urgency of articulating 'woman's relationship to herself, women's relationships among themselves, and especially the relationship between mother and daughter' (66). As we have seen, the cultivation of such relations is vital to effect a shift from a horizon in which women are reduced to the 'other' of the male subject (and hence to the other of the Same), to one in which they can see themselves as similar yet different to other women, and hence as belonging to their sex without losing their singularity.

Perhaps the most famous essay in which Irigaray explores such female–female relations is 'When Our Lips Speak Together', examined earlier in this chapter. Of all Irigaray's works, this is the one that is usually seen as the most explicit celebration of erotic relations between women. In its images of sensuous touch and 'two lips kissing two lips', its rhetoric affirms the fecundity of lesbian pleasure and desire (*TS*, 210). Nonetheless, as indicated above, I would still read this essay in terms of a more general affirmation of female auto-affection, and hence as primarily concerned with woman's relation to her own sex: whether that sex is manifest in her own body, that of the mother, or the loving bodies of other women. While these bodies are always uniquely different from one another, what matters here is that a woman can take up a relation to her own sex – to the many different ways of being female – without having to define herself against a male norm. Thus, Irigaray seeks figures for a distinctive female morphology while recognizing that no two women will embody that morphology in exactly the same way.[79] The affirmation of lesbian erotics takes place within this wider project of forging figures for an autonomous female subjectivity and desire. Conversely, such a figuring of female specificity is essential for erotic relations between women to be articulated in ways that do not involve mimicking the heterosexual norms that have hitherto been governed by *male* subjectivity and desire. As Grosz puts it, Irigaray's explorations of female intimacy imply 'the possibility of women loving each other as women, not as male substitutes'.[80]

This brings us to a crucial point brought out by Grosz's essay, 'The Hetero and the Homo: the Sexual Ethics of Luce Irigaray'.[81] For Irigaray, our existing culture is not hetero-normative: on the contrary, the problem is that the hetero-geneity of hetero-sexual relations has yet to be adequately thought. Instead, male–female relations are firmly embedded in a hom(m)osocial order that takes

the male subject (*l'homme*) as norm and ideal. As Whitford
sums up, pointing to a critical difference between Irigaray and
Butler, 'what Judith Butler identifies as a heterosexual matrix,
Irigaray sees as a patriarchal hom(m)osexuality'.[82] And as Irigaray
herself notes, 'it's essential not to confuse ... this ideological and
cultural *hom(m)osexualité* with the practice of homosexuality'.[83]

As we have seen in previous chapters, for Irigaray, western
culture is typified by the ways in which woman's 'otherness' is
recognized not in terms of an autonomous female specificity but
only insofar as she is 'other' to the male subject, reducing her to an
other of the Same. This hom(m)osocial order is of course not
particularly welcoming of male homosexuality – as Grosz notes,
from an Irigarayan perspective: 'the oppression of gay men may
well be a consequence of the male homosexual openly avowing
what is in fact implicit, and a social norm, for all patriarchal forms
of exchange. The male homosexual says and does what remains
unspoken, a disavowed condition of social functioning.'[84] But
within a hom(m)osocial culture, the position of the lesbian is doubly
disavowed: not only because she breaks with the patriarchal norms
which define women according to their sexual and reproductive
relations with men, but because this culture lacks the resources to
articulate women's love for other women in terms of their female
specificity (see *S*, 101–4).

Insofar as the call for a culture of two is a call for women to be
recognized as subjects in their own terms, it is the condition for
women to love one another *as* women – whether this involves
lesbian eroticism, sisterly friendships, collegial support, or mother-
daughter relations. Cultivating the difference between the sexes
makes it possible for there to be female/female relations that are
not based on male/female ones. This is why it is crucial to read
Irigaray's later work on relations between the sexes in terms of her
earlier and primary demand for the cultural recognition of female
autonomy and specificity. For Irigaray, the possibility of any positive relation *between* the sexes – where 'positive' implies a relation
which allows for genuine difference between them – is conditional
upon woman finding the terms with which to relate to herself and
to articulate her (female) specificity in ways that no longer define
her against man. As Whitford summarizes: 'For exchange to take
place between the two terms of sexual difference, there must first
be two terms.'[85] Irigaray's later investigations into the question of
how two sexuate subjects might listen and speak to each other are
thus centrally informed by the answers she has already begun to

develop to her earlier question, 'what if the "object" [woman] started to speak?' Far from reinscribing an existing heterosexual norm, Irigaray's demand for a culture of two seeks to displace an existing hom(m)osociality in favour of a heterosexuality (and het- erosociality) that has not yet existed, and that would allow for two, different but non-opposed, subjects. Such a culture would make space for the heterogeneity of female and male homosexuality, such that both could be cultivated without either being modelled on the other, and without either coming to constitute the violently repressed 'other' that is always required when one subject seeks to attain the status of the universal.

A further key point which needs to be added here is that, as others have noted, for Irigaray, the sexuate is not the same as the sexual,[86] where the latter is understood as referring to one's sexual 'object' choice (and which Irigaray is seeking to reconfigure as erotic relations between desiring *subjects*). Thus she insists that: 'it's important not to confuse sexual choice with sexual difference. For me sexual difference is a fundamental parameter of the socio-cul- tural order; sexual choice is secondary. Even if one chooses to remain among women, it's necessary to resolve the problem of sexual difference. And likewise if one remains among men.'[87] By prioritizing our existence as sexual (in the sense of *sexuate*) subjects, Irigaray is in no way seeking to prescribe our *sexuality*, that is, whether we are hetero-/homo-/bi-sexual, though a philosophy of being as two would require a rethinking of all of these categories (as well as their intersections with transgendered, transsexual, and intersexed individuals). As we have seen, there are a number of texts in which Irigaray does focus specifically on refiguring woman's sexuality; but as we have also seen, this refiguring of woman's pleasure is never separable from the wider project of rethinking woman's relation to herself as well as the processes through which she is constituted as a woman, that is, as a sexuate female subject. Irigaray's main concern is not with sexual orienta- tion, but with releasing woman from the phallocentric tradition in which all modes of sexuality are defined in relation to one and the same sex. A culture of two sexuate (male and female) subjects leaves it entirely open what the sexual preferences of these subjects might be – as long as they are no longer modelled in ways that take a male body and subject as the universal norm.

Thus, while one way in which sexuate subjects can relate to one another is in sexual (i.e. erotic) relations, the call for a culture of sexual – in the sense of sexuate – difference is much broader than

this and involves the recognition of two different kinds of beings
– male and female – regardless of their sexual preferences. As Heidi
Bostic argues, one of the reasons Irigaray's project is sometimes
misconstrued is because of 'a misunderstanding of this privileging
of the relation between men and women':

> Nowhere does Luce Irigaray make the claim that someone of the
> other sex must be my life partner. Love between men and women
> need not mean a sexual relationship. ... In fact, Irigaray encourages
> us to theorize love 'within social relations and with cultural media-
> tions' instead of simply within the 'immediacy' of genital sex. ...
> Irigaray suggests that we all, regardless of sexual orientation, must
> learn to love across the lines of gender in order to build a new social
> order.[88]

While I think that the privileging of the male–female couple in texts
such as *I love to you* is sometimes more problematic than this suggests, nonetheless, I agree with Bostic that Irigaray situates the
necessity of reworking the male–female relation within a much
wider project. The relations between men and women that need to
be transformed are not merely sexual, but also civic, legal, cultural,
familial, political and professional. For this to happen, the relations
between public and private, particular and universal, nature and
culture will also need to be transformed: for men and – differently
– for women. Only then will women be able to participate actively
in a social order in which they are fully recognized as both desiring
and political subjects.

Gender/Genre and the Ontological Status of
Sexuate Difference

To appreciate the kind of transformation Irigaray has in mind, we
need to examine her notion of 'genre' and its relation to sexuate
difference. First, however, it is worth clarifying further the notion
of the 'sexuate', to see why sexuate difference is neither simply
biological nor sexual, though it is certainly manifested in bodily
relations and thus always inflects our sexual encounters. In the
previous section, I suggested that attending to sexuate difference
means recognizing two different kinds of *beings*. This is why Irigaray refers to sexuate difference as 'ontological': ontology traditionally refers to the study of being (from the Greek, *ontos*). Irigaray

deploys this term in its Heideggerian sense where it is contrasted with 'ontic'. As Michael Gelven puts it: 'An inquiry about what it means to be is called "ontological", whereas an inquiry about an entity is called "ontic".'[89] Thus, Heidegger's distinction between Being and beings draws our attention to the way that '[B]eing – the sheer fact that there is (es gibt) existence, that existence unfathomably surges up – is not itself an entity'.[90] From this perspective, sexual preferences are 'ontic': specific features of a particular individual's way of being in the world. But sexuate difference is 'ontological': it concerns the way Being 'surges up' such that we come to be.

For Heidegger, the history of western thought has concentrated on identifying human beings as subjects of knowledge over against a world of objects, thereby forgetting to ask the more elusive question about the nature of Being itself, and our relation to it. In so doing, it has forgotten 'the ontological difference or the relation between Being and beings'.[91] This difference cannot be directly approached because, while Being is not reducible to any particular being (i.e. existing entity), nonetheless, we never encounter Being as such – it is only revealed to us in and through particular beings in the world. Being allows each of these beings to be, but only by withdrawing so as to allow their particular way of being to emerge. For the Heidegger of Being and Time, what is special about the kind of being that human beings are (Dasein) is that this kind of entity is thrown (geworfen) into the world in such a way that it is uniquely capable of asking the question of its own being (its being-here, its Da-sein) and hence, of raising ontological questions about what it means to be – about Being as such, rather than just about particular entities.[92]

As we have seen, Irigaray's claim is that, despite reminding us of our capacity to ask such questions, Heidegger himself perpetuates a fundamental act of 'forgetting' by forgetting that Being is two. At this point, it is helpful to remember that the ontological difference for Heidegger concerns a relation between Being and beings. This is important because it helps us to see that when Irigaray claims that sexuate difference is ontological, she does not mean it is anything like an essence: sexuate difference is not a special kind of substance (biological or otherwise) that makes some beings men and others women. Heidegger himself reminds us that questions about substance and essence are questions about what something is and how it exists as the specific kind of being that it is, rather than about its coming to be and hence its relation to Being as such.[93] So, for Irigaray sexuate difference is ontological insofar as it concerns an originary *relation*: if Heidegger asks us to recall the ontological difference between Being and beings, Irigaray asks to remember that the relation between Being and beings unfolds in two different ways, disclosed in our differing relations to the mother through whom we are brought into being: for in being born of a mother who is also a woman, each of us is born from someone either of the same or of a different sex to ourselves.[94]

The sexuate being disclosed in our originary relations to the body of the mother is increasingly emphasized by Irigaray in her later works, as the following passage from *Between East and West* illustrates:

> The subjectivity of man and that of woman are structured starting from a *relational identity* specific to each one ... This specific relational identity ... is based on different irreducible givens: the woman is born of a woman, of someone of her gender, the man is born of someone from another gender than himself ... The first relational situation is thus very different for the girl and the boy. And they build their relation to the other in a very different way. (*BEW*, 129)[95]

This passage attests to Irigaray's commitment to thinking two sexuate subjects whose constitution (or possibilities of being-in-the-world, to put it in more Heideggerian terms) begins with their differing relations to the mother, which in turn engender different ways of relating to the other. Each of these relations brings its own distinctive risks of appropriation and loss. For the girl, the originary relation to the other is non-agonistic insofar as a female child and her mother share the same sex;[96] thus the challenge for the girl will be to develop a sufficiently differentiated sense of self, while at the same time cultivating a relation to the different other of the male subject without losing a constitutive relation to her own sex. For the boy, born of someone of a different sex, the risk is of becoming locked in agonistic relations that tend to reinforce an oppositional and appropriative approach to others, rather than developing appropriate relations to himself (as a natal, and hence sexuate and singular being). Thus, if there is to be a non-appropriative relation between the sexes, the subjectivity of each must be articulated in its own terms. A 'double subjectivity, a double "being-I" ' is required (*BEW*, 98).

The ontological status of sexuate difference reinforces the point that Irigaray is not a biological essentialist: far from arguing that our biology determines our existence, Irigaray's position implies that sexuate difference is expressed in our bodies because it is a fundamental condition of our being. As Stone succinctly puts it, for Irigaray sexual (in the sense of sexuate) difference is 'a difference in *being*, not in biology.'[97] Moreover, if we are transported into being through birth, then it is our originary relation to the mother which makes relations to other beings possible; thus if, for Heidegger, the world is that openness which makes relationality possible, for Irigaray, relationality is made possible by our originary, sexuate relations with the mother who brings us into the world. Nonetheless, the sexuate Being disclosed in human beings' originary relations to the mother is not on its own enough to secure a culture of sexuate difference in which the 'double being-I' of two sexuate subjects would be fostered and sustained. For this to happen, we need to take up an active relation to these originary sexuate relations, which need to be cultivated so as to allow each sex to develop ways of relating to others to whom they are similar (with whom they share a sex) as well as others of a different sex. Sexuate difference needs to be elaborated into a *genre*: a style or mode of being which elaborates the sexuate difference implicit in male and female infants' differing relations to the mother.[98]

As an active elaboration of these originary relations of similarity and difference, Irigaray's notion of '*genre*' is neither a simple expression of our biology, nor a wholly socio-cultural construction imposed on blankly malleable bodies (and hence in some sense entirely arbitrary). *Genre* is neither a matter of 'natural immediacy' nor a 'simple projection' (*ILTY*, 39). Thus, in response to the question of whether gender is an effect of biology ('nature') or social conditioning ('nurture'), Irigaray argues that posing the issue in these dichotomous terms 'fails to take into account the fact that being or becoming a woman means acquiring a civil dimension which is appropriate to "feminine identity", a culture which corresponds to one's own body and specific genealogy, one's own way of loving and of procreating, of desiring and of thinking' (*DBT*, 36–7). *Genre* is a question of how we take up our originally sexuate relations to the mother by elaborating modes of being that involve more or less affirmative, more or less destructive relations to our own sex as well as those who belong to a different sex (whose being is articulated in a different *genre*).[99]

To elucidate Irigaray's concept of *genre*, it is worth returning briefly to her relation to Heidegger. For Heidegger, an authentic mode of existence, that is, one characterized by the fullest inhabiting of what it means to be, involves taking up an active relation to the possibility of one's not-being and appropriating the (always ungraspable) possibility of one's own death *as* one's own in what he calls 'being-towards-death'.[100] However, as we have seen, Irigaray's sexuate ontology takes birth, rather than death, as the horizon of Being, as reflected in her comment that: 'Although life, obviously, is always sexed, death on the contrary no longer makes this distinction' (*DBT*, 37). Within this horizon, we need to take up an active relation to the sexuate being that is disclosed in our own birth, and in particular in our relation to the mother from whom we are born. Irigaray thus describes the active appropriation of our own sexuate possibilities in terms of *genre* as something to be accomplished. This accomplishment depends both on 'becom[ing] aware of *being* a woman or a man, and *wanting to become* one' (*ILTY*, 39; my emphasis). Thus whereas de Beauvoir famously claimed that 'one is not born, but becomes a woman', Irigaray is concerned with how a woman can become the woman she is by birth.[101] To be a woman by birth is to be born into a particular relation to the body of the mother; to become a woman means elaborating the terms for a female *genre* that (among other things) makes it possible for a daughter to take up an active relation to her mother *as* a woman, and thereby to take up a positive relation to her own sex.

Like de Beauvoir, Irigaray thinks of the process of becoming as a 'project', thereby insisting that women are not tied to immanence in the sense of being passively determined by their bodies (locked into 'natural immediacy'). And like de Beauvoir, Irigaray seeks a process of becoming which would release woman from being the 'Other' for a male subject. However, unlike de Beauvoir, for Irigaray this process does not involve overcoming the female body,[102] but on the contrary, cultivating women's bodily being into ways of acting, living, and relating to others that do not deny her sexuate specificity. To articulate that specificity, what is required is the poetic inventiveness outlined above. The 'project-ive naming' of the two lips is one way of cultivating a female *genre*. Another is found in the propositional expressions that allow us to articulate relations between two subjects rather than subject and object, as in Irigaray's translation of 'I love you' into 'I love *to* you'.[103] Other possibilities are found in the generative erotic relations – released from the imperative of reproduction – recovered from Diotima's speech, as well as the cultivation of breath, as outlined at the end of Chapter 4. The latter examples show that, in keeping with

Irigaray's view of the body as active and generative matter, the transcendence involved in cultivating a female subject would consist not in freeing oneself from matter, but in materially embodied becomings that cultivate the active matter that we are. Thus, for woman to elaborate her own *genre* involves a constant movement between origin and horizon: between her originary relation to her mother, as an other of the same sex, and the projection of modes of being which elaborate a positive relation to this sex, and allow her to relate to the mother (and herself) as a woman.

The necessity of a sexuate 'horizon' is taken up in Irigaray's writings on the divine: by affirming the value of woman's sexuate being, a female divine operates as a horizon orienting women in relation to the positive value of being female. Between the body of the mother in which their being begins, and the affirmative space opened up by such a horizon, women can elaborate ways of living that nurture and cultivate their sexuate being. In keeping with Irigaray's writings on *genre*, a female divine would not transcend the material world. Instead it stands for the spiritual value of woman's sexuate materiality, and for a horizon located not at the border with some other-worldly realm, but within every woman insofar as she is able to affirm and cultivate the value of her own sex. It is in this sense that a 'female divine' engenders 'divine women'.[104]

By linking together notions of transcendence (understood as embodied becoming) and infinity, the divine also helps us see why the process of becoming a subject would be necessarily different for each sex: insofar as a woman is of the same sex as her mother, and hence, can relate to the sex that gives birth as her own (whether she herself gives birth or not), she is able to situate herself within a mode of being that is capable of becoming other to itself (transcending) by bearing otherness within through the processes of pregnancy and generation. Such processes are one way of realizing the notion of the in-finite which Irigaray recovers from Diotima's speech, as an infinity of becomings folded into finite life. Insofar as men have a different relation to the body that births, being of a different sex, their relation to this infinity of becomings will need to be taken up in a different way. To negotiate the passage of becoming a subject, each sex will have to negotiate the relations between finite and infinite, matter and spirit; to do so without neglecting their sexuate specificity, each sex will have to negotiate these relations differently.

Displacing (Hetero)Sexism through the Sexuate

To conclude this chapter, I wish to return once more to the issue of Irigaray's purported heterosexism in light of the above discussion of the ontological status of sexuate difference. As should by now be clear, sexuate difference for Irigaray is not a matter of our sexual preferences, but of the ontological difference between men and women disclosed in their differing relations to the mother who gave birth to them. These dissymmetrical *relations* manifest the alterity between the sexes, not a simple opposition between 'men' and 'women': indeed, the originary relation to the mother determines only that some are of the same sex, others of a different sex to her. This is not, on its own, enough to determine the full meaning of what 'men' and 'women' might be or become. But if this alterity is to be preserved, the sexuate specificity of each sex needs to be elaborated on its own terms, in ways taking their differing originary relations to the mother as a starting point; neither should be defined in terms of, or by means of opposition to, the other. Within a culture that has only fully elaborated the journey to selfhood in terms of the male subject, the most urgent task in this regard is to cultivate the female *genre* allowing women to accede to the status of subjects in their own right, without sacrificing their sexuate specificity. This specificity can and indeed needs to be cultivated in female/female relations just as much as female/male ones. Sexuate difference does not mean the difference of one sex *from* the other; rather, it means acknowledging the existence of two different modes of being, each of which faces different challenges in traversing the passage to mature subjectivity.

Once understood in these terms, it does not make sense to think of sexuate difference as either 'more' or 'less' present in relations between two women than in relations between a man and a woman (whether sexual, in the sense of erotic, or not). Relations between women are just as 'sexuate' as those between women and men. Both female/female and male/female relations need to be cultivated in ways that recognize sexuate difference as it is expressed in the sexuate specificity of each and every human being. It is true that, on Irigaray's model, there is an irreducible difference or alterity *between* men and women of a different kind to that found between those who belong to the same sex. However, Irigaray makes it clear first, that this alterity is expressed (and needs to be cultivated) in all relations between men and women, including but not just sexual (erotic) relations; and second, that the positive cultivation of this alterity is dependent on each sex being recognized and cultivated in its own terms. Such cultivation is no less a feature of homosexual erotic relations than heterosexual ones. Finally, Irigaray also repeatedly affirms the irreplaceable singularity of each human being which is itself rooted in the singular event of their birth: as we have seen in her reading of Plato, it is because of our originary relation to the mother that we are constituted '(as) an original' (S, 293). In keeping with this, her later work emphasizes that the cultivation of a *genre* appropriate to the sexuate being we are by birth remains a task 'for each person in his or her own unique singularity' (*ILTY*, 27). Thus, the existence of a different kind of alterity *between* the sexes does not mean that those of the *same* sex are any less irreducible to one another.

It might be thought that the emphasis on birth as safeguarding both sexuate difference and singularity itself leads to an inevitable privileging of the male–female couple involved in generation: but again, this is not as simple as it might seem. While Irigaray does insist that generation depends on two – on 'sexual difference meant as the dissymmetry between the sexes'[105] – she is also clear that neither woman nor the generative relation between the sexes should be reduced to a merely reproductive function (as we saw in her analysis of Diotima's speech). Moreover, as Pheng Cheah observes, our connection to this generative power of sexuate difference does not depend on our own involvement as adults in either heterosexual relations or reproduction:

> [Irigaray] suggests that we need to affirm and tap into the generative power of the interval of sexual difference because, for her, this is the source or necessary condition of possibility of our being. At this very general level, her argument is not heterosexist. If I could phrase it this way, she seems to be saying, 'we may not all be mothers and fathers, but all of us have been children once. And until the cloning of humans is successful, in order for us to be born, in order for us to *be*, there must be two sexes or at least the genetic material from two sexes.' ... this is the trace of the other in us, the constitutive trace of sexual alterity.[106]

Thus, Cheah also emphasizes that Irigaray's position 'is not phrased in terms of sexual preferences at all or different configurations of child-rearing and sexuality in different cultures or racial communities'.[107] Through both cultural differences and technological developments, the relations between men and women necessary for birth and generation can take place in many different ways: such relations can, and should, be acknowledged and valued without having to be mapped onto the form of the male/female couple – even the radically re-imagined couple which Irigaray seeks.

Putting all of this together, I would argue that Irigaray's philosophy of sexuate difference does not necessarily imply that heterosexual relations have any kind of ontological or ethical priority. And yet: there are places where Irigaray does seem to privilege the heterosexual couple as a site where difference is manifest and can be cultivated, over and above both other kinds of relations between men and women, and other kinds of (same sex) erotic relation, such as where she writes that:

> Sexual desire demands a realization appropriate to its matter, its nature. This realization takes place in the body proper and in the couple that man forms with the other sex – woman. This couple forms the elementary social community. It is where sensible desire must become potentially universal culture, where the gender of the man and of the woman may become the model of male human kind or of female human kind while keeping to the singular task of being *this* man or *this* woman. (*ILTY*, 28)

Despite emphasizing singularity, this passage does seem to accord heterosexual relations a privileged status, as a potential 'model' for not only sexuate but social relations generally. That male and female *genres* do need to be elaborated within the context of heterosexual relations is undoubtedly an urgent task; but for the reasons outlined above, Irigaray's notion of sexuate difference neither requires nor legitimates making heterosexual relations the site where these *genres* are elaborated in an *exemplary* way. As Deutscher notes, there is a significant difference between wishing to create 'alternative possibilities' for heterosexuality and taking heterosexuality as 'the privileged emblem' of what the open space of sexual difference could be.[108] It is this privileging which understandably troubles some of Irigaray's interlocutors, insofar as it seems to make same-sex relations the excluded 'other' of Irigaray's later writings. Such concerns are reinforced by the following passage:

> [W]hat part of life, of love and truth is left to one side when relations stop at relations between those who are alike? How then to maintain the two? ... No doubt some features distinguish those who are the same at a sexuate level, but that often blind attraction determined by sexuate difference no longer exists between them, an attraction

which often becomes destructive for lack of cultivation of its transcendental dimension. A transcendence, then, which not only stays
beyond and outside ourselves and to which we ought to submit our
desire, but rather that the desire for the different other can awaken
in ourselves.[109]

This passage occludes the way that sexuate difference exists not
only *between* the sexes, but also as a positive expression of female
specificity.

It is uncharacteristically dismissive of differences and desires
between those of the same sex, and out of keeping with many other
passages in which Irigaray emphasizes the importance of other
kinds of difference alongside sexuate difference. Indeed, for reasons
I will explore in the next chapter, the cultivation of sexuate difference is crucial according to Irigaray *because* it is the condition for
properly valuing other differences. This passage also runs against
the strong emphasis on the irreplaceable singularity of each human
being to be found throughout Irigaray's work, as noted above. Such
singularity means that 'the different other' can be found in the
unique and singular being of another of the same sex as myself, as
well as in someone of the other sex.

Thus, when Irigaray does seem to privilege heterosexual relations in an unwarranted way, I would argue that her own thinking
about sexuate difference has given us some of the strongest
resources for questioning and displacing such privilege.[110] Some
readers have suggested that the problem is not so much with what
Irigaray *does* say about heterosexual relations as what she *does not*
say about homosexual ones. On the more generous version of this
view, although some of Irigaray's texts do seem to occlude the
value of homosexual relations, this lacuna can be filled in by other
readers, who can write Irigaray's notion of sexuate difference into
accounts of 'queer' or homosexual desire – or indeed, 'any human
relationship that seeks to move beyond the model of domination
and appropriation, toward love and respect in difference.'[111] Some
have already begun to undertake this project: thus, while Sarah
Cooper expresses concerns about the 'excluded others' of Irigaray's
own theorizing, she nonetheless finds in Irigaray's thought the
resources for a 'queering of sexual identity' which 'may influence
readers to perform queer readings of texts (by Irigaray and others)
whose desires appear to be more straightforward.'[112] While I appreciate the ethics of generosity that underpins such readings, I am
not sure that this is quite enough: Irigaray herself is one of the
thinkers who has taught us how the tradition has excluded women

through its choice of examples and images, regardless of its (sometimes) good intentions of affirming inclusiveness or difference. Along parallel lines, the sometimes alienating effect of the (relative) absence of attention to the specific value of homosexual relations in Irigaray's later texts is problematic (particularly perhaps with regard to lesbian relations, which one might think would have a particularly important role to play in the cultivation of female subjectivity). We cannot write for or as everywoman (or man), but Irigaray herself has taught us the importance of writing in ways that manifest our own specificity *and* hold open passages to other modes of being, without seeking either to exclude or to appropriate them.

The centrality of an ethics of *non*-appropriation to Irigaray's thinking has already been indicated in her reading of Descartes on wonder. It will be examined in more depth in the next chapter, in the context of her readings of Hegel and Levinas, and her development of an ethics of sexuate difference. In this chapter, I hope to have laid the ground for approaching these issues by showing how Irigaray's notion of *sexuate* difference should be equated neither with the *sexual*, understood as a matter of sexual orientation, nor with the heterosexual. If, as Irigaray claims, an ethics of sexuate difference is the condition for ethics in general, this cannot be on the basis of a generalization from sexual – in the sense of erotic – relations (heterosexual or otherwise), but because unless we recognize the ontological difference between men and women, we will continue to inscribe a model of sameness even where we try to attend to other kinds of differences. I also hope to have shown why the sexuate is not simply a matter of biological sex, and how Irigaray's notion of *genre* differs from the model of gender as cultural construction. Instead, Irigaray's position involves what we might call a *relational* ontology, for at least two reasons: first, because female specificity is cultivated in terms of contiguous relations capable of bearing otherness within rather than a split dividing self from other; and second, because sexuate difference is ontological insofar as it concerns the originary difference between men and women manifest in their differing relations to the body of the mother. It is to the ethical implications of this relational ontology that we will now turn.

7

An Ethics of Sexuate Difference

In the previous chapter, I argued that Irigaray's philosophy of sexuate difference does not entail that ethical priority must necessarily be given to heterosexual relations. Nonetheless, it remains the case that sexuate difference itself *does* hold both ontological and ethical priority for Irigaray. Her unambiguous statements on this point have led to concerns about the way in which she privileges sexuate difference over other kinds of difference, including race. This chapter will examine those concerns, as well as the implications of Irigaray's position on sexuate difference for the ways in which we might approach other kinds of difference. As we will see, for Irigaray, an ethics of sexuate difference is the necessary condition for ethical relations in general.

To understand why Irigaray makes this claim, we need to attend to her critical dialogue with Levinas around the notion of 'alterity', or the irreducible otherness of the other. Before doing so, however, we will return to *Speculum* once more, this time focusing on Irigaray's reading of Hegel, as this frames her approach to the ethical and helps open the way towards both an ethics of sexuate difference and an appeal for sexuate civil rights. While Irigaray does engage with the specific details of Hegel's writings on woman and the ethical, she also positions him as representative of the western tradition, insofar as woman has typically been excluded from the status of a fully fledged ethical subject. As with her reading of Freud, Irigaray treats Hegel as in some ways offering an acute analysis of this exclusionary logic: just as Freud shows that subjectivity takes shape through sexuate relations, so Hegel helps us to see how the relation between the sexes is a privileged site for the historical unfolding of both ethics and citizenship. But Hegel, like Freud, is also seen as insufficiently critical of the processes he diagnoses, and as legitimating women's subordination as both moral subjects and potential citizens by inscribing it as historical necessity. If Heidegger forgets to think Being as two, Hegel fails to consider what it might mean for women to enter history – and ethics – as fully fledged subjects themselves.

Irigaray and Antigone: Disrupting a Hegelian Dream

As we have seen throughout this book, Irigaray argues that western thought and culture has silenced sexuate difference. Even when philosophy seems to speak of this difference and to accord it an ethical status, woman has been trapped back into a logic of the same that denies her sexuate specificity. As Irigaray shows, this is the trap that characterizes Hegel's account of the ethical, which seems to accord woman a privileged role in the figure of Sophocles' Antigone. Yet as Irigaray and others have observed, in the end Hegel does not escape the logic of the original drama in which Antigone is walled up alive.[1]

In Sophocles' play, Antigone buries her dead brother Polyneices, against the explicit edict of the King, Creon. For Creon, Polyneices is a traitor and his body is to be left to rot outside the city walls. For Antigone, he is an irreplaceable brother who should be accorded the appropriate funeral rites. Antigone undertakes to perform these rites, knowing that Creon has determined to punish by death anyone who goes against his word. Antigone is caught and Creon condemns her to be walled up in a cave alive. Despite Creon's last minute change of heart, brought about by the dire warnings of the soothsayer, Antigone dies in her cave-tomb, taking her life with her own hand. She is followed by Creon's wife and son (Haemon, Antigone's betrothed), and in the end, Creon too says he is 'no more a live man than one dead'.[2]

As both victim of patriarchal power, and courageous rebel against its worst excesses, Antigone has unsurprisingly become an emblematic figure for feminist thinkers. Irigaray's analysis in *Speculum* focuses on Hegel's appropriation of the play in his account of ethical consciousness in *Phenomenology of Spirit*.[3] In this text, the ethical is presented as a key stage in the dialectical unfolding of consciousness through history, albeit a stage that is itself transcended in the movement of spirit (or *Geist*) towards the absolute, where thought and reality are fully reconciled. Once again the epigraphs are crucial to Irigaray's approach, for the chapter on Hegel begins not with *Phenomenology*, but two framing passages from Hegel's *Philosophy of Nature*. In the first, Hegel broadly repeats the Aristotelian view of woman, contrasting the passivity of the clitoris with the activity of the male sex organ, and positioning woman as the passive receptacle for the semen of the male which constitutes the active (re-)productive principle. In conception, Hegel affirms, woman provides the matter, man the subjectivity.[4]

The passage attunes the reader, sensitizing them to the ways in which this gendering is repeated in Hegel's account of the ethical. For Hegel, Sophocles' *Antigone* is archetypal because its chief protagonists embody the two modes of ethical consciousness, that is, two different ways of taking up a relation to the universal. This generates a series of dissymmetries between the sexes which is indicative of their difference as well as of the limits of each of their perspectives. This in itself is not a problem for Irigaray, given that she also seeks to affirm both dissymmetrical difference between the sexes and the intrinsic limit of each sexuate mode of being. The problem with Hegel's account is that these dissymmetries are mapped in terms of a clear hierarchy or progression, in which female ethical consciousness is sublated in the higher ethical order represented by the male subject. Moreover, the limit intrinsic to the ethical perspective of each sex is seen as rendering their relation necessarily destructive; such limits are not only regarded as something to be overcome in the fullest unfolding of spirit: the irresolvable conflict between them inevitably generates their own overcoming.

Both this mutual destructiveness, and the hierarchical ordering of dissymmetrical differences, are exemplified in Hegel's account of the relation between Creon and Antigone. Creon is the representative of human (i.e. civil) law, which enables the male citizen to work towards the universal by consciously determining and acting for the good of the community as a whole. Antigone represents divine law, which is rooted in kinship relations and the life of the family. Divine law does not need to be consciously determined: Antigone thus represents woman as unconscious ethical being. Nonetheless, insofar as they are ethical, woman's actions still have a relation to the universal: Antigone acts not because of her feelings for Polyneices as a particular individual, but simply because he is her brother. For woman, the particular becomes the universal.[5]

As Hegel says, the natural division between the sexes thereby gains a spiritual and ethical dimension.[6] But as Irigaray shows, this also means that the (hierarchical) dissymmetries that mark Hegel's account of the 'natural' difference between the sexes also mark his account of spiritualized nature. Just as females are aligned with the passive material required for active males to reproduce themselves, so woman is identified with unconscious ethical life while man represents self-conscious ethical activity. Hegel does accord woman a relation to the universal and a distinctive ethical value allied with her sexed specificity; but he also repeats a familiar pattern in which women are subordinated and sacrificed to support man's journey of spiritual development.

As Irigaray emphasizes, women's ethical being is essential to the well-being of the community, above all, because of the way divine law demands that one care for the dead. By burying the dead with the proper rites and rituals, woman turns a natural event into one that is consciously taken up: 'Man is still subject to (natural) death, of course, but what matters is to make a movement of the mind out of this accident that befalls the single individual and, in its raw state, drives consciousness out of its own country, cutting off that return into the self which allows it to become self-consciousness' (S, 215). Woman thus restores the dead to the self-conscious life of the spirit. Yet she does so unconsciously: she does not take up a self-conscious relation to the ground of her own actions. She is thus excluded from the development of spirit her actions serve to protect.[7] Indeed, as Irigaray notes, civil law places a negative meaning on woman's ethical actions (S, 215). While she honours the particular as universal, from the perspective of the city, these bonds of kin are *merely* particular in comparison with the 'truly universal' which is found in the life of the community.[8]

Thus woman is appropriated twice over: first, because she takes care of the substance of family life, releasing man to work for the *polis* while protecting him from the blind forces of irrational matter; second, because the more abstract universality for which the male citizen works is formed only by transcending the life of the family whose ethical law she embodies. In this movement of sublation, the development of ethical self-consciousness in the male subject relies on woman's position as unconscious ethical being which he is able to overcome. Thus, on Hegel's model, (ethical) man requires (ethical) woman, so as to draw new strength from her, a new form, whereas the other [woman] sinks further and further into a ground that harbors a substance which expends itself without the mark of any individualism. ... Hence, woman does not take an active part in the development of history, for she is never anything but the still undifferentiated opaqueness of sensible matter, the store (of) substance for the sublation of self. (S, 223–4)

Irigaray shows how this dissymmetry unsettles even the relation between man and woman that, for Hegel, is most ethically ideal. One reason Antigone epitomizes the ethical life of the family for Hegel is because she acts to honour her brother. The brother–sister relation is ideal because untainted by desire.[9] It might seem as if in this ideal equilibrium, if nowhere else, woman might find herself recognized as one individual in relation to another. But as Irigaray notes, even this relation is marked by dissymmetry:

as Hegel admits when he affirms that the brother is for the sister that possibility of recognition of which she is deprived as mother and wife/woman [femme], but does not state that the situation is reciprocal. This means that the brother has already been invested with a value for the sister that she cannot offer in return, except by devoting herself to his cult after death. (S, 217; translation modified)[10]

As a man, the brother is destined to become a citizen and gain recognition from his fellow citizens in community, whereupon his familial relations become markers of his particularity. By contrast, for the sister, her relation with her brother is the only one in which she can be recognized as an individual; because she is not recognized as a citizen in the public sphere, her relations as mother, woman and wife remain unparticularized and indistinguishable, lost in the darkness of what Hegel calls the 'nether world'.[11] Thus while the sister may find herself reflected in the brother, 'the reverse is not necessarily true' (S, 220): once he passes from adolescence into adulthood, the brother will no longer find his self-conscious being reflected in his sister's more shadowy form.

The idealized brother–sister relation is thus no more than 'a consoling fancy': a 'Hegelian dream' of equilibrium in the midst of the dissymmetries between the sexes that the unfolding of spirit demands (S, 217). By drawing on a different reading of Sophocles' play, Irigaray robs Hegel of even this consolation by suggesting that, far from being an expression of pure ethical love, Antigone's actions are full of desire from the start, in ways that remind us of the incestuous blood-line to which she belongs (as the daughter of Oedipus and his own mother, Jocasta). This Antigone finds her *'jouissance'* in acting with a perverse 'nocturnal passion' for her brother, her mother's son (*S*, 218). The repeated references to Antigone's *jouissance* provide a textual clue to Irigaray's approach, which operates by weaving traces of Lacan's interpretation of the play through her more overt Hegelian frame.

Hegel versus Lacan: Doubling Dialectics for a Female Subject

Like Hegel, in his three lectures on Sophocles' play Lacan aligns Antigone with the ethical.[12] However, against Hegel, Lacan argues that Antigone acts not in obedience to divine law, but out of love for the unique singularity of her irreplacable brother.[13] Her action is ethical because she acts in the name of a uniqueness to which no law can do justice. Such uniqueness cannot be represented without erasing its unrepeatable singularity. Nonetheless, it can be marked only from *within* language, as that which the symbolic order can only fail to capture.[14] Once again, woman is aligned with the unconscious: not as divine law, but as singular desire that language cannot help but occlude. For Lacan, Antigone's position constitutes a radical limit marking an irrecuperable remainder that ruptures the symbolic from within.[15]

Lacan's reading not only destabilizes the brother–sister relation. The Hegelian balance between two ethical powers is also rewritten, in favour (it seems) of Antigone, whose actions are compelled by a singular desire that Creon's universalizing edicts simply cannot touch. Lacan makes the mother central to the drama, insofar as he reads Antigone's perverse attachment to her brother – her mother's son – as a repetition of her mother's desire (that is, Jocasta's desire for Oedipus): 'Think about it. What happens to her desire? Shouldn't it be the desire of the Other and be linked to the desire of the mother? The text alludes to the fact that the desire of the mother is the origin of everything.'[16] This thread of Lacan's reading allows Irigaray to disrupt the Hegelian frame in which woman is defined against man by reintroducing Antigone's relation to her mother. However, her retelling makes it clear that Lacan, no less than Hegel, fails to allow women to exist as individualized selves:

But how are mother and wife/woman [femme] to be distinguished? This is the dreadful paradigm of a mother who is both wife [*épouse*] and mother to her husband. Thus the sister will strangle herself in order to save at least the mother's son. She will cut off her breath – her voice, her air, blood, life – with the veil of her belt, returning into the shadow (of a) tomb, the night (of) death, so that her brother, *her mother's desire*, may have eternal life. She never becomes a woman. (*S*, 219; translation modified)

In this over-determined scene, one thing is clear: insofar as she is aligned with the excess of an unrepresentable desire, there is no way to distinguish between Antigone and her mother. Woman remains identified with the maternal and both mother and daughter are sacrificed to the singular desire that marks the limit of the symbolic. Echoing Sophocles' Antigone, who laments that she must die before entering womanhood, Lacan entombs Antigone (and her mother) in an excessive desire that forecloses the possibility of living as a woman.

This is of course in keeping with Lacan's account of feminine *jouissance* as mystical excess, as well as his claim that woman cannot exist as such – that is, as a subject in the symbolic order. This is not to say that Irigaray does not value Lacan's emphasis both on Antigone's relation to her mother, and on her commitment to a singular alterity that inhabits and exceeds the symbolic, a singularity that is lost altogether from the two universals that govern the Hegelian frame. But Irigaray's reading also shows that this ethical commitment to irreducible alterity comes at the price of sacrificing Antigone's own specificity as a woman. In this regard, Hegel's reading has the advantage, insofar as the attachment between brother and sister expresses a desire for a relation that is *sexuate*, even if, in this case, it is (sexual) desire itself that must be sacrificed (*S*, 220).

In this way, as Christine Battersby puts it, Irigaray 'sets Hegel and Lacan to destroy each other. They fight to the death, as do Polynices and Eteocles, Oedipus's twin sons and Antigone's brothers, in the Theban legend.'[17] The two readings work dramatically against each other, each helping to reveal the other's blindspots, yet they do not simply cancel out. On the one hand, what both have in common is the alignment of woman with an ethics rooted in the unconscious in ways that make it impossible for her to become an individualized subject. On the other, Irigaray exacerbates the differences between these two warring interpretations to open up a further perspective, irrecuperable to either.

206 An Ethics of Sexuate Difference

As Battersby shows, this perspective depends on Irigaray's problematization of the Hegelian link between woman and the blood ties of kinship. As we have seen, Irigaray emphasizes Antigone's incestuous blood-line to suggest that in this sister's relation to her brother, 'the balance of blood' has already been upset (*S*, 221). However, she also puts pressure on what is at stake in Hegel's claim that brother and sister are of 'the same blood' by introducing a distinction between red blood associated with the mother and white blood, the father's sperm.[18] This distinction links back to the epigraphs and runs through the chapter, destabilizing both Hegel's and Lacan's frameworks.

The second epigraph is especially significant here. In it, Hegel cites a description which claims that the finer arteries of the eye no longer contain red blood. In conjunction with Hegel's ethics, Irigaray uses this passage to suggest that the visible realm – where one appears as a citizen – is distanced from the 'nether world' associated with the mother's blood. By playing on the way that the French for that which appears (*semblant*) is homophonic with *sang blanc* (white blood), Irigaray's reading connects the two epigraphs to link the world of appearances to the 'white blood' of the father, the sperm. This allows her to emphasize that it is an active male principle that determines who is permitted to appear and gain recognition in the city, or (to put it in more Lacanian terms) that it is the symbolic law of the father that determines who gains representation as a subject.[19]

Irigaray's playful deployment of the epigraphs allows her to show how, on Hegel's account, human law distances itself from the red blood of the mother to produce the de-sanguinated forms of representation that secure the activities of male citizens. Woman's role is 'care of the *bloodless*' (*S*, 214): not just the dead, but all those who cut themselves off from the mother's blood to appear in the *polis*. Her blood is sacrificed to feed this community, which appropriates her sons as future citizens: 'the color of blood fades as more and more semblances are produced' (*S*, 221–2). In the end, woman herself becomes a 'bloodless shadow' confined to the 'nether world' of the unconscious:

> Woman is the guardian of the blood. But as both she and it have had to use their substance to nourish the universal consciousness of self, it is in the form of *bloodless shadows* – of unconscious fantasies – that they maintain an underground subsistence. ... This enables us to understand why femininity consists essentially in laying the dead

man back in the womb of the earth, and giving him eternal life. For the *bloodless one is the mediation that she knows in her being*, whereby a being-there that has given up being as a self here passes from something living and singular and deeply buried to essence at its most general. (*S*, 225)

Drained of her own life's blood, woman has an affinity with the dead who she recalls to consciousness, for she too has had to give up being a 'living and singular' self so as to sustain the universal. However, the spectre of Lacan's Antigone should make us wary of reading Irigaray as idealizing the red blood of the mother as if it embodied some kind of lost essence of woman. If left as an undifferentiated flow, this blood will continue to erase the difference between being a mother and being a woman, and woman's singularity will be lost once again.

Thus, Irigaray insists that red blood requires its own processes of mediation, allowing its unconscious flow to be translated into symbolic forms that permit women to appear as individualized subjects. For this to occur, it would not be enough to allow women entry to the public realm on the same terms as the male citizen: as we have seen, his activity is constituted via the transcendence and suppression of woman. Instead of making one sex bear the weight of being the unconscious life required to sustain the self-conscious development of the other, Irigaray suggests that each sex requires the terms to make the transition from unconscious to conscious life, to translate the singularity of desire into the specificity of a sexuate subjectivity:

> Unless each of these/its terms is doubled so radically that *a single dialectic is no longer sufficient to articulate their copulation*. For if it is asserted that the one character and the other are split into a conscious and an unconscious, with each character itself giving rise to that opposition, there remains the question of how it will be possible to *translate* the laws of the unconscious into those of the conscious, the so-called divine laws into the laws of philosophy, the laws of the female into those of the male. What will be the passage of their *difference* in the subsequent movement of the mind? (*S*, 223–4; translation modified)

In keeping with her project of articulating being (as) two, Irigaray calls for two dialectical processes, allowing two different movements of becoming a subject and two sexuate subjects to co-exist within the *polis*. Such a double dialectic would be capable of articulating the relation of family to *polis* and nature to culture twice over, in terms specific and appropriate to each of the sexes.

Irigaray's engagement with Hegel thus plays a key role in the development of her notions of sexuate being and *genre* examined in the previous chapter. If men and women were each allowed their own relation to both consciousness and the unconscious, everything would have to be redoubled: there would be two different ways of mediating relations between human and divine, desire and language, bodily life and political representation. There would no longer be two universals related hierarchically, as in Hegel's model of the divine law of kinship and the more 'truly universal' human law. Instead there would be two relations to the universal understood as sexual difference itself, which articulates human beings as two and is thus embodied in two different *genres*, each requiring its own dialectic of self-formation. These dual dialectical processes would allow for the singularity of different desires, those of women as well as men. The relation between male and female would itself be doubled, for each sexuate subject would need to articulate its own relation to the other, rather than this relation being determined by the laws or desires of only one of the two.

As the title of Irigaray's chapter reminds us, for Hegel, woman becomes the 'everlasting irony [in the life] of the community'.[20] By constructing its own universal against hers and thereby redefining her concerns as merely 'particular', human law produces its own internal enemy. Woman will henceforth be a possible threat, as well as support, to the life of community, especially if she stirs up her adolescent sons and brothers, those not-quite-yet citizens. Yet as Irigaray suggests, such is the power of the city that it will absorb even these '*seeds* of revolt', by appropriating for its own defence the young men's readiness to be persuaded into battle and to wage war on one another. Whatever threat woman poses is always already 'reduced to nothing by being *separated from the universal goal* pursued by the citizens' (S, 226).

By playing Hegel off against Lacan, Irigaray redoubles the ironies to generate the resources for a different kind of revolt, one which would rely on mothers and daughters being able to relate to one another as women, instead of mediating their desires and frustrations through men. For Hegel, the two ethical powers of divine and human law are equally one-sided: each offends the other such that the only right outcome is their mutual destruction.[21] By contrast, Irigaray's reassessment of Hegel allows us a glimpse of two sexuate beings who might live alongside one another, each recognizing the other *as* other by accepting the limited and specific way in which they themselves embody sexual difference.

Antigone's Call

Irigaray returns to the figure of Antigone throughout her work. Antigone thus operates as a guiding thread, allowing us to draw together several of the key themes examined so far and to link them with developments in Irigaray's later texts. For Irigaray, Antigone calls on us to seek the conditions under which she might have acted as a woman, in the singularity of her desire, without having to die for it. In response, Irigaray continues to emphasize the need for an ethics of sexual difference and a 'double dialectic' allowing both men and women to accede to subjectivity on their own terms.[22] Thus, in *I love to you* (a text which Irigaray explicitly positions in terms of her ongoing engagement with Hegel), she writes that the aim of *Speculum* was to facilitate:

> a dialectic proper to the female subject, meaning specific relations between her nature and her culture, her same and her other, her singularity and the community, her interiority and her exteriority, etc; *Speculum* and my other works insist upon the irreducibility – either subjective or objective – of the sexes to one another, which requires us to establish a dialectic of the relation of woman to herself and of man to himself, a double dialectic therefore, enabling a real, cultured, and ethical relation between them. (*ILTY*, 62)

Instead of aligning woman with material nature and man with the forms of civil and ethical advancement, as has been the general pattern in the western tradition, this dialectic requires each subject to work through his or her relation to their own material nature and to take up an active relation to the forms through which their sexuate being is represented in political and ethical life. This requires man to re-address his own bodily specificity, which has been repressed in the illegitimate equation of the male subject with the universal (see *ILTY*, 35–41). Taking up an active relation to his own sexuate being would release man from a natural immediacy which he has not previously escaped, but simply projected onto woman. Antigone serves as a constant reminder of the need for woman to be released from such projections and have her own place in the *polis*. In her later work, Irigaray argues that such a *polis* would be informed by a conception of sexuate rights rather than a single set of supposedly universal human rights.[23] The latter are necessarily limited by virtue of taking one kind of subject (the male) as the model for all human beings, instead of attending to sexual difference itself as universal, and thus to the ways in which human being is articulated in two different *genres* (see in particular *ILTY*, 35–57).

Antigone also helps explain why Irigaray attaches such importance to the construction of female genealogies, a central theme in several texts after *Speculum*. As we have seen, for Hegel and Lacan, Antigone's fate is determined either by an apparently inevitable conflict with Creon, or by an equally inevitable and unconscious repetition of her mother's incestuous desire. Either way, she ends up 'walled up in a cave on the border of the world of citizens', without a place in the *polis* or a home in the world (*ESD*, 107). By contrast, Irigaray suggests that, if women are not to keep re-living Antigone's fate, we need to establish female genealogies involving both *vertical* relations between mothers and daughters and *horizontal* relations between women (*ESD*, 108). Such genealogies would allow women to relate directly to one another without mediation via the desires of (or for) a male subject. Instead, they would register both the differences between mothers and daughters (in terms of their respective positions in a generative order) and their likeness (their shared sex). In turn, this would allow women to relate to those who gave birth to them as both mothers *and* women, and thus to relate to their origins in their own sex without simply identifying themselves with a maternal function. As we have seen, Irigaray considers such reconfigured relations between women, and in particular, between mothers and daughters, as necessary conditions for the development of a female *genre*: 'If we are not to be accomplices in the murder of the mother we also need to assert that there is a genealogy of women.'[24]

As well as emblematizing the need for female genealogies, in Irigaray's later work, increasing emphasis is also placed on Antigone's links with the natural life (and death) of the body. Antigone reminds us that rethinking woman's place in the political order is inseparable from rethinking human beings' relations to material nature more generally.[25] In contrast to western culture's tendency to objectify and exploit both nature and women, Antigone's care for her brother's body reminds us of human beings' place within a cosmic order that encompasses birth, life and death. In the wake of Chernobyl in 1986 (an event to which several of Irigaray's essays explicitly respond), and in light of the global environmental crisis now facing us, this strand of Irigaray's work takes on an increasingly poignant urgency. A dual dialectic, in which each sex both recognizes its own material nature and acquires its own way of negotiating the passage between nature and culture, would help us break away from the damaging struc-ture in which nature is aligned with 'feminine' immediacy and opposed to culture as a realm of rational 'masculine' activity. Such a model reinforces the objectification of material nature and legiti-mates its treatment as a resource for rational subjects who either implicitly repress or actively seek to escape the ways in which they too are part of the material world. The cultivation of sexuate difference to which we are called by Antigone's fate thus also promises to help us rethink the relation between nature and culture in ways that are attentive to human beings' own material-ity as well as their place in a greater ecological whole.

By pointing towards these conjoined projects, Antigone reminds us that rethinking woman's sexuate specificity, and hence, her rela-tion to herself, cannot happen without a more thoroughgoing transformation of our culture. Hence the importance for Irigaray of the ways in which Antigone spans the natural, the political and the religious. With regard to the latter, Antigone signals the need for woman to have her own relation to the divine, rather than being made the care-taker of human beings' relation to the gods in ways that sustain men by releasing them for the active work of citizen-ship.[26] Some may be uncomfortable with Irigaray's insistence on the importance of a female divine, given the many ways in which religious belief has served to legitimate women's subordination and oppression. However, as indicated in the previous chapter, Irigaray's fundamental point does not commit her to any specific religious creed, but is ontological and existential: if woman is to become a subject in her own right, she needs to be able to situate herself within a horizon that projects and protects the value of her own sex. Moreover, as Lacan reminds us, as long as woman *is* 'Other', she has no 'Other' to herself (there is no 'Other' of the 'Other'); but, as Irigaray reminds us, for woman to become a subject, she needs to be able to take up a relation to those 'other' to her in ways that do not repeat the exclusionary or hierarchical logic of the masculine order: otherwise she will accede to subjectiv-ity only by mimicking the male subject position. The notion of a female divine plays a key role in enabling woman to figure her own relation to that which is radically Other, without this relation either being subsumed in the service of man or modelled on the male subject's terms. Thus, Irigaray's female divine is allied not with immaterial transcendence but with a continual becoming that animates the infinite potential within material life.

In keeping with the need to elaborate woman's relation to *her* other, Antigone's relation to Creon reminds us that the project of releasing woman from her role as *man's* 'other' is inseparable from rethinking the relation *between* the sexes. As I argued at length in the previous chapter, Irigaray's increasing attention to the need to rework this relation does not signal a retreat from her commitment to finding the terms in which woman might speak as an autonomous subject, *without* being defined in relation to man: on the contrary, it is a necessary condition of transforming the relation *between* the sexes that woman's relation to herself first be transformed. If men and women are to relate to each other in their sexuate specificity, then woman must become a sexuate subject in her own right. In turn, this will entail that the male subject is recognized as sexuate too.

This points to a further way in which a reworking of Hegel becomes crucial to Irigaray's later thinking. As we have seen, Irigaray argues that, in the history of western thought, woman is aligned with all that the subject must renounce, transcend or exclude so as to secure his own identity. The supposedly 'universal' subject becomes male, and vice versa, via the negation of female 'otherness'. This negation itself negates the possibility of thinking female difference as anything other than the 'other of the Same'. Thus if two sexuate subjects are to co-exist, the male subject will have to renounce the 'dreams of being the whole' sustained via the negation of woman (*ILTY*, 40). Instead, Irigaray argues for the acceptance of the negative as a constitutive limit placed on all human beings by their sexuate specificity, a limit which means that neither sex can lay claim to the whole of being: 'The negative in sexual difference means an acceptance of the limits of my gender and recognition of the irreducibility of the other. It cannot be overcome but it gives a positive access ... to the other' (*ILTY*, 13; see also 35–41). If the male subject were to accept the negative as a limit proper to his own gender, this would secure the possibility of relating to an other (female) subject who cannot be defined in his own terms – terms which would thereby be recognized as having limited rather than universal application. This 'positive access' to the other – on the part of both (ontologically limited) sexes – is what needs to be cultivated through the double dialectic of two sexuate *genres*.

Only this double transformation will allow the sexes to relate to one another as irreducibly different. Thus, the male subject's acceptance of the negative must be matched with the cultivation of woman as a sexuate subject. This point can be restated in terms of the image of the two lips. As Irigaray notes, the 'two' of the lips is not the same as the 'two' of 'being two', where this is understood as the sexuate nature of human being expressed in the dissymmetrical (but non-hierarchical) difference between the sexes. Nonetheless, these non-equivalent 'twos' are intimately related, insofar as nurturing the sexuate specificity of woman via figures such as the 'two lips' is a condition making it possible to cultivate being (as) two:

> the expression 'two lips' tries to express a basic way of self-affection for the feminine subject, while 'being-two' refers to a relation between two subjects. Self-affection is a determining factor in reaching 'being-two' but cannot amount to relation itself. Turning one's attention or one's feeling only to 'the two lips' remains in the perspective of one and alone subject. Of course this subject now is in the feminine but we have not yet reached a culture of two subjects.[27]

Only if woman accedes to the status of a sexuate subject herself can she begin to relate to the male subject as a (sexuate, non-symmetrical) other – and he to her. Unless such relations are developed, female auto-affection risks repeating a hom(m)osocial logic which values only one kind of subject. A culture of two would acknowledge not only the sexuate specificity of two different subjects, but also the ways in which that specificity informs each subject's (different) modes of relating to the other. Thus, cultivating the fluid relations to 'otherness within' that constitute a specifically female subject also permits women to relate to the alterity of 'otherness without': to male subjects, formed by a very different process of (self-)constitution. The spacing *between the lips* that allows woman to relate to herself thereby opens up a spacing *between men and women* that allows each to relate to the other without negation, assimilation, or appropriation. Instead, this spacing shelters an irreducible difference.

Cultivating Alterity

The female specificity figured in the two lips opens into a sexuate culture of *being two* that in turn permits the cultivation of the irreducible difference *between* two and thus, a 'culture of alterity' (*BEW*, 126). Such alterity is in many ways the counterpart of the singularity which Irigaray seeks to retain from Lacan's reading of *Antigone*. However, just as she reinscribes this singularity within the horizon of sexuate difference, such that it refers to the irreducible singularity of the two genders that incarnate being as two, so she also reinscribes alterity within this horizon: for Irigaray, the cultivation of sexuate difference is the condition of an ethics capable of doing justice to the irreducible otherness of the other.

The notion of alterity is drawn in part from Immanuel Levinas who, like Heidegger, becomes an important interlocutor in Irigaray's work after *Speculum*. As with Heidegger, Irigaray's relation to Levinas is both generative and profoundly critical. In the final essay of *An Ethics of Sexual Difference*, 'The Fecundity of the Caress', she seeks to draw out what she sees as an unrealized ethical potential from the account of *eros* in Levinas' *Totality and Infinity*.[28] She achieves this by entwining Levinas with both Diotima's account of love, and the sense of wonder at the forever unknowable other that she reclaims from Descartes.

As Chanter explains, in *Totality and Infinity* Levinas positions the erotic as equivocal: somewhere between the ethical encounter with alterity and immersion in the everyday life of consumption and enjoyment.[29] While love initiates a relation to the Other in their alterity, it also 'reverts into need'. Thus: 'Not only does desire, as eros, transcend, it also falls short of genuine transcendence', even becoming 'the underside of transcendence'.[30] Yet for Irigaray, it is love's in-between status which holds the greatest potential for an ethics of sexual difference insofar as it offers the possibility of an encounter with alterity which is nonetheless carnate.

On Irigaray's reading, Levinas' account of the erotic makes us attentive to the caress as a touch(ing) that occurs both before any subject position is secured and as an undoing of any such self-certainty. The caress 'binds and unbinds two others in a flesh that is still and always untouched by mastery' – of self, or of other (*ESD*, 186). As a non-objectifying touch, the caress offers an alternative to the specular logic which opposes (male) subject to (female) object.[31] Just as the two lips touch on each other without becoming one, the caress allows a relation between two who renew one another in an intimate proximity where neither seeks to possess or appropriate. Thus each remains other to the other, and each gives new life to the other in their otherness: 'Prior to any procreation, the lovers bestow on each other – life. Love fecundates both of them in turn, through the genesis of their immortality. They are reborn, each for the other' (*ESD*, 190).[32]

As in the reading of Diotima, this immortality is found not beyond but within mortal life, in the ceaseless passage of rebirth incarnated in the lovers' touch and in the in-finite which pulses and quivers in their encounter (*ESD*, 194). Irigaray thus finds in the caress a realization of Diotima's teaching: an encounter between two as a repetition of birth in which the carnal and the spiritual remain constantly entwined. Instead of a nostalgia for a lost fusion with the mother, the fecundity of the lovers' encounter evokes one's first (maternal) dwelling as a place where one is able to live and move with(in) another, touching and being touched without ever merging into a single being (*ESD*, 188–91). Like the intimate proximity of the lips, through which a woman has always already been touched, is always already touching (on) herself, the caress allows for a *jouissance* in which the lovers are constantly regenerated without wholly absorbing each other or completely losing themselves.

Entwined with Irigaray's poetics of the caress is a call to Levinas that implores him to see how his philosophy betrays its own potential for refiguring an ethics of alterity that would no longer be founded on the one. Irigaray draws attention to the way that Levinas does not write of male and female lovers, both active and both undone – and remade – in their mutual encounter. Instead, in a disheartening repetition of the tradition, a male lover is counterposed with a female beloved who is aligned with animality and infancy in ways that block her from acceding to the properly ethical encounter with a transcendent Other: 'The beloved woman would be cast down to the depths so that the male lover could be raised to the heights. The act of love would amount to reaching the inordinate limits of discourse, so that the woman is sent back to the position of fallen animal or child, and man to ecstasy in God. Two poles that are indefinitely separate' (*ESD*, 198). While the sensuality of the beloved is like an abyss in which the male lover loses himself, he is left 'a solitary call to his God' that allows him to be called out of the depths of erotic intimacy (*ESD*, 202).

The danger here is not only that woman lacks a relation to the divine, or an ethical relation to a transcendent Other, but that this loss forecloses any path 'back to herself, to herself within herself' (*ESD*, 199). The encounter with the Other, for Levinas, is an encounter with an absolute alterity whose irreducible otherness means the call of the Other can never be adequately answered; instead, the

Other places the subject under an infinite obligation. Yet in calling the 'I' into question, the encounter with the Other also singularizes the subject, making it aware of itself as an 'I' distinct from the other subjects and objects that constitute its world. For Levinas, ethics precedes ontology because only the encounter with an Other calls the subject into being as such: the subject is first and foremost response-able.[33]

Like Levinas, Irigaray seeks an ethics which is attentive to irreducible otherness. But by positioning woman as a beloved object of desire, rather than a lover who can be called out of erotic intimacy by the absolute alterity of the Other, Levinas effectively cuts woman off from full participation in the ethical and therefore from the singularizing movement of becoming a responsible subject. On Irigaray's reading, this neglect of woman is not something that can be easily rectified because, in the end, it makes Levinas' project self-defeating. Despite his attentiveness to irreducible otherness, so long as the other is an absolute Other that singularizes only one kind of subject, this other will inevitably be trapped back into a position as the 'Other of the same' (ESD, 213).

For Irigaray, genuine alterity can only be preserved between two, where each attends to an otherness that is irreducible to either, and that cannot be polarized by its relation to only one subject. Instead, as each is called upon to attend to the irreducible alterity of the other, each is also inhabited by this alterity, though neither is inhabited by it absolutely. In this way, woman is no longer aligned with the Other as she so often has been in the past, but neither is Otherness that which stands over and above the one; rather, Irigaray insists on 'the irreducible strangeness of the one *and* the other. *Between* the one and the other' (ESD, 210–11; my emphasis).

Both in her essay on the caress, and in her more recent essay 'Approaching the Other as Other' (BEW, 121–30), Irigaray, like Levinas, is concerned with the ways in which 'we make our own what we approach, what approaches us. ... we reduce the other to ourselves, we incorporate the other' (BEW, 121–3). However, contra Levinas, she suggests that it is only by being positioned as an irreducible otherness *between two* that alterity is protected from being an 'Other of the same'. It is therefore in the caress, rather than Levinas's account of the Other, that she finds the potential for a genuine ethics of alterity which would arise from and be nurtured within an ethics of sexuate difference. In this 'ethical fidelity to incarnation' (ESD, 217), the transcendence of the other would be found within and between carnate beings. Such beings would be singularized not by an absolute alterity, but by their sexuate specificity and the fecund relations this permits between them in their irreducible strangeness to one another.

Refounding Ethics on Sexuate Difference

For Irigaray, refounding society and culture on sexuate difference means: 'to learn, at the most intimate, at the most passionate and carnal level of the relation to the other, to renounce all possession, all appropriation, in order to respect, in the relation, two subjects, without ever reducing one to the other' (*BEW*, 128). An ethics of sexuate difference which seeks to cultivate being (as) two is thus the condition not only of a just *polis*, but of an ethics capable of attending to both singularity and alterity. The recognition of two sexuate subjects means that neither is absolute: neither absolutely Other nor absolutely self-sufficient as a subject. Both are limited, but these limits are what give their encounters form, allowing them to be transformative without either wholly appropriating the other. In her later writings, Irigaray suggests that, if we can learn to relate to those who belong to a different gender without seeking to assimilate them to ourselves, we can learn to encounter other kinds of difference – of race, class, age, ethnicity – without appropriation too. The ambiguity in the above passage, and throughout the essay 'Approaching the Other as Other' from which it is taken, can thus be read not as a weakness but a strength of Irigaray's approach: whether we are talking of the difference between two *sexuate* subjects, or two subjects who differ in other ways, what matters is not reducing one to the other. In this way, Irigaray extends her argument that an ethics of sexual difference is required so as to foster dissymmetrical difference between the sexes, and suggests that cultivating sexuate difference is a necessary condition for developing ethical relations to difference of all kinds.

At this point, it is worth recalling that Irigaray's model of a dual dialectic involves not only two different processes of becoming a subject, but also two different journeys through which each sexuate subject learns how to negotiate relations with others. The key point here is not that others are only irreducible to us if they are of a different gender, but that different sexuate subjects develop different ways of relating to otherness, of whatever kind. Nonetheless, it is clear that Irigaray *does* give priority to sexuate difference, such as when she writes that 'no one can be reduced to anyone else,

An Ethics of Sexuate Difference

but the most fundamental locus of irreducibility is between man and woman'; for Irigaray, this 'most universal and irreducible difference' is 'the ultimate anchorage of real alterity' (*ILTY*, 139; *BEW*, 98; *ILTY*, 62). Likewise, in the concluding section of 'Approaching the Other as Other', sexual difference is positioned as 'the foundation of alterity' (*BEW*, 127). The context of this essay makes it particularly clear that Irigaray does not intend this priority to devalue other kinds of difference: on the contrary, the text to which it belongs, *Between East and West*, explicitly foregrounds the importance of non-appropriative relations to all kinds of difference. And despite Irigaray's own wording at times, it is also clear that it does not make sense to think of this priority as a quantitative matter: it cannot be that there is somehow 'more' alterity between men and women than between those of different races, because irreducibility does not come in degrees in this way. A difference – of whatever kind – is either irreducible or it is not: for something to be 'less irreducible' means it is partly reducible, and hence is not irreducible at all. Moreover, as indicated in the previous chapter, Irigaray emphasizes the singularity not only of each gender, but of each human being, as given in the singular event of their birth; thus, each is irreducible to any other 'in his or her totality' (*BEW*, 124).

Thus, when Irigaray describes sexuate difference as the 'foundational' or 'most fundamental' locus of alterity, we need to hear this as signalling a *qualitative* difference and a *transcendental* status. To explain: the alterity between the sexes is of a different kind than other kinds of difference because – on Irigaray's account – sexuate difference is ontological difference. As we have seen, for Irigaray, sexuate difference is inscribed into our very being by the way we come to be in the world: both because we are born of man *and* woman, and because we are born through and into an originary sexuate relation to the body of the mother. Thus, the alterity between the sexes is a manifestation of the sexuate difference which is the condition of our very being and informs our differing constitution as sexuate subjects. Cultivating a non-appropriative relation to this originary and constitutive difference will inflect our whole mode of being, thereby allowing us to relate non-appropriatively to other kinds of difference: it is 'a gesture which will then permit all the various forms of alterity to be respected without authority or hierarchy, whether one is dealing with race, age, culture, religion, etc.' (*DBT*, 141).

Thus, it is not only that if we cannot deal adequately with sexuate difference, then there is not much hope of our being able to deal with other (for Irigaray, ontic or empirical) differences in a non-appropriative way; nor even that unless we cultivate an ethics that respects sexuate difference, we will not be able to respect other kinds of difference, because sexuate difference runs through and inflects them all. Even more importantly, our relation to sexuate difference runs through and inflects *us* – and hence, the way we form relations of all kinds. This is not to say that, in different situations, at different times, some differences may be much more important – politically, existentially, ethically – than sexuate difference. But it is to say that, for Irigaray, cultivating a non-appropriative approach to alterity between the sexes is a *condition* for being able to relate in non-appropriative ways to other kinds of difference. It is in this sense that sexuate difference is 'transcendental' (albeit, of course, a sensible transcendental, manifest in our sensuate, bodily modes of being): 'It appears as the empirical as well as transcendental condition for guaranteeing the possibility of a new epoch of History or, more simply, for assuring for humanity a becoming' (*BEW*, 98–9). And it is in this transcendental and ontological sense that sexuate difference has priority for Irigaray.

This might clarify the issue, but seems to reinforce the original concern: why consider only sexuate difference as ontological? Why not allow that other kinds of difference can also be constitutive of our mode of being, and hence fundamental to the constitution of our subjectivity? This is a question that has arisen with particular urgency in relation to Irigaray's views on race.[34] In *I love to you*, for example, she explicitly states that: 'The problem of race is, in fact, a secondary problem ... and the same goes for other cultural diversities – religious, economic and political ones' (*ILTY*, 47). Such passages make Irigaray's position clear, but taken in isolation, they do not do enough to show why (or indeed, whether) race should be treated as an 'ontic' matter of cultural diversity akin to different religious beliefs or political systems, rather than an 'ontological' issue in its own right. Before returning to this issue, it is worth contrasting such unequivocal statements about the secondary status of race and other differences with Irigaray's later text, *Between East and West*. Here issues of race and cultural diversity take centre stage. The intimate alliances made possible at a personal level in an inter-cultural, multi-cultural society are presented by Irigaray as a promising site for the emergence of non-appropriative relations to otherness: 'Marriage between a white woman and a black man, between a Catholic woman and a Muslim man' have the potential to be 'an extraordinary seed for growth for our civilizations' (*BEW*,

144).[35] Such non-appropriative modes of relating to others are urgently needed in an increasingly culturally mixed global context in which, Irigaray suggests, our ethical and political frameworks tend to lag behind the multi-cultural, multi-racial realities of living together in difference (*BEW*, 133).

Nonetheless, there are places where this text seems to perform an appropriative gesture of its own. This is reflected in the passage cited above, in which differences of race, culture and religious belief are reinscribed in a frame positioning the heterosexual couple as the basis for renewing family and community life. In the previous chapter, I argued that such a privileging is not in fact legitimated by Irigaray's own account of sexuate difference. It is also at odds with the implications of Irigaray's view that racially and culturally mixed families 'disturb our mental habits, our common laws, our legislative criteria' (insofar as these habits and laws tend to privilege sameness over difference), and 'compel us to transformations of desire, of thinking, to civil forms of meeting and cohesion of which we have hardly an idea' (*BEW*, 144–5). If families in which diverse races and cultures meet are a particularly fecund site for cultivating non-appropriative relations to difference, there is no reason why the 'transformations of desire' involved might not lead to radical re-imaginings of the family itself, along with the civil forms in which different kinds of marriages and kinship bonds are recognized.

To aid such re-imagining, we might supplement Irigaray's approach with a different feminist response to the figure of Antigone, that offered by Judith Butler. For Butler, by troubling relations between kinship, gender and the state, Antigone calls into question the norms that govern cultural intelligibility, and thus calls on us to re-examine 'which social arrangements can be recognized as legitimate love, and which human losses can be explicitly grieved as real and consequential loss.'[36] By challenging us to rethink the kinds of family and kinship relations to which we are prepared to give social and political recognition, Butler offers some of the resources required to fully realize Irigaray's own commitment to difference.

Approached in this way, the increased emphasis in *Between East and West* on the transformative potential of differences of all kinds – age, sex, race, culture, religion – can be seen to undercut Irigaray's continued if intermittent privileging of the heterosexual couple. Irigaray's own insistence on the importance of cultivating diversity implies that we should also cultivate diverse models of family life, involving different kinds of extended families as well as same-sex couples. Moreover, these diverse, non-nuclear families not only can, but should, continue to be sites where sexuate difference is cultivated: there is no reason to limit the site of that cultivation to the heterosexual couple.

In a somewhat surprising way, in *Between East and West* it some-times seems as if the priority of sexuate difference over other kinds of difference has if anything been reversed: as Deutscher notes, '*Between East and West* argues that we should recognize and culti-vate relations of sexual difference *because* they will contribute to a plural and multicultural community.'[37] Sexuate difference thus seems to be in the service of multiculturalism in this text in ways that appear to be in tension with Irigaray's continued positioning of sexuate difference as the 'foundation of alterity'. However, I would suggest that if we understand this foundational status in the terms outlined above, there is no real tension, either within *Between East and West* or with Irigaray's comments on race in earlier texts such as *I love to you*: sexuate difference does continue to have prior-ity insofar as cultivating sexuate difference is the *condition* of devel-oping non-appropriative relations to otherness in general. It is as such a condition that sexuate difference is 'in the service' of other kinds of difference. Thus, Deutscher's formulation helps show why according sexuate difference this kind of (ontological and transcen-dental) priority is not the same as saying it is always the most important kind of difference: on the contrary, we should cultivate the condition (sexuate difference) *for the sake of* the conditioned (non-appropriative relations to differences of all kinds) that it allows to come into being.

Irigaray, Cultural Difference, and Race

One of the difficulties of reading *Between East and West* is that – as we have seen in relation to its continued privileging of heterosexual relations – this text does not always seem entirely to live up to the non-appropriative standards it unequivocally espouses. In her careful and detailed work on this text, Deutscher shows how Irigaray tends to both homogenize and idealize Eastern cultures.[38] While it is clear that Irigaray seeks to displace the assumed value of western norms and to approach other cultures with an openness to what she (and other westerners) may have to learn, nonetheless, as Deutscher suggests, she does not adequately reflect on the potential appropriativeness of such an approach. It is not that Irigaray is unaware of such risks: at one point, she counsels against severing the Buddha from his context in spiritual practice and 'using him to critique Western discursivity – while forgetting his gestures' (*BEW*, 36). But despite this, in *Between East and West*, Irigaray does not sufficiently interrogate the ways in which her positive valuation of 'Eastern' cultures 'can read as an appropriation that bolsters her own depreciation of the West'.[39] As Deutscher shows, this is not to say that Irigaray is entirely uncritical of the Eastern cultures and practices to which she refers.[40] Nor is it to underestimate the importance of the extension of Irigaray's own critique of the logic of 'the same' in ways that make it explicit that the male subject who has served as norm and ideal in western culture is a *white* male subject.[41] But it is to suggest, following Deutscher, that Irigaray is not always attentive enough to the ways in which her own figuring of 'the East' remains trapped by oppositional and appropriative structures of thought, even as she argues so powerfully against them.

Deutscher's critique is generous, suggesting that Irigaray's own approach to sexual difference provides the resources to see what is still lacking in her approach to differences of both race and culture, and how she (and we) might approach such differences otherwise: 'Directed at her own writing, Irigarayan questions about difference are still good questions to ask.'[42] In *A Politics of Impossible Difference*, Deutscher argues that Irigaray's account of the way 'sedimented subjects are produced by difference', as well as of a politics appropriate to such subjects, allows her to make a contribution to 'a philosophy of race and cultural difference that goes beyond the actual comments about multiculturalism made in the late work.'[43] In her philosophy of sexual difference, Deutscher suggests, Irigaray emphasizes how western thought and culture has constitutively excluded the possibility of figuring this difference positively (such that woman would be 'something more than opposite, complement or same').[44] Sexual difference must therefore be approached as an impossible difference and in anticipation of alternative female (or male) identities: existing differences between men and women tend to reflect 'the absence, not the existence, of a culture of sexual difference'.[45]

It is the conjoined figures of impossibility and anticipation which Deutscher finds to be missing in Irigaray's approach to cultural difference. Whereas Irigaray shows how the west has *failed* to think sexuate difference, *Between East and West* tends to take existing cultural traditions as the already present site of *positive* differences that we should cultivate further. A more productive – and more properly 'Irigarayan' – approach, Deutscher suggests, would be to subject existing representations of race and cultural difference to the same kinds of questions that Irigaray has already posed in relation to sexual difference. Such an approach would thus seek to identify the formulations of race and cultural difference on whose exclusion western thought has depended. As well as investigating 'how cultural difference can *not* be represented today', it would also encourage us to ask how the 'non-depiction' of cultural difference in Irigaray's own writing 'connect[s] with the patterns in its non-depiction through the histories of philosophical and cultural treatments of race'.[46] Through such an approach, positive notions of race and cultural difference would be re-positioned as something to be anticipated and worked towards, rather than located in (inevitably idealized) aspects of existing cultural relations.

While my understanding of Irigaray's overall project of sexuate difference differs from Deutscher's in some key respects, I nonetheless think she is right to suggest that a properly 'Irigarayan' approach would need to involve the same kind of detailed critical analysis of the depiction of race and cultural difference as Irigaray has undertaken with regard to sexual difference, generating 'a genealogy not just of what has been said about race and cultural difference throughout the history of philosophy, but of what that history has not wanted to say about race and cultural difference.'[47] As Deutscher indicates, philosophers and critical race theorists have already undertaken extensive work along these lines.[48] Being aware of the different, if intersecting, genealogies of racial exclusion can help feminists avoid the homogenizing gesture of assuming that the exclusions of race can be approached *in the same way* as the exclusions of sexual difference.[49] Otherwise, feminism risks repeating the logic of sameness it seeks to resist, by treating the struggles of all excluded 'others' as fundamentally 'the same'.

Such equations make it impossible to account for the ways in which racism and sexism intersect. They thus blind us to the ways in which feminism itself has been constituted by the repression of racialized others, insofar as it has taken the experience of one group of women (white, western, largely middle class) as the norm in ways that make their own racial identity ('whiteness') invisible.[50] Thus, as Ellen Armour argues, we need to break down the divide between race and gender, not to conflate them, but in order that 'whitefeminism' can confront and take responsibility for the ways in which it 'has erected itself in and through the exclusion of its raced others and its own race'.[51] Given their own imbrication in histories of colonization and oppression, white western feminists have to give up the privileged position of '*the* other' and learn to listen to the voices of other women, whose different journeys of exclusion and 'othering' have forged different critical perspectives. Armour thus suggests that white feminists not only need to engage in critical self-reflection, but to read and actively engage with work by women of colour.[52] While recognizing that this strategy 'begins as a gesture of appropriation', Armour suggests that if followed through to its end, it can reveal the centrality of whiteness to what has counted as feminist in ways that displace a falsely unifying concept of woman in favour of 'woman as site of contestation'.[53] In this way, the appropriating gesture ends up dis-appropriating whitefeminism of its own identity, and helps generate a feminism better able to resist 'the multiple oppressions women face'.[54]

Armour engages extensively with Irigaray, insisting on her non-essentialism and reading her alongside Derrida in ways that (knowingly) privilege Irigaray's earlier work for offering an account of woman as 'essentially' differing/deferring. This 'holds out substantial promise for allowing the difference race makes to women to register, and for a different mode of relationality among differing women.' In the end, Armour suggests, Irigaray falls short of fulfilling this promise: 'The power of her insistence that women resist the form of oppression that most affects them is undercut by her own failure to attend to any salient difference in oppression.'[55] Nonetheless, this means not that Irigaray's work should be rejected, but that it 'needs supplementation by an analysis that carries racial difference to the same depth in the specular economy'.[56]

While woman as differing/deferring is one of the many figures that appears in Irigaray's texts, I would argue that this figure alone does not adequately capture Irigaray's project of cultivating the specificity of a sexuate (female) subject.[57] I nonetheless agree with Armour (and Deutscher) that Irigaray's critical analysis of woman as 'other' of a male subject needs to be matched by an equal attentiveness to processes of racial othering, as well as with further reflection on the ways in which such attentiveness might re-inflect and transform an Irigarayan approach to difference. The work of Armour and Deutscher suggests two specific ways in which this approach could be supplemented and developed. First, by more explicitly acknowledging that the desire to learn from our cultural 'others' inevitably involves the risk of appropriation, we can more actively seek out ways to negotiate, displace and avoid such appropriations. Second, by more fully acknowledging the different voices and other 'others' within our own cultures, we can become more responsible for our own roles in their 'othering', while moving away from an implicit model of cultures as internally homogeneous. The notion of 'otherness within' is of course central to Irigaray's own thinking about an alternative female model of (non-oppositional) identity; however, Irigaray herself does not sufficiently extend this as a way of thinking about other cultural, racial, and historical 'others within'. To see how this might be done, we could turn to the work of Christine Battersby.

In *The Phenomenal Woman*, Battersby develops a distinctive feminist metaphysics for a female body that births, starting out from the question of 'what would have to change were we to take seriously the notion that a "person" could normally, at least always potentially, become two.'[58] As this suggests, Battersby's project is informed by Irigaray's work, though her position also differs from Irigaray's in significant ways. Rather than repeating the feminist rejection of essence, Battersby seeks a reworked model that does not involve the Aristotelian paradigm of 'underlying sameness of substance'.[59] Instead she re-positions essence in terms of a 'historically and socially emergent norm that changes over time'.[60] This model of 'fluid essence' means that, while Battersby agrees with Irigaray that being female 'involves a necessary reference to bodily morphology', she places more emphasis than Irigaray on the ways in which the 'bodily/sexual categories of male and female ... are historically and culturally variable'.[61] Thus, rather than positioning sexual difference in terms of either biological essence or ontological difference (in Irigaray's post-Heideggerian sense), Battersby argues that 'for us (in our culture) to be a female human is tied to a body that could birth' in ways that 'result[s] in a specific positioning in terms of the social networks of power and the conceptual networks by which identity is determined'.[62] A key factor in this socio-historical positioning is the way that an embodied female subject, capable of bearing otherness within, need only be seen as paradoxical 'if the male subject is taken as norm.'[63] In response, Battersby develops an alternative model of the self that takes the capacity to birth as both normal and constitutive and links the female subject-position 'to ways of thinking identity as emerging out of patterns of becoming. On such a model, "self" grows out of "otherness", and "sameness" is gradually patterned from "difference".[64]

In her later book *The Sublime, Terror and Human Difference*, Battersby can be seen as drawing on this model in which identity is shaped by fluid inter-relations with otherness (both 'within' and 'without') to account for the different kinds of 'others' who inhabit the folds of history. The book begins by undertaking exactly the kind of critical genealogy which Deutscher advocates, offering a detailed examination of Kant's views on both women and race (as well as the complex relations between them) in relation to the privileged aesthetic category of the sublime. As Battersby emphasizes, her approach does not involve arguing that all female or non-European subjects occupy identical positions in relation to such categories, but paying attention to 'the *specificity* of the exclusions relating to human differences' in a tradition that takes the European male subject as both norm and ideal.[65] Drawing on Nietzsche, Battersby goes on to develop an account of a 'radical otherness' which is 'not simply a construct of the I' and hence is not merely the other *of* the (European, male) subject. Nonetheless, this otherness is 'not negated': it disappears from the subject's gaze *without* thereby disappearing from the 'multifaceted complexities' of reality or history.[66] Historical time harbours a multiplicity of differences and 'others within', who cannot all be seen from within a single space-time frame. Such 'forgotten differences' have the capacity to re-erupt in ways that transform established conceptual frameworks by forcing us to recall that which does not belong to them as they stand.[67]

Battersby's approach means taking seriously the need to rethink the metaphysical categories with which we conceptualize both the female subject and other kinds of 'others' whose exclusion has played a constitutive role in the western philosophical tradition. By extending the valence of Irigaray's attention to the existence of 'others within', her work provides a way of re-approaching the issue of race as ontological – not in the Heideggerian sense of originary difference which Irigaray deploys, but as a category that is 'constitutive of reality', as outlined in Linda Martín Alcoff's analysis of race and racial identity.[68] Although as Alcoff notes, by the end of the twentieth century a consensus had emerged that 'race is a myth, that the term corresponds to no significant biological category', this does not affect the manifold ways in which racial categories continue to have real effects in lived experience.[69]

Alcoff thus argues that we should think of race as an 'ontological category':

> [W]hen I say that race is an ontological category I am using ontology here to refer to basic categories of reality which are within history, at least partly produced by social practices, and which are culturally various. Race itself signifies differently and is lived differently between different discursive and cultural locations. ... the traditional ontological project of ascertaining certain basic categories can be reconfigured as the attempt to ascertain those elements of reality which, although mutable, currently intersect and determine a wide variety of discourses and practices, and thus are more fundamental not because of their ahistorical or transcendental status but because of their central intersectional position.[70]

For Battersby and Alcoff, both race and sexual difference 'can be understood to figure in identity formation not as a *metaphysical* necessity but as a necessity with a given *historical* context.'[71] Such approaches offer positive responses to Irigaray's call for an attentiveness to difference based on non-appropriative relations to otherness. But neither Alcoff nor Battersby position race or sexual difference in terms of the originary ontological difference which I have suggested is central to Irigaray's position, and which I suspect both thinkers would see as making difference constitutive in ways that are troublingly ahistorical.

One thinker who does seek to position race as having the kind of originary ontological status that Irigaray accords to sexuate difference is Penelope Ingram, who draws on Frantz Fanon's phenomenological writings on race, as well as both Heidegger and Derrida, to supplement Irigaray and develop an ontology of racial and sexual difference capable of thinking alterity positively in all its forms. Implicitly recalling Irigaray's dialogue with Levinas, Ingram argues that the ontological *is* the ethical insofar as 'Being is disclosed in the ethical encounter with the Other'.[72] Like Irigaray, she also suggests that the form/matter distinction must be undone if the logic of Othering that sustains representational thought is to be overcome. Ingram's analysis leads to a rich discussion of the non-representational operations of racially and sexually signifying bodies in both film and literature, and shows how the challenge of rethinking sexual alongside racial difference is crucial to how we take up and develop Irigaray's work. Nonetheless, in the end it remains unclear in what sense the 'sexual' and 'racial' are themselves ontological on Ingram's account: the ethical relations she seeks to cultivate seem to be enabled by a material ontology which gives ontological status to difference itself, reconceived as something like self-differentiating matter, in ways that allow multiple differences to be affirmed at the ontic (bodily) level. While such an ontology has a strong appeal to those interested in questions of difference (of all kinds), from an Irigarayan perspective, the concern would be that the specifically *sexuate* nature of originary difference – and hence, the sexuate nature of our being – has once again been lost, in favour of a proliferation of multiple differences.

One significant feature of Ingram's discussion is that she does not link Irigaray's account of sexuate difference as ontological specifically to Irigaray's concern with our beginnings in birth. However, I have suggested that for Irigaray, sexuate difference is constitutive of our being *because* it is the condition of our coming into being, in ways that are disclosed in our originary relations with the body of the mother. For Irigaray, we all begin as 'others within', while the sexuate specificity of our relations to the mother provides different (sexuate) starting points for building relations to 'others without'. Thus, before deciding whether we would wish to give race the same kind of originary ontological status as Irigaray gives to sexuate difference, it would be necessary to work through the complex and troubled genealogy that connects concepts of race to those of genesis and origin, particularly given the ways in which such concepts have been historically conjoined with notions of 'purity' so as to legitimate not only hierarchical exclusions but the worst kinds of genocidal violence. This is not to say that there could not be ways of according race ontological status – Alcoff and Battersby show how this might be done, albeit in ways that require a concept of the ontological that differs from Irigaray's, while Ingram's work demonstrates the generative potential of seeking an originary ontology of racial and sexual difference. But it is a further reminder that to do ontological justice to race alongside sexuate difference does not necessarily mean positioning them in exactly the same ways.

The ominous resonances of the conjunction of race with the discourse of origin reminds us (by way of contrast) that difference figures largely as a positive value in Irigaray's work; difference is what we have failed to think, and what an ethics of sexuate difference will help us think otherwise. But this does not mean that all differences are always positive: her work reflects the fact that differences can structured in ways that are oppressive, hierarchical, and exclusionary. As a final reflection on Irigaray's development of an ethics of sexuate difference, I would suggest that one of its strengths is the way in which it gives us a touchstone for differentiating differences: those which lead to exclusion, oppression, and the devaluation of human beings in their irreducibility should be resisted and wherever possible overcome; those which allow not only the sexuate specificity but the singular uniqueness of each irreducible being to flourish should be cultivated and nurtured.

Conclusion

The Incalculable Being of Being Between

> If we are to get away from the omnipotent model of the one and the many, we have to move on to the *two*, a two which is not two times one itself, not even a bigger or a smaller one, but which would be made up of *two* which are really different. (*DBT*, 129)

One of Ingram's concerns about Irigaray's own position is that her conception of sexuate difference in terms of 'being two' is unnecessarily limiting. Thus Ingram suggests that, while Irigaray is clear that the terms for both a female subject and an ethical relation between the sexes have yet to be adequately articulated, her emphasis on being two means that: 'the theorization of such an ethics is firmly lodged in our present conceptions of a relation, albeit a future one, between *male* and *female* subjects.'[1] As Ingram's concern is shared by other feminist readers, I wish to conclude by suggesting that before coming to this judgement, we need to ensure we have fully taken on board just how transformed and transformative Irigaray's notion of the 'two' is. It is not just that as Ingram rightly says, this two 'is not binarized or hierarchized':[2] it is not even 'two', in any recognizable sense.

As we have seen, Irigaray's project involves working towards an account of sexuate difference in which there are not only two subjects, but two different and non-symmetrical processes of (self-) constitution. This is crucial if the sexuate subjects who articulate being (as) two are not simply to collapse back into two 'ones': two versions of the same kind of subject, each making the other into an 'other of the Same'. Hence Irigaray's suspicion of calls for the multiple: if we multiply the number of different subjects we are prepared to recognize without multiplying their processes of constitution at the same time, we will end up reproducing further versions of the self-identical unity that constitutes the traditional male subject. For Irigaray, sexuate difference as ontological difference structures an opening for thought, leading us to consider two necessarily different processes of constitution producing subjects with constitutively different ways of building relations to others.

The significance of these differing processes of constitution is reflected in Irigaray's emphasis, throughout her elaboration of the terms for a female subject, on a 'two' that cannot be a duality or doubling in any simple sense: 'For the/a woman, two does not divide into ones. Relationships defy being cut into units' (S, 236). As we have seen, figures such as the two lips and the placental economy allow Irigaray to present woman in terms that escape a logic that pits one against its other. In contrast to such a logic, in which identity is secured via a split with the other that ensures the replication of the self-same, Irigaray writes of the way that: 'within herself, she is already two – but not divisible into one(s) – that caress each other. ... Whence the mystery that woman represents in a culture claiming to count everything, to number everything by units ... *She is neither one nor two*. Rigorously speaking, she cannot be identified either as one person, or as two' (TS, 24, 26). As noted above, the space between men and women as sexuate subjects is not the same as the space between the two lips that figure woman in her sexuate specificity. Nonetheless, it is *because* women's lips cannot be simply divided, so that she is neither one nor two, that she cannot be simply added together with the male subject to make two 'ones'. Instead, she is 'without common measure with the one (of the subject)' (S, 238).

In this way, Irigaray escapes specular oppositions by turning duality (of lips and thus of subjects) into dis-symmetrical difference that strictly speaking can no longer be counted as two at all: 'two syntaxes. Irreducible in their strangeness and eccentricity one to the other. ... In fact, of course, these terms cannot fittingly be designated by the number "two" and the adjective "different", if only because they are not susceptible to comparison' (S, 139). We need to take Irigaray seriously when she says that the number 'two' is inadequate to designate sexual difference, and when she reminds us, as she repeatedly does, that this difference is properly speaking incalculable: 'What does the difference between woma(e)n and ma(e)n consist of? The error has been to want to quantify or enumerate a difference which is of another nature than one which can be described, evaluated, counted' (*DBT*, 150). Unlike the indifferent logic that 'speak[s] of the "other" in a language already systematized by/for the same' (*S*, 139), an ontology founded on 'being two' remains attentive to the incalculable difference that makes it impossible to quantify beings *as* two, if 'two' denotes anything like two ones, or a binary, doubling, or duality. In the end, whether we are talking of two lips, two women, or a woman and a man, the 'two' marks an incalculable difference between beings who are irreducible both to each other, and to two times one: 'we are more than one. And two. The accounts overflow, calculation is lost. *If* neither I nor you are appropriated by the one or the other' (*EP*, 58–9; my emphasis).

As this passage reminds us, this irreducible difference can be articulated with differing degrees of cultivation or denial. Irigaray calls on us to cultivate difference by making space for woman as a sexuate subject as well as for a relation between the sexes in which neither seeks to appropriate the other. Re-orienting ourselves in terms of such non-appropriative relations would transform our relations to differences of all kinds; in ways that Irigaray's work suggests but does not always fully develop, it would also mean allowing the diversity of those differences to transform *us*, along with our models of family, community and political life. And in all these forms of life, an attentiveness to sexuate difference and our beginnings in birth would call on us to nurture the singular irreducibility of each (sexuate) being. To undertake this shared project of cultural transformation, we will require not only attentiveness, but also imagination, immense patience, and a capacity for laughter:

> Neither one nor two. I've never known how to count. Up to you. In their calculations, we make two. Really, two? Doesn't that make you laugh? An odd sort of two. And yet not one. Especially not one. Let's leave *one* to them ... And the strange way they divide up their couples, with the other as the image of the one. [...] Whereas we are always one and the other, at the same time. (*TS*, 207, 217)

Notes

Introduction: Towards a Sexuate Philosophy

1 While Irigaray has emphasized the philosophical grounding of her project, she is uneasy about any simple identification of her work as 'feminist' (see the interview, 'Je – Luce Irigaray', 97, 100).
2 Kant, *Critique of Pure Reason*, 22 [Bxvi–xvii].
3 Burke, 'Translation Modified', 257. For a perceptive essay on the different kinds of reading relationship invited by Irigaray's texts, see Still, 'Poetic Nuptials'.
4 Foucault argues that 'sex' is itself a construction, a 'fictitous unity' which operates to regulate behaviour, while Butler develops his ideas to position both 'sex' and gendered identity as retroactive effects, 'illusions of substance' fabricated via repeated gendered performances. See Foucault, *The History of Sexuality: Volume 1*, 154; Butler, *Gender Trouble: Feminism and the Subversion of Identity*, 186.
5 On this point, see Gatens, *Feminism and Philosophy: Perspectives on Difference and Equality*, 115; Stone, *Luce Irigaray and the Philosophy of Sexual Difference*, 9–10; Battersby, *The Phenomenal Woman: Feminist Metaphysics and the Patterns of Identity*, 18–23.
6 The rubric 'New French Feminisms' derives from Marks and Courtivron's 1981 collection of the same name. While problematic because of its homogenizing effects, this label does carry historical significance insofar as it marks the moment when the work of a number of French feminist thinkers impacted on Anglo-American feminist thought. Alongside Irigaray, the two thinkers most commonly invoked under this rubric are Hélène Cixous and Julia Kristeva.
7 See Gatens' critique of the sex/gender distinction in *Imaginary Bodies*, 3–20.

8 See Chanter, *Ethics of Eros: Irigaray's rewriting of the Philosophers*, preface and ch. 1; Fuss, *Essentially Speaking: Feminism, Nature and Difference*, ch. 4; Gatens, *Feminism and Philosophy*, ch. 6; Grosz, *Sexual Subversions: Three French Feminists*, ch. 4; Schor, 'This Essentialism Which is Not One'; Stone, *Luce Irigaray and the Philosophy of Sexual Difference*, chs 1 and 3; Whitford, *Luce Irigaray: Philosophy in the Feminine*, and 'Reading Irigaray in the Nineties'.

9 Cimitile and Miller, *Returning to Irigaray*, 1–2; 4.

10 Whitford's introduction in *The Irigaray Reader*, 12.

11 Ibid., 11; see also Burke, 'Translation Modified', 257.

12 Burke, 'Translation Modified', 250.

13 Whitford, *Luce Irigaray*, 3.

14 Chanter, *Ethics of Eros*, 9.

15 Stone's original and productive interpretation explores Irigaray's relation to the German Romantic philosophers (particularly Hölderlin and Schelling) in ways that allow her to read Irigaray in terms of a philosophy of self-differentiating nature which demands expression in a self-critical sexuate culture.

16 Deutscher, *A Politics of Impossible Difference: The Later Work of Luce Irigaray*, 29.

17 Both of these collections include essays reflecting on the state of play within Irigaray scholarship: see Schor's 'Previous Engagements: The Receptions of Irigaray' and Whitford's 'Reading Irigaray in the Nineties' in *Engaging with Irigaray*, and Cimitile and Miller's introduction to *Returning to Irigaray*, along with Gail Schwab's essay 'Reading Irigaray (and her Readers) in the Twenty-First Century'. Taken together, these provide a helpful picture of key developments in Anglo-American readings of Irigaray over the past 30 years.

18 Burke, 'Translation Modified', 251.

19 On the challenges of translating Irigaray, see Burke's 'Translation Modified'.

1 Approaching Irigaray: Feminism, Philosophy, Feminist Philosophy

1 See for example the opening paragraph of 'Questions' in *Ce sexe qui n'en est pas un*. See also Whitford, *Luce Irigaray*, 49.

2 See for example Irigaray's use of this phrase in 'The Other: Woman' in *ILTY*, a good starting point for those engaging with Irigaray's thought for the first time.

3 On the female philosopher and commentator as the 'dutiful daughter' whose work tends to be seen as both too faithful and not faithful enough, see Deutscher, '"Imperfect Discretion": Interventions into the History of Philosophy by 20th Century French Women Philosophers'.

4   See for example Moi's account in *Sexual/Textual Politics*, 126–48.
5   See for example Lloyd's classic text, *The Man of Reason: 'Male' and 'Female' in Western Philosophy*.
6   Grosz, *Sexual Subversions*, 179.
7   This forms the core of Irigaray's critique of Heidegger (who recalls the earth but forgets the fluid maternal-materiality of air) and Nietzsche (who celebrates feminine seas of becoming while forgetting the amniotic waters of birth). See *The Forgetting of Air* and *Marine Lover*, respectively; along with *Elemental Passions*, these texts form part of Irigaray's project of rethinking the elements, one of the ways in which she seeks to escape the confines of the hylomorphic tradition.
8   See Gatens, *Feminism and Philosophy*, 9–26.
9   Ibid., 24.
10 For a succinct statement of Irigaray's position on this issue, see *je, tu, nous*, 12–14.
11 Irigaray reaffirms her commitment to issues that are often raised under the banner of 'equality' in several places (for example, *je, tu, nous*, 11; *TS*, 165–6), though for the reasons outlined in this chapter, she argues that addressing such issues in the name of equality alone is at best inadequate and at worst counter-productive.
12 For Irigaray's call for sexuate rights, see in particular 'Each Sex Must Have Its Own Rights', in *Sexes and Genealogies*; 'How do we Become Civil Women?' and 'Civil Rights and Responsibilities for the Two Sexes' in *Thinking the Difference: For a Peaceful Revolution*; and 'Why Define Sexed Rights?' in *je, tu, nous*.
13 Deutscher, *A Politics of Impossible Difference*, 10.
14 See the Introduction to de Beauvoir's *The Second Sex*.
15 See Irigaray, 'A Personal Note: Equal or Different?', in *je, tu, nous*.
16 For a careful discussion of the relations between Irigaray, Cixous and Kristeva, see Oliver, *Reading Kristeva: Unravelling the Double-Bind*, ch. VII. Irigaray herself has noted the resonances between her work and some radical feminist thought in the Anglo-American tradition (*DBT*, 125); in this regard, it is worth comparing Irigaray's analysis of phallo-centrism with Frye's analysis of phallism in *The Politics of Reality*.
17 For clear accounts of Cixous on *écriture féminine* and *l'autre bisexualité*, see the relevant chapters in Sellers, *Hélène Cixous: Authorship, Autobiography and Love*, and Sarah Cooper, *Relating to Queer Theory: Rereading Sexual Self-Definition with Irigaray, Kristeva, Wittig and Cixous*.
18 For an account of Cixous which foregrounds the positive resonances between her project and Irigaray's, see Gatens, *Feminism and Philosophy*, 111–21.
19 See *ILTY*, 63: 'In my case, it was more a question of inverting myself. I was the other of/for man ... . I carried out an inversion of

the femininity imposed upon me in order to try to define the female corresponding to my gender: the in-and-for-itself of my female nature.'

20 For a clear introduction to Kristeva's thought, including the distinction between the semiotic and the symbolic, see Grosz, *Sexual Subversions*, chs 2 and 3.

21 Hence McAfee argues that, because Kristeva's work instantiates a kind of process philosophy, it cannot be essentialist, as it explodes the very category of essence; this parallels the line taken in this book with regard to Irigaray, namely, that her work is not essentialist because of her re-conceptualization of matter as active, and hence fluidly generative of form. See McAfee, *Julia Kristeva*, ch. 5.

22 Oliver, Introduction, *Ethics, Politics and Difference in Julia Kristeva's Writing*, 13.

23 For an account of Kristeva's work which shows how her critique of identity as exclusionary leads to an equally critical relation to many forms of feminism, see Grosz, *Sexual Subversions*, chs 2 and 3; Grosz problematizes the ways in which Kristeva severs femininity and maternity from having any specific link to *women*, thereby showing how her position ends up being in tension with Irigaray's. For an account placing the emphasis more on the possibilities of Kristeva's thought for the generation of a non-totalizing 'outlaw ethics' of alterity, see Oliver's *Reading Kristeva*. For an important essay in which Kristeva's position comes closer to Irigaray's, see Kristeva, 'The Meaning of Parity'.

24 See Irigaray, 'Sexual Difference as Universal' in *ILTY*.

25 Lloyd, 'Feminism in History of Philosophy', 246–7.

26 Ibid., 248–9.

27 Lloyd offers the example of Hannah Arendt, who 'thinks with' Kant in ways that extend his thought and hers by using Kant's concepts to interrogate her own present; Lloyd, 'Feminism in History of Philosophy', 253–6, 260–1.

28 For the claim that Irigaray homogenizes the history of western thought, see Battersby, *The Phenomenal Woman*, 56, 101–2, 119. Battersby emphasizes the value and import of Irigaray's project and thus her criticism is not dismissive, but raises a serious concern regarding the ways in which feminist philosophers are able to engage with and re-appropriate resources from the philosophical tradition. A related concern is raised by Deutscher regarding some of Irigaray's later work: see *A Politics of Impossible Difference*, 142–63. Deutscher contrasts the emphasis Irigaray places on the inconsistencies and instabilities within philosophical texts in her early work (including *Speculum*), with a tendency in some later work (her specific example is *To Be Two*) to read for a consistent masculinism in ways that close down the possibilities for destabilizing texts from within. Thus on Deutscher's analysis the 'myth' that the history of

philosophy has been homogeneously masculine is consolidated in Irigaray's later work (*A Politics of Impossible Difference*, 162).

29   Deutscher, *A Politics of Impossible Difference*, 191.

30   See for example Irigaray's transformative readings of Diotima's speech from Plato's *Symposium*, Descartes on wonder, or Levinas on the caress, discussed in Chapters 3, 4, and 7.

2   Re-Visiting Plato's Cave: Orientation and Origins

1   Plato, *Timaeus*, 63–4 [46a–c]; cited in *S*, 147.

2   For an account of Irigaray's notion of productive mimicry which situates it in relation to her critical and transformative approach to mimesis, see Robinson, *Reading Art, Reading Irigaray* (ch. 1). Robinson also offers helpful sections on the role of the mirror and the speculum in Irigaray's thought (ch. 2).

3   See 'The Other: Woman', in *ILTY*, where Irigaray discusses the title of *Speculum* in detail and notes that she intended the Other in the subtitle to be understood as a substantive (*ILTY*, 61), indicating the way that 'the other' is not neutral but has been identified as and with woman.

4   Plato, *Republic*, 187 [515a].

5   There are two standard English translations of the Greek term Plato uses for these archetypes (*eidos*): Ideas and Forms. Irigaray uses the French *l'Idée*, foregrounding the ideal, non-material status of the archetypes, which belong to a realm accessible only via the intellect; however their causal role in *giving form* to the sensible world is just as important for her interpretation. As the more common rendering of this term in modern English translations and commentaries is 'Forms', for the most part, I will refer to the Forms, doubling up with Idea (with a capital I) where this is more appropriate to Irigaray's argument.

6   Plato, *Republic*, 180 [506e–507c]; the word used for 'father' is *patros*.

7   As well as refering to dialogues such as *Laws*, *Phaedrus*, *Symposium* and *Theaetetus*, Irigaray also moves between the Myth of the Cave and passages from *Timaeus* (which are spoken not by Socrates but in the much less reliable voice of Timaeus himself; see Chapter 3) and a section of *Alcibiades* (on the eye as a mirror) whose status as a genuine Platonic dialogue is dubious (see Taylor, *Plato: The Man and his Work*, 12–13).

8   Plato, *Meno*, 80a–d, in *Collected Dialogues*.

9   Plato, *Theaetetus*, 149a–51d, in *Collected Dialogues*.

10   Plato, *Phaedo*, 66b–67b, in *Collected Dialogues*.

11   Stone, *An Introduction to Feminist Philosophy*, 125.

12   See Plato *Phaedo*, 67c–68b, in *Collected Dialogues*.

13   Irigaray shifts between the concepts of topography [*topographie*] and topology [*topologie*] in her reading of the myth (see *S*, 244, *Sf*, 302). The two terms are closely related: topography refers to the science of describing a particular place, focusing on its particular features; similarly, topology can be used to mean the scientific study of a particular locality, but also refers to a branch of mathematics concerned with spatial properties unchanged by any deformation that is continuous. Irigaray is concerned both with the spatial organization of Plato's myth, and with the way the myth relies on a structure of mimicry which preserves sameness through change. She is also playing on the literal meaning of these terms, from the Greek roots for place (*topos*), to write (*graphein*) and discourse, speech or reason/ing (*logos*); the cave's 'topography'/'topology' is the 'logic of place/space' it inscribes and relies upon.

14   Elsewhere Irigaray notes that the Greek tradition includes another model of mimesis which allows that mimesis is productive, rather than reproductive; Irigaray's own brand of disruptive mimicry is thus seeking to play the former tradition off against the latter. See *TS*, 131.

15   Plato, *Republic*, 187 [515a].

16   Ibid., 266 [596d–e].

17   Ibid., 266 [596e].

3   The Way Out of the Cave: A Likely Story ...

1   See Plato, *Republic*, 190 [518c].

2   See Taylor, who notes that 'Owing to the fact that the first two thirds of it were continuously preserved through the "dark ages" in the Latin version and with the commentary of Chalcidius, it was the one Greek philosophical work of the best age with which the west of Europe was well acquainted before the recovery of Aristotle's metaphysical and physical writings in the thirteenth century; it thus furnished the earlier Middle Ages with their standing general scheme of the natural world' (Taylor, *Plato*, 436).

3   Plato, *Timaeus*, 42 [29e–30a].

4   Ibid., 41 [29a–b].

5   Ibid., 43 [30d–31b].

6   Ibid., 41 [28e].

7   Ibid., 69 [50d].

8   Ibid., 122–3 [90e–91d]. The passage goes on to give an account of sexual desire as a kind of 'living creature' that possesses both men and women, making men's genitals 'naturally disobedient and self-willed, like a creature that will not listen to reason' while the womb (*hystera*) in women so longs to bear children that 'if it is left unfertilized long beyond the normal time, it causes extreme unrest, strays about the body, blocks the channels of the breath and causes in con-

sequence acute distress and disorders of all kinds' (122–3 [91c]). This image of men taken over by sexual impulses they cannot control still finds echoes in commonplace clichés about male sexuality. Even more significant for Irigaray's analysis of Freud in particular is the way in which the image of the roaming *hystera* is taken up in the nineteenth-century notion of hysteria, a psycho-sexual disorder thought to be particularly prevalant in women.

9 Plato, *Timaeus*, 69 [50c–d]; translation modified.
10 Ibid., 69–70 [50b–51a].
11 Ibid., 71 [52b].
12 Ibid., 72 [52c].
13 Ibid., 69 [50d].
14 Ibid., 70 [51a–b].
15 Ibid., 71 [52b].
16 Ibid., 123 [91c].
17 See Braidotti, 'Of Bugs and Women', 123; Mortensen, 'Woman's (Un) truth and *le féminin*: Reading Luce Irigaray with Friedrich Nietzsche and Martin Heidegger', passim; and Butler, *Bodies that Matter: On the Discursive Limits of 'Sex'*, 31.
18 Timaeus tellingly compares the receptacle to gold in which someone might mould geometric figures of all kinds; Plato, *Timaeus*, 69 [50a–b].
19 Plato, *Timaeus*, 42 [29d].
20 See *je, tu, nous* where Irigaray writes: 'One of the distinctive features of the female body is its toleration of the other's growth within itself without incurring illness or death for either one of the living organisms', and of 'the model of tolerance of the other within and with a self that this relationship manifests' (45).
21 See in particular Irigaray's interview with Hélène Rouch, 'On the Maternal Order', as well as 'The Culture of Difference', both in *je, tu, nous*.
22 In the English version of *Speculum*, '*contiguïté*' is here translated as 'conception'; elsewhere it is often translated as 'contact' (see *S*, 346, 348, 351; *Sf*, 434, 437, 439) or 'immediate contact' (*S*, 209; *Sf*, 260), a rendering which captures the important connotations of proximity and touch. However, a disadvantage of not translating '*contiguïté*' as 'contiguity' is that this obscures the way that Irigaray's project of thinking a female subject is bound up with rethinking the kinds of *relations* which constitute that subject.
23 In Plato's *Symposium*, Aristophanes tells how human beings began as circular creatures of three kinds (male, female, and an androgynous mix of the two), who Zeus punished by cutting them in half. From that time on, each sundered being sought its other half; in this way, erotic desire was born. See Plato, *Symposium*, 130–4 [189d–93a].
24 *Sexes and Genealogies*, 18–19.
25 Plato, *Symposium*, 155 [210a–d].

26 Ibid., 150 [206b].
27 See Dover ed., *Plato: Symposium*, 147. The French with which Irigaray is working renders it *'un enfantement'* from the verb to give birth, *'enfanter'*. See Irigaray, 'L'Amour sorcier', in *Éthique de la différence sexuelle*, 31–2: "Et Diotime de répondre: *'C'est un enfantement dans la beauté et selon le corps et selon l'âme.'"* Irigaray is quoting the Pléiade edition of *Symposium, Le Banquet*, in *Oeuvres Complètes* [205, 206].
28 Plato, *Symposium*, 150 [206c–d].
29 Ibid., 153 [208e–209b].
30 I borrow this formulation of sexual difference as a 'generative interval' from Pheng Cheah, in Cheah and Grosz, 'The Future of Sexual Difference: An Interview with Judith Butler and Drucilla Cornell', 27–8.
31 As Irigaray notes, 'The wisdom of love is perhaps the first meaning of the word "philosophy." ' *The Way of Love*, 1.

4 Woman as Other: Variations on an Old Theme

1 This phrase is taken from the title of the first section of *Speculum*, 'The Blind Spot of an Old Dream of Symmetry'.
2 The term 'metaphysics' originated as a way of referring to the parts of Aristotle's work that were collected together after (*meta*) those on material nature (*physis*). It has since come to refer to a branch of philosophy concerning that which goes beyond ('comes after' in the sense of transcends) the physical, material world.
3 Ackrill, *Aristotle the Philosopher*, 32.
4 Aristotle's definition of formal cause can be found in *Physics*, II.3.194b lines 27–9, in *The Complete Works of Aristotle*, vol. 1; and *Metaphysics*, I.3.983a lines 24–29, in *Complete Works*, vol. 2.
5 Politis, *Aristotle and the 'Metaphysics'*, 53.
6 The notion of onto-theology is drawn from Heidegger's use of this term, which contributes to his analysis of the forgetting of Being in western philosophical thought; as discussed in Chapter 6, Irigaray extends this analysis by suggesting that it is not just Being, but the sexuate nature of Being that has been forgotten.
7 Aristotle, *Generation of Animals* in *Complete Works*, vol. 1, 1130 [728a17–18] and 1144 [737a27–9]. See also Freeland, 'Nourishing Speculation' and Tuana, 'Aristotle and the Politics of Reproduction'.
8 Aristotle, *Generation of Animals*, in *Complete Works*, vol. 1, 1133 [728a32–3].
9 Gerson, Introduction, *The Cambridge Companion to Plotinus*, 3.
10 O'Meara, 'The Hierarchical Ordering of Reality in Plotinus', 77.
11 Gerson, Introduction, *The Cambridge Companion to Plotinus*, 6.

12 As noted, all quotations from this section of *Speculum* are direct citations from Plotinus' *Enneads* (specifically, the Sixth Tractate), as indicated in Gill's translation of *Speculum*, which uses Plotinus' *Enneads*, trans. S. MacKenna, 201–22. For full reference, see *S*, 168.

13 See Brandhorst, *Descartes' 'Meditations on First Philosophy'*.

14 Descartes, *Optics*, in *The Philosophical Writings of Descartes: vol. 1*, 166.

15 Descartes, *Optics*, cited in *S*, 180. As the version of *Optics* I am using here, from *The Philosophical Writings of Descartes: vol. 1*, is abridged, the passage Irigaray cites is not included; however, Descartes makes a similar point in the *Treatise on Man*, also in *The Philosophical Writings of Descartes: vol. 1*, 106. The original French text can be found in *La Dioptrique*, in René Descartes, *Oeuvres et Lettres*, 216; see the translator's note, *S*, 180.

16 Not only did Descartes' female contemporaries take up and debate his philosophy, but Descartes himself taught and admired some of them, dedicating his *Principles of Philosophy* to one of the most famous, Princess Elisabeth of Bohemia. See also note 24 below.

17 The passage cited as an epigraph also continues the tradition of reducing maternal generative power to a reproductive function which woman passively fulfils. In strong contrast to Irigaray's own elaboration of a placental economy (see Chapter 6), the subtle interactions between mother and foetus are here reduced to mechanical processes over which neither has any control.

18 On this point, see also Lloyd, *The Man of Reason*, 44–50. For a feminist analysis that positions Descartes' philosophy as part of a distinctively seventeenth-century 'masculinization of thought', see Bordo, *The Flight to Objectivity: Essays On Cartesianism and Culture*.

19 See for example Husserl, *Cartesian Meditations*, 35–7.

20 See also Descartes, *Discourse on the Method*, Part One, in *The Philosophical Writings of Descartes: vol. I*, 111–16, and the opening paragraph of the 'First Meditation', *Meditations on First Philosophy*, in *The Philosophical Writings of Descartes: vol. II*, 12.

21 See Descartes, *Meditations on First Philosophy*, in *The Philosophical Writings of Descartes: vol. II*, 31–2.

22 For a succinct and compelling analysis of the way Cartesian mind–body dualism has contributed to making the body a conceptual blindspot in western philosophical thought, together with its implications for feminism, see Grosz's *Volatile Bodies: Towards A Corporeal Feminism*, 3–24.

23 Descartes, *Meditations on First Philosophy*, in *The Philosophical Writings of Descartes: vol. II*, 56.

24 One of the first readers to put significant critical pressure on the relation of mind and body was Elisabeth of Bohemia (see note 16 above). Descartes exchanged an important series of letters with Elisabeth on this topic (see Shapiro, ed., *Princess Elisabeth of Bohemia and René Descartes*), and wrote *The Passions of the Soul* partly in

response to her questions. More recently, Erica Harth has drawn attention to the genealogy linking Irigaray back to Elisabeth and other seventeenth-century female readers and critics of Descartes, suggesting that Irigaray's own 'methodical doubt' of philosophical history may make her 'the last of the Cartesian women'. Harth, *Cartesian Women*, 235.

25 Descartes, *The World*, in *The Philosophical Writings of Descartes: vol. 1*, 90.

26 Ibid., 92.

27 Ibid., 91–2.

28 Ibid., 92; Descartes explicitly equates nature with matter at this point. See also *Meditations on First Philosophy*, in *The Philosophical Writings of Descartes: vol. II*, 44.

29 Descartes, *The Passions of the Soul*, art. 53, 358; this reference is to the Haldene and Ross translation in *The Philosophical Works of Descartes, vol. 1*, as cited in Irigaray, *ESD*, 73.

30 Kant, *Critique of Pure Reason*, 22 [Bxvi–xvii].

31 Ibid., 245–47 [B275–79].

32 There are two key aspects to this process (what Kant calls the two 'fundamental sources' of knowledge, see *Critique of Pure Reason*, 92–3 [A50–52 B74–76]). First, nothing can appear to human beings unless it does so within a space-time frame. Sensible intuitions are not strictly speaking 'raw data' but always already framed by the forms of intuition, space and time. These forms are the a priori condition of anything appearing to us at all. The spatio-temporal flux of appearances is then organized or synthesized according to a priori conceptual rules so as to constitute recognizable objects. These rules or categories, which are provided by the understanding, are thus the second component of the transcendental frame making experience and knowledge of objects possible.

33 These essays can be found Kant, *Werke vol. 1: Vorkritische Schriften I 1747–1756*, 415–72. The passage cited from *Speculum* seems to refer to the third essay, where Kant is particularly scathing of those who think the earthquake was caused by the earth going off course and moving closer to the sun.

34 For Kant's early ('pre-critical') account of the sublime, see *Observations on the Feeling of the Beautiful and Sublime*. His more mature philosophy of aesthetics, informed by the Copernican turn made in the *Critique of Pure Reason*, is presented in the *Critique of Judgment*.

35 Kant, *Prolegomena to Any Future Metaphysics*, 37–8 [4:285–6], cited in *S*, 203.

36 As Kant puts it: 'there are no inner differences here that any understanding could merely think, and yet the differences are inner as far as the senses teach, for the left hand cannot, after all, be enclosed within the same boundaries as the right (they cannot be made congruent)', *Prolegomena*, 37–8 [4:286].

37   Kant, 'What is Orientation in Thinking?', 295 [8:135], cited in S, 203. The final sentence of the passage Irigaray cites (which is missing from the English translation of *Speculum*) reads as follows: 'This happens at night when I walk and make the proper turns in a street which I know but in which I cannot distinguish any houses.'

38   For the technical distinction between determinative and reflective judgement, see Kant, First Introduction to the *Critique of Judgment*, §V, 399–404 [XX:211–16]; and Second Introduction, §IV, 18–20 [5:179–81].

39   See for example Kant, Second Introduction, *Critique of Judgment*, §VI and VII, 26 and 30 [5:186 and 190].

40   For Kant's account of the mathematical and dynamic sublime (provoked by nature's apparent infinity or its might respectively), see *Critique of Judgment* §25–8, 103–23 [5: 248–64].

41   See Kant, *Critique of Judgment* §28, 123 [5:264].

42   For Irigaray's use of this term, see ESD, 32; *To Speak is Never Neutral*, 243; and 'Women-amongst-themselves', in *The Irigaray Reader*, 190.

43   On Kant's inability to 'intelligibly explicate' either inner bodily spaces or 'otherness within the self, the foetus in the womb', see Battersby, *The Phenomenal Woman*, 71. Battersby's analysis, which it is extremely helpful to read alongside Irigaray, draws on a comment Kant makes in a letter to Schiller in 1795, where he describes sexual difference as a 'chasm of thought' (Kant, cited in Battersby, 71).

44   BEW, 73–91; for Kant's essay, 'An Answer to the Question: What is Enlightenment?', see *Immanuel Kant: Practical Philosophy*, 11–21 [8:33–42].

5   Freud, Lacan, and Speaking (as a) Woman

1   For a more extensive analysis of the psychoanalytic dimensions of Irigaray's work, see Whitford's unparalleled *Luce Irigaray*. Whitford offers a detailed account of the way Irigaray critically entwines philosophical and psychoanalytic frames to transform both while generating the terms for an alternative feminine subject.

2   The unconscious thus has what Kant would call a transcendental status. This is particularly clear in Freud's 1915 paper 'The Unconscious', in *On Metapsychology*, 167–73.

3   This passage echoes Kant's famous claim that two things fill the mind with ever-increasing awe, *'the starry heavens above me and the moral law within me.'* Kant, *Critique of Practical Reason*, 258 [5:161].

4   Freud, 'Femininity', in *New Introductory Lectures on Psychoanalysis*, 169.

5   Ibid., 147; cited in S, 15.

6   Ibid., 152; cited in S, 31.

7   Freud 'Dissolution of the Oedipus Complex', in *On Sexuality*, 320; cited in *S*, 32.

8   Ibid., 320–1.

9   This means that in the case of the little girl, as Freud himself notes, the order of the Oedipus complex and the castration complex is reversed (in comparison to their role in the little boy's development). See Freud, 'Some Psychical Consequences of the Anatomical Distinction Between the Sexes', in *On Sexuality*, 341. As the castration anxiety propels the little girl into the Oedipal complex rather than resolving it, further problems arise as to how this phase can ever be adequately resolved into 'normal' sexuality for the girl, who Freud argues will be prone to neurosis (characterized, unsurprisingly, by a general suppression of her sexual instincts) or 'masculinism' (that is, female homosexuality considered as an 'abnormal' sexual type). See Freud, 'Femininity', in *New Introductory Lectures on Psychoanalysis*, 160–4; and *S*, 98–104.

10 Recalling Aristotle's description of woman as a kind of mutilated male, at one point Freud describes how the little boy sees the mother as a 'mutilated creature'. Freud, 'Some Psychical Consequences of the Anatomical Distinction Between the Sexes', in *On Sexuality*, 336; cited in *S*, 59.

11 Freud, 'Femininity', in *New Introductory Lectures on Psychoanalysis*, 159; see also *S*, 57–8.

12 See Chapter 3, note 8.

13 *S*, 69, citing Freud, 'Mourning and Melancholia', in *On Metapsychology*, 257.

14 *S*, 67–8, citing Freud, 'Mourning and Melancholia', in *On Metapsychology*, 254.

15 Freud, 'Female Sexuality', in *On Sexuality*, 373; cited in *S*, 64. In this essay, Freud goes so far as to draw an analogy between the early pre-Oedipal stage in girls and the archeological discovery of 'the Minoan-Mycenaean civilization behind the civilization of Greece.' 'Female Sexuality', 372; cited in *S*, 64.

16 Freud, 'Female Sexuality', in *On Sexuality*, 372, cited in *S*, 63–4.

17 See Lacan, *Encore: On Feminine Sexuality: The Limits of Love and Knowledge*, 15, and *The Four Fundamental Concepts of Pyschoanalysis*, 149, 203.

18 Footnote 26 of *Speculum* (*S*, 43; *Sf*, n28, 47) refers to 'foreclosure' (*forclusion*) as a specifically 'Lacanian' term; thus the only appearance of Lacan's name (one that does not quite name him, but refers to the mode of psychoanalysis arising from his thought) is consigned, appropriately enough, to the margins of Irigaray's text.

19 Lacan, 'The Mirror Stage', in *Écrits*, 75–81; 75–6.

20 On the parallel between the mis-identification of the mirror stage and the split that takes place in the *cogito*, see for example 'The Function and Field of Speech and Language in Psychoanalysis [The Rome

Discourse]', where Lacan refers to 'the passivating image by which the subject makes himself an object by displaying himself before the mirror' (*Écrits*, 208).

21 Lacan, 'The Mirror Stage', in *Écrits*, 75. See also Lacan's radical rewriting of the *cogito* in 'The Instance of the Letter in the Unconscious': 'I am thinking where I am not, therefore I am where I am not thinking' (*Écrits*, 429–30).

22 See Lacan, 'The Mirror Stage', in *Écrits*, 76.

23 Ibid.

24 See Lacan, 'The Instance of the Letter in the Unconscious': 'language, with its structure, exists prior to each subject's entry into it at a certain moment in his mental development. ... And the subject, while he may appear to be the slave of language, is still more the slave of a discourse in the universal movement of which his place is already inscribed at his birth, if only in the form of his proper name' (*Écrits*, 413–14).

25 'There isn't the slightest prediscursive reality, for the very fine reason that what constitutes a collectivity – what I call men, women, and children – means nothing qua prediscursive reality. *Men, women and children are but signifiers.*' Lacan, *Encore*, 33; my emphasis. On the constitution of the subject as signifier, see in particular 'The Function and Field of Speech and Language' and 'The Instance of the Letter in the Unconscious', both in *Écrits*.

26 Stavrakakis, *Lacan and the Political*, 28.

27 See *TS*, 101, where Irigaray aligns the symbolic with the intelligible as 'the place of inscription of forms'.

28 Lacan, *Encore*, 72.

29 Ibid., 72–3; for the French, see *Le Seminaire de Jacques Lacan, XX: Encore*, 68.

30 Lacan, *Encore*, 81.

31 Ibid., 72; *Le Seminaire de Jacques Lacan, XX: Encore*, 68.

32 My rendering of these lines is informed by that offered by David Macey in *The Irigaray Reader* (57), where the relevant chapter of *Speculum* appears under the title 'Volume without Contours'. It is worth keeping Macey's alternative title in mind alongside that used in the Gill translation ('Volume-Fluidity'). Each captures a different aspect of the thought Irigaray seeks to convey (in the original French, *L'incontournable volume*, lit. the uncircumscribable volume). Where I have modified translations of this chapter, this is always in consultation with Macey's version.

33 See for example Lacan, *Encore*, 6: 'Love is impotent, though mutual, because it is not aware that it is but the desire to be One, which leads us to the impossibility of establishing the relationship between "them-two" (*la relation d'eux*). The relationship between them-two what? – them-two sexes.'

34 Gallop, *Feminism and Psychoanalysis: The Daughter's Seduction*, 40.

35   See Lacan, *Encore*, 15, and *Four Fundamental Concepts*, 149, 203.
36   See Lacan, 'The Function and Field of Speech and Language': 'the subject's unconscious is the other's discourse', *Écrits*, 219.
37   See for example Lacan, *Encore*, 81.
38   See Lacan, *Four Fundamental Concepts*, 203–5: 'The Other is the locus in which is situated the chain of the signifier that governs whatever may be made present of the subject ... the subject depends on the signifier and ... the signifier is first of all in the field of the Other.'
39   Lacan, *Encore*, 76.
40   Ibid., 74–6.
41   See the translator's note, *S*, 191.
42   For another reading that emphasizes the intensely 'double-edged' language of the 'Volume-Fluidity' chapter, see Rawes, *Irigaray for Architects*, 79, which foregrounds Irigaray's use of the term *'écart'* (gap, space, distance).
43   See *S*, 143–5 and *S*, 191 the epigram from Ruysbroeck the Admirable.

6   The Status of Sexuate Difference

1   I borrow this formulation of sexual difference as a radical dissymmetry between the sexes from Braidotti, 'Of Bugs and Women', 121–2.
2   Irigaray, *je, tu, nous*, 45.
3   Mortensen, 'Woman's (Un)truth and *le féminin*', 212.
4   See in particular 'Volume-Fluidity' (*S*, 227–40) and 'The "Mechanics" of Fluids' (*TS*, 106–18).
5   For a detailed analysis of *EP*, see Canters and Jantzen, *Forever Fluid: A Reading of Luce Irigaray's Elemental Passions*.
6   Nonetheless, as Vasseleu shows in *Textures of Light: Vision and Touch in Irigaray, Levinas and Merleau-Ponty*, Irigaray's project does not simply denigrate vision, but implies a rethinking of the relation between sight, light and touch. This is reflected in a number of recent texts that take up the potential of Irigaray's work for filmic analysis: see Constable, *Thinking in Images: Film Theory, Feminist Philosophy and Marlene Dietrich*; Bainbridge, *Feminine Cinematics: Luce Irigaray, Women and Film*; and Bolton, "'But what if the object started to speak?': The Representation of Female Consciousness On-Screen".
7   On the lips as those of both mouth and labia, as well as the relation of lips to touch, see *To Speak Is Never Neutral*, 240–44. Here and in *An Ethics of Sexual Difference*, Irigaray links the lips to mucous, another figure drawn from the female body which could have been included in this chapter, and which Irigaray deploys across a number of texts

to help articulate the fluid self–other relation characterizing the female subject.

8 Irigaray, *The Way of Love*, 11.
9 On this point, see *Sexes and Genealogies*, 14–19.
10 This charge is made for example by Toril Moi and by Monique Plaza, in the following terms: 'Irigaray's attempt to establish a theory of femininity that escapes patriarchal specul(ariz)ation necessarily lapses into a form of essentialism. Her efforts to provide woman with a "gallant representation of her own sex" (S 130) are likewise doomed to become another enactment of the inexorable logic of the Same ... She thus comes to analyse 'woman' in idealist categories, just like the male philosophers she is denouncing' (Moi, *Sexual Textual Politics*, 142, 147–8). '[Luce Irigaray's] approach remains fundamentally naturalist and completely influenced by patriarchal ideology. For one cannot describe morphology as if it presented itself to perception without ideological mediation. The positivism of Irigaray's construction is here doubled by a flagrant empiricism. ... The whole mode of existence that ideology imputes to women as dependent on the Eternal Feminine, and which Irigaray seems for a moment to have posed as the result of oppression, from now on is woman's essence, woman's being. All that "is" woman comes to her in the last instance from her anatomical sex, which touches itself all the time' (Plaza, ' "Phallomorphic" Power and the Psychology of "Woman" ', 97).
11 Schor, 'This Essentialism Which Is Not One', 60. Schor nuances the debate by showing that *'essentialism is not one'* and distinguishing four different critiques of essentialism. This helps show how Irigaray can be aligned with some critiques of essentialism, while simultaneously being the target of others.
12 Schor, 'This Essentialism Which Is Not One', 59.
13 See for example hooks, *Ain't I a Woman* and Spivak, *In Other Worlds: Essays in Cultural Politics*.
14 See Braidotti, 'Of Bugs and Women', 112.
15 Chanter, *Ethics of Eros*, 175.
16 Pregnancy can also be represented as a form of alienation of course, as happens in de Beauvoir's depiction of the pregnant woman as 'tenanted by another' (*The Second Sex*, 55). However, the point is that pregnancy need not be depicted in this way. Part of what Irigaray seeks to show is that descriptions of the female body are never neutral but reflect, reinforce, and (sometimes) disrupt specific conceptual frameworks. Hence her attentiveness to aspects of pregnant embodiment which do not readily fit an oppositional self/other model, for which she seeks more appropriate conceptual terms.
17 The term 'strategic essentialism' was coined by Spivak, in the context of her work on Subaltern Studies; see Spivak, *In Other Worlds*, 205.

18 See in particular Fuss, *Essentially Speaking* and Whitford, *Luce Irigaray*. I am indebted to both Whitford and Fuss, whose readings inform my own throughout; see in particular the discussion of the two lips earlier in this chapter, and of contact and contiguity in Chapter 3.

19 Fuss, *Essentially Speaking*, 72.

20 By 'traditional', I mean broadly those inherited from the Aristotelian tradition outlined in Chapter 3, whereby something is made what it is by its formal cause – or 'essence' – which contains and determines its possibilities for being. For a feminist analysis which makes the case for a historicized (non-Aristotelian) model of essence as emergent (rather than determining), see Battersby, *The Phenomenal Woman*, ch. 2.

21 Whitford, *Luce Irigaray*, 103.

22 Ibid., 94.

23 Ibid., 103.

24 Ibid., 143. On the notion and necessity of 'language work' see for example *TS*, 78–80.

25 Schor, 'Previous Engagements', 11–12.

26 See for example Fuss, *Essentially Speaking*, 66; Whitford, *Luce Irigaray*, 177–85.

27 Fuss, *Essentially Speaking*, 66.

28 Whitford, *Luce Irigaray*, 182.

29 Ibid., 180–2.

30 Ibid., 173. See also 170–3 on feminist readings of the 'two lips'.

31 Gatens, *Feminism and Philosophy*, 118. See also Grosz: 'Whether male or female, the human body is thus already coded, placed in a social network, and given meaning in and by culture, the male being constituted as virile or phallic, the female as passive and castrated. These are not the result of biology, but of the *social and psychical meaning of the body*.' *Sexual Subversions*, 111.

32 Gatens, *Feminism and Philosophy*, 115. Irigaray uses the term morphology from an early stage in her work, deploying it throughout *Speculum* (see for example, *S*, 27, 229, 320) and explicitly distinguishing it from anatomy: 'we must go back to the question not of the anatomy but of the morphology of the female sex' ('Women's Exile', 64); see also Grosz, *Sexual Subversions*, 110–13.

33 Grosz, *Sexual Subversions*, 116.

34 Gatens, *Feminism and Philosophy*, 115; see also Grosz, *Sexual Subversions*, 113–17.

35 These tensions perhaps help to explain why the conceptual language of psychoanalysis and appeals to a feminine imaginary or symbolic recede in Irigaray's later works, in favour of a more philosophical language that seeks to articulate an ontology of 'being two'.

36 Whitford, *Luce Irigaray*, 91.

37 Kant, *Critique of Pure Reason*, 93, A51/B75.

38 Irigaray signals the importance of the specifically Kantian notion of the schematism to her work in the interview, ' "Je – Luce Irigaray" ', 101–2.

39 Grosz, *Sexual Subversions*, 112.

40 This is clear not only in their readings of Irigaray already cited but in their later work; see for example Gatens' critique of the sex/gender distinction in *Imaginary Bodies*, 3–20; or Grosz's account of sexual difference in *Volatile Bodies*, 17–19. In these texts, both Gatens and Grosz develop rich accounts of the body as an *active* site of self-constitution, in ways that build on and move beyond their readings of Irigaray.

41 Grosz, *Sexual Subversions*, 111; my emphasis.

42 Ibid., 117, *Volatile Bodies*, 18.

43 Stone, *Luce Irigaray and the Philosophy of Sexual Difference*, 36.

44 In her insightful analysis, Stone suggests that Irigaray's concept of 'morphology' shifts from an emphasis on cultural imagery in her earlier work, towards an active unfolding of forms shaped by sexuate bodily rhythms in her later work (*Luce Irigaray and the Philosophy of Sexual Difference*, 108–9); I would suggest that these two different ways of thinking morphology – as a product of cultural representation on the one hand, and of an actively self-shaping matter on the other – are both already present, and to some extent in tension, in Irigaray's earlier work.

45 Stone, *Luce Irigaray and the Philosophy of Sexual Difference*, 36.

46 Ibid., 99.

47 My reading here diverges from that of Stone, who argues that Irigaray's later work does in fact move towards a form of realist essentialism. Stone clearly differentiates this from the biological essentialism which has been my main critical focus here: thus, although she argues that Irigaray does think of bodies as having 'naturally different characters which require expression', she also suggests that Irigaray understands these 'inherent characters' in terms of two natural sexuate rhythms which realize themselves in a fluid unfolding of bodily forms. In turn, these (sexually differentiated) bodily forms strive to express themselves at a cultural and symbolic level (*Luce Irigaray and the Philosophy of Sexual Difference*, 106). I agree with Stone that Irigaray's project involves rethinking matter as active and self-expressive. However, rather than thinking of sexuate beings as grounded in natural (rhythmic) difference, I would argue that for Irigaray, natural bodily differences (and even the sexuate rhythms of nature) are themselves the expression of 'being (as) two' (that is, of sexuate difference understood as originary ontological difference).

48 Irigaray comes close to the notion of projective announcement in *Sharing the World*, where she writes of: 'A between-us for which we must care, like for some star, some prophecy, some announcement

being the sign of a new horizon, new progressions and ways of Being that will introduce us, alone or together, into a world until now unknown. Nevertheless, this world is more our own than what we lived as familiarity itself' (47).

49 See *The Forgetting of Air in Martin Heidegger* (originally published in 1983) and more recently, *The Way of Love* (2002) and *Sharing the World* (2008).

50 Heidegger, 'The Origin of the Work of Art', in *Poetry, Language, Thought*, 69.

51 Ibid., 35. Heidegger is here drawing on the Greek term *aletheia* (literally, non-forgetting), which Plato uses for the process of learning as recollection. See also Heidegger, *The Essence of Truth*, 6–13. Aletheia figures in Irigaray's reading of Plato in *Speculum* in ways that are in critical dialogue with both Plato and Heidegger (see *S*, 253).

52 Heidegger, 'The Origin of the Work of Art', in *Poetry, Language, Thought*, 60.

53 Ibid., 43. In ways there is not room to explore here, but which are obviously relevant to Irigaray's wider project, for Heidegger, the setting up of a world is inseparable from the way the work also 'sets forth the earth ... *The work lets the earth be an earth*' (45).

54 Heidegger, 'The Origin of the Work of Art', in *Poetry, Language, Thought*, 44.

55 Ibid., 43.

56 Drawing on both Heidegger and Hölderlin, Irigaray expands on the possibilities of building such a world through poetic language in *Sharing the World*, where she focuses on the question of how to approach the (sexuate) other as other. For an analysis which translates the implications of Irigaray's work on poetic dwelling into a sexuate approach to architecture, see Rawes, *Irigaray for Architects*, especially chapters 7 and 8.

57 For this formulation of the ontic-ontological distinction, see Gelven, *A Commentary on Heidegger's 'Being and Time'*, 24. I use the capitalized term 'Being' throughout this section to distinguish questions of Being as such from those about beings (i.e., specific entities), despite the risk of thereby re-substantializing 'Being' in ways that are at odds with both Heidegger's and Irigaray's projects. On this point, see Irigaray, *The Way of Love*, xiii–xiv.

58 *Poiēsis* is one of the words Diotima uses for the making/creating fostered by *eros*; see *Symposium* 205b-c.

59 Heidegger, 'The Origin of the Work of Art', in *Poetry, Language, Thought*, 71.

60 For Heidegger's comments on the figure in relation to the artwork, see 'The Origin of the Work of Art', in *Poetry, Language, Thought*, 62.

61 See in particular *The Way of Love*, which is in explicit dialogue with Heidegger's *Unterwegs zur Sprache* (*On the Way to Language*). Irigaray

seeks to resituate Heidegger's emphasis on 'the way to language' in the context of our originary relation to sexuate difference such that it becomes possible for language to become the site of a genuine (that is, non-appropriative) way of speaking with an other.

62 Heidegger, 'The Way to Language', in *On the Way to Language*, 127; 'Der Weg zur Sprache', in *Unterwegs zur Sprache*, 258.

63 Ibid., 128; 'Der Weg zur Sprache', in *Unterwegs zur Sprache*, 259.

64 On Irigaray's engagement with Heidegger, see Hodge, 'Irigaray Reading Heidgger', and Cimitile, 'Irigaray in Dialogue With Heidegger'.

65 Heidegger, 'A Letter on Humanism', in *Pathmarks*, 254.

66 See *Sharing the World*, 121–6.

67 See Irigaray's analysis of Heidegger in *The Forgetting of Air*, as discussed in Cimitile, 'Irigaray in Dialogue With Heidegger', 275–6.

68 Heidegger, 'The Way to Language', in *On the Way to Language*, 126; *Der Weg zur Sprache*, in *Unterwegs zur Sprache*, 257.

69 For another transformative feminist approach to philosophy – inspired in part by Irigaray, but also by Hannah Arendt – which makes the case for reorienting our thought and culture around birth, see Cavarero, *In Spite of Plato: A Feminist Rewriting of Ancient Philosophy*.

70 Heidegger, 'The Way to Language', in *On the Way to Language*, 128; 'Der Weg zur Sprache', in *Unterwegs zur Sprache*, 259.

71 Irigaray's more recent work expands on this to argue that, if Being is originally two, then the speaking of Being that can take place in poetic language 'first of all exists in a present dialogue with an other different from myself.' *The Way of Love*, xi.

72 Butler, in Cheah and Grosz, 'The Future of Sexual Difference', 28.

73 See Butler's extensive critical engagement with Irigaray in the opening chapter of *Bodies that Matter* (reprinted in *Engaging with Irigaray*). This chapter signals the very different frames within which these two thinkers are working, despite their many shared points of contact (especially Hegel and Lacan). Butler is concerned with feminist appeals to sexual difference which take the matter of bodies as unconstructed and given; she thus seeks to problematize the (discursively, normatively) constructed nature of this apparently 'unconstructed' matter. Irigaray by contrast seeks to rethink matter *as* constructive, in the sense of active and generative. Nonetheless, as Stone argues, and as I signal in the next chapter, it is not impossible to combine Irigaray's philosophy of sexuate difference with Butler's acute analysis of the socio-cultural norms that regulate gender, sexuality, and kinship, in ways that would strengthen an Irigarayan approach.

74 Cooper, *Relating to Queer Theory*, 35.

75 Schwab, 'Sexual Difference as Model: An Ethics for the Global Future', 82.

76 On this point, see the opening pages of Schwab's 'Sexual Difference as Model'; this article offers a nuanced reading of the wider implications of Irigaray's rethinking of romantic and conjugal relations by generalizing these to include couples of all sexual orientations.
77 Deutscher, *A Politics of Impossible Difference*, 78; see also 127–8; and Bostic 'Luce Irigaray and Love', 605.
78 Grosz, 'The Hetero and the Homo: The Sexual Ethics of Luce Irigaray', 335.
79 See *To Speak is Never Neutral*, 243.
80 Grosz, 'The Hetero and the Homo', 339.
81 Ibid., 335–50. On this issue, see also Whitford, *Luce Irigaray*, 154.
82 Whitford, 'Reading Irigaray in the Nineties', 27.
83 ' "Je – Luce Irigaray" ', 112.
84 Grosz, 'The Hetero and the Homo', 340.
85 Whitford, *Luce Irigaray*, 154.
86 See for example Bostic, 'Luce Irigaray and Love', 606; Pheng Cheah in Cheah and Grosz, 'The Future of Sexual Difference', 28.
87 ' "Je – Luce Irigaray" ', 112.
88 Bostic, 'Luce Irigaray and Love', 605, quoting *ILTY*, 82.
89 Gelven, *A Commentary on Heidegger's 'Being and Time'*, 24; see sections I and II of Gelven's book for a clear introduction to the key Heideggerian notions of the ontic, the ontological, and *Dasein*.
90 Stone, *Luce Irigaray and the Philosophy of Sexual Difference*, 96.
91 Chanter, *Ethics of Eros*, 127; Chanter offers an excellent in-depth account of Irigaray's relation to Heidegger, as well as of sexual difference to ontological difference, see 127–51 in particular.
92 Heidegger, *Being and Time*, 32: 'Dasein is an entity which does not just occur among other entities. Rather it is ontically distinguished by the fact that, in its very Being, that Being is an *issue* for it.' On Dasein and thrownness, see *Being and Time*, 174.
93 See Heidegger, *The Basic Problems of Phenomenology*, 119–20.
94 This neglects the issue of those who are intersexed, a problem which neither Irigaray nor this book sufficiently addresses. Rather than taking the existence of intersexed individuals as immediate disproof of Irigaray's position, it would be worth exploring, first, what her critique of the forgetting of Being as two might be able to contribute to an understanding of the crisis such individuals often face, at least in modern western cultures; and second, whether her account of sexuate difference is capable of fostering a positive existential space for such individuals. Tentatively, I would suggest that, if sexuate difference is 'the ultimate anchorage of real alterity' (*ILTY*, 62), those whose sexed specificity embodies both male and female could perhaps be seen as occupying a privileged (if highly complex) ethical position in terms of their embodiment of alterity (of course, such a positioning could not happen without a wholesale transformation

of our cultural norms, otherwise ethical 'privilege' becomes little more than a rationalization of suffering). For a discussion of inter-sexed bodies in relation to Irigaray, see Stone, *Luce Irigaray and the Philosophy of Sexual Difference*, 49, 113–21.

95   See also *DBT*, 151; ' "Je – Luce Irigaray" ', 107–8, 110.
96   Such originary relations are of course entirely different to the often highly conflictual relationships between mothers and daughters that tend to develop in a culture which refuses to recognize women as autonomous subjects; while they are ontologically primary, such originary relations are empirically at their most minimal and always stand in need of cultivation.
97   Stone, *Luce Irigaray and the Philosophy of Sexual Difference*, 87; see also 94–6, 104–13. Whereas my account of sexuate difference as ontologi-cal places the emphasis on the *relational* nature of this difference, Stone characterizes it in terms of bodily differences that need to be understood as two different (sexuate) *rhythms* informing the whole of nature (construed as *physis*).
98   As Deutscher notes, the French word *genre* can refer to the 'gender' of a term in grammatical contexts; or to 'an artistic style or type'; or 'a category, a class, or a subdivision'; see *A Politics of Impossible Dif-ference*, 203–4, which also discusses English translations of *genre* and the problems of equating *genre* with the concept of gender as deployed in the sex/gender divide.
99   On this point, see Deutscher, *A Politics of Impossible Difference*, 75.
100   See Heidegger, *Being and Time*, 279–311.
101   See *Conversations*, 155–6; *ILTY*, 107.
102   On the ways in which, for de Beauvoir, the female body operates as a barrier to female subjectivity and freedom which must be over-come, see Lloyd, *The Man of Reason*, ch. 6.
103   See Irigaray's essay 'I love to you' in the volume of the same name, and Schwab's discussion in 'Sexual Difference as Model', 85–90.
104   See 'Divine Women' in *Sexes and Genealogies*, especially 61–4.
105   Braidotti, 'Of Bugs and Women', 122.
106   Cheah and Grosz, 'The Future of Sexual Difference', 28.
107   Ibid., 28.
108   Deutscher, *A Politics of Impossible Difference*, 127.
109   *Conversations*, xii.
110   For a parallel approach to this issue, see Deutscher, *A Politics of Impossible Difference*, 137–41.
111   Bostic, 'Luce Irigaray and Love', 606.
112   Cooper, *Relating to Queer Theory*, 139; it is perhaps telling that the key text for Cooper is 'When Our Lips Speak Together', though her reading invites us to develop queer readings of Irigaray's later texts as well.

7   An Ethics of Sexuate Difference

1   For other feminist analyses of Hegel's reading of *Antigone*, see Lloyd, *The Man of Reason*, chs 4–6; Mills, 'Hegel's *Antigone*'; and Butler, *Antigone's Claim: Kinship Between Life and Death*. For detailed analyses of Irigaray's response to Hegel, see ch. 3 in Chanter, *Ethics of Eros* and ch. 5 in Stone, *Luce Irigaray and the Philosophy of Sexual Difference*; ch. 4 in Hutchings, *Hegel and Feminist Philosophy* offers a helpful critical comparison of Irigaray, Mills and Butler alongside an alternative feminist reading of Hegel.

2   *Antigone*, in *Sophocles I*, ed. Grene and Lattimore, 211, c.line 1321.

3   Hegel, *Phenomenology of Spirit*, 266–89 [§444–76].

4   See *S*, 214; *Sf*, 266. The English translation of *Speculum* omits the final lines of the passage Irigaray cites, which read: '*Conception* must not be regarded as consisting of nothing but the ovary and the male semen, as if the new formation were merely a composition of the forms or parts of both sides, for the female certainly contains the material element, while the male contains the subjectivity. Conception is the contraction of the whole individual into the simple self-abandoning unity of its representation. The seed is precisely this simple representation; it is a wholly singular point, as is its name and its entire self.' Hegel, *Philosophy of Nature*, ed. and trans. Petry, 175. In the French version of this passage which appears in *Speculum*, the earlier part of the extract refers explicitly to the female as the passive principle ('*le principe passif*') rather than the 'principle of conception', while the uterus is described as a receptacle ('*simple réceptacle*') rather than in terms of the 'retention of the conception'. This French rendering of the text more strongly draws out aspects of the original German which reflect the tradition Irigaray is critiquing (for example, by translating receptivity, *das Empfangende*, in terms of passivity). See Hegel, *System der Philosophie. Zweite Teil. Die Naturphilosophie*, 672 [vii, 646]₁.

5   See Hegel, *Phenomenology*, 274 [§457].

6   Ibid., 275–6 [§459].

7   Antigone thus embodies the alignment of woman with the unconscious as described in an earlier section of *Speculum*: 'Unconsciousness she is, but not for herself, not with a subjectivity that might take cognizance of it, recognize it as her own. Close to herself, admittedly, but in a total ignorance (of self).' *S*, 141.

8   Hegel, *Phenomenology*, 269 [§451].

9   Ibid., 274–5 [§457].

10   Here and at a number of other points in this section of *Speculum* it is helpful to bear in mind that the French *femme* can denote both woman and wife. Irigaray keeps both in play to encourage us to separate them in our thinking.

11   Hegel, *Phenomenology*, 276 [§460].

12 Lacan's lectures on Antigone appear as part of a series published as *The Ethics of Psychoanalysis (1959–1960), The seminar of Jacques Lacan Book VII*, 243–87.

13 Lacan, *Ethics of Psychoanalysis*, 279.

14 On Lacan's reading, Creon's tragic error is to think he can extend human law – the law that subsumes particulars under the universal, the law governed by the name of the father – to incorporate this necessarily *irrecuperable* and unrepresentable remainder.

15 Lacan, *Ethics of Psychoanalysis*, 278–9.

16 Ibid., 282–3.

17 Battersby, *The Phenomenal Woman*, 114.

18 On the 'equilibrium' of the 'same blood' shared between brother and sister, see Hegel, *Phenomenology*, 274 [§457]. For Battersby's illuminating reading of 'red' and 'white' blood as the key to Irigaray's response to both Hegel and Lacan on Antigone, see *The Phenomenal Woman*, 112–116.

19 The link to Lacan is reinforced by the final (untranslated) part of the first epigraph (see note 4 above). Here Hegel describes the seed or sperm (*la semence* in the French translation Irigaray uses) as a simple representation of the individual and 'a single point, like the name and the entire self.' (See *Sf*, 266; and Hegel, *Philosophy of Nature*, trans. Petry, 175; translation modified drawing on A.V. Miller's translation, 413–14.) The sperm is thus presented as a representation of the individual that quite literally embodies 'the name of the father'.

20 Hegel, *Phenomenology*, 288 [§275].

21 Irigaray suggests that even this necessary undoing of each ethical power by the other is marked by the dissymmetry between the sexes. This is because, while the basis of the feminine ethical essence that is expressed in divine law remains unconscious, the mode of the ethical manifested in (masculine) civil law demands self-conscious participation. Thus (following the logic of Hegel's interpretation), Antigone, not Creon, commits the greater fault, because she 'knew in advance what law and power [she] was *disobeying*' (*S*, 223; my emphasis); hence the severity of her punishment.

22 On Antigone's significance as a provocation to an ethics of sexual difference, see *ESD*, 97–129, and 'The Female Gender', in *Sexes and Genealogies*. Irigaray's ongoing dialogue with Hegel and the need for a dual or sexuate dialectic runs throughout *ILTY*; see also *BEW* (e.g.16); 'The Universal as Mediation', in *Sexes and Genealogies*; and 'How do we become Civil Women?' in *Thinking the Difference*.

23 On sexuate rights, see: the introduction to *Sexes and Genealogies*, 'Each Sex Must Have Its Own Rights'; *DBT*; and *Thinking the Difference*, especially the essay 'Civil Rights and Responsibilities for the Two Sexes'. In several of these texts, Irigaray returns to the figure of

Antigone to consider rights and responsibilities from a sexuate perspective.

24   *Sexes and Genealogies*, 19. On female genealogies, see also 'The Neglect of Female Genealogies', in *je, tu, nous*; and 'The Forgotten Mystery of Female Ancestry', in *Thinking the Difference*.

25   See 'A Chance for Life' in *Sexes and Genealogies*; this essay also appears, in a different translation, as 'A Chance to Live', in *Thinking the Difference*. On this issue, see also 'Between Us, A Fabricated World' and 'She Before the King', in *To be Two*.

26   See 'Love of Self' and 'Love of Same, Love of Other', in *ESD*; and 'Divine Women' and 'The Female Gender', in *Sexes and Genealogies*.

27   *Conversations*, 66.

28   Irigaray's essay is a close reading of the section 'Phenomenology of Eros', in *Totality and Infinity*, 256–66.

29   See Chanter, *Ethics of Eros*, 204–6. Chapter 5 of this book offers a detailed account of Levinas on ethics and the Other in relation to Irigaray, to which I am much indebted.

30   Chanter, *Ethics of Eros*, 205.

31   As Irigaray notes at the beginning of her essay, in Levinas' phenomenology of eros, the look itself remains both tactile and carnal (*ESD*, 185); it no longer belongs to a subject that stands opposed to objects of knowledge which it views from a distance and seeks to master through a purely specular act. On rethinking vision and/as touch, see Vasseleu on Levinas and Irigaray in *Textures of Light*.

32   This phrase is a knowing echo of Irigaray's earlier description of Diotima's teaching, 'Love is fecund prior to any procreation'; *ESD*, 25–6.

33   Again, see Chanter, *Ethics of Eros*: 'it is through the other that the I both becomes an I – identifies itself as such – and is able to generate the categories of being, or to universalize. The other produces the I by putting it in question' (190; see also 222–3).

34   For a critical discussion of Irigaray's privileging of sexuate difference over race, see Stone, *Luce Irigaray and the Philosophy of Sexual Difference*, 48–9, 215–19.

35   It should be noted that Irigaray is clear that, if differences are *not* actively and positively cultivated, such inter-cultural, inter-racial alliances can easily become sites for the regressive re-inscription of repressive power relations of domination and subordination.

36   Butler, *Antigone's Claim*, 24.

37   Deutscher, *'Between East and West* and the Politics of "Cultural Ingé-nuité"*: Irigaray on Cultural Difference', 137, my emphasis.

38   For example, Irigaray tends to present a generalized figure of 'the East', sometimes aligned specifically with India, which she praises for harbouring 'feminine aboriginal cultures' whose traces have been allowed to persist alongside the post-Ayran patriarchal tradi-

tions privileged by the West. See *BEW*, 10, 15, 29, 39. See also Deutscher, *A Politics of Impossible Difference*, ch. 10.

39   Deutscher, 'Between East and West and the Politics of "Cultural Ingé-nuité"*, 142.

40   Deutscher, *A Politics of Impossible Difference*, 174.

41   Deutscher, 'Between East and West and the Politics of "Cultural Ingé-nuité"*, 138; see for example *BEW*, 127.

42   Deutscher, 'Between East and West and the Politics of "Cultural Ingé-nuité"*, 143.

43   Deutscher, *A Politics of Impossible Difference*, 186, 191.

44   Ibid., 29.

45   Deutscher, 'Between East and West and the Politics of "Cultural Ingé-nuité"*, 141.

46   Ibid,, 143.

47   Deutscher, *A Politics of Impossible Difference*, 194.

48   Ibid., 193. One example Deutscher cites is the work of Charles Mills on the racial contract, which complements Pateman's classic study of the ways in which the social contract implicitly depends upon a sexual contract.

49   Deutscher elaborates this point by staging a critical dialogue between Spivak and Irigaray; see *A Politics of Impossible Difference*, 180–4.

50   See hooks, *Ain't I a Woman*, on the relation of racism and sexism and the way white feminists have perpetuated the former even as they have challenged the latter; and Spivak on the subaltern and the 'Native Informant', in *A Critique of Postcolonial Reason: Toward a History of the Vanishing Present*. For a self-critical perspective on approaching differences of race as a white feminist, see Frye 'On Being White', in *The Politics of Reality*.

51   Armour, *Deconstruction, Feminist Theology, and the Problem of Differ-ence: Subverting the Race/Gender Divide*, 166. 'Whitefeminism' is a term coined by Armour 'to highlight the fact that what counts as "feminist" is always already racially marked', 185, n.6.

52   In her own study, Armour focuses particularly on African American feminist literary theory; see Armour, *Deconstruction, Feminist Theol-ogy, and the Problem of Difference*, chs 1 and 6.

53   Ibid., 167, 183.

54   Ibid., 168.

55   Ibid., 134, 133.

56   Ibid., 134.

57   Armour is aware of this, but sees it in terms of a break between Irigaray's earlier and later work, suggesting that 'this differing and deferring woman virtually disappears from much of Irigaray's later work' which is concerned with 'thinking *genuine* sexual difference' (Armour, *Deconstruction, Feminist Theology, and the Problem of Differ-ence*, 130). I have suggested that this focus on sexual difference runs

right through Irigaray's work; while I think this reading does more justice to Irigaray's project, it also heightens the point that the lack of significant attention to race is not just a problem in the later texts that are explicitly concerned with cultural difference; instead, to be true to Irigaray's own call to attend to differences of all kinds, we would need to re-read her earlier texts for the potentially constitutive role played by the absence of raced difference.

58 Battersby, *The Phenomenal Woman*, 2. For another feminist thinker who seeks to develop a relational ontology rooted in both birth and sexual difference, see Cavarero, *In Spite of Plato* and *Relating Narratives*. Lisa Guenther makes a further distinctive contribution by offering a rethinking of our beginnings in birth that draws on an extended reading of Levinas. Via Levinas, Guenther argues that birth is a gift *of* the Other which in turn gives each of us over into responsibility *for* Others; and via feminism, she argues that this account of birth nonetheless needs to be supplemented with a feminist politics of maternity. See Guenther, *The Gift of the Other*.

59 Battersby, *The Phenomenal Woman*, 37.

60 Ibid., 23.

61 Ibid., 35, 21.

62 Ibid., 7, 21.

63 Ibid., 8.

64 Ibid., 209.

65 Battersby, *The Sublime, Terror and Human Difference*, 103.

66 Ibid., 185.

67 Ibid., 188.

68 Alcoff, 'Philosophy and Racial Identity', 20. This essay was originally published in *Radical Philosophy* 75, Jan/Feb 1996, and is also reprinted in *Race*, ed. Bernasconi.

69 Alcoff, 'Philosophy and Racial Identity', 15. On the emergence of race as a scientific concept at the end of the seventeenth and across the eighteenth century, see Bernasconi, 'Who invented the Concept of Race? Kant's Role in the Enlightenment Construction of Race'; on the debunking of the biological basis of race, the work of Anthony Appiah is central, see his key article 'The Uncompleted Argument: Du Bois and the Illusion of Race', originally published in 1985. For further discussion of race and racial identities, see also the later dialogue between Appiah and Gutmann, in *Color Conscious*.

70 Alcoff, 'Philosophy and Racial Identity', 17.

71 Ibid., 28; my emphasis. A key reference point for both Alcoff and Battersby is *Black Atlantic: Modernity and Double Consciousness*, Paul Gilroy's ground-breaking exploration of concepts of racial, and specifically, black identity in the context of the Atlantic slave trade, which simultaneously sets out the critique of the western Enlightenment made possible from the slaves' perspective.

72 Ingram, *The Signifying Body: Towards an Ethics of Sexual and Racial Difference*, 120.

Conclusion

1 Ingram, *The Signifying Body*, xxviii.
2 Ibid.

Bibliography

For a more complete list of works by and on Irigaray, see the Bibliography prepared by Kaisa Kukkola in Luce Irigaray, *Key Writings*. Whereas I have limited myself here for the most part to books by Irigaray translated into English, Kukkola lists articles not collected in books, as well as interviews and Irigaray's contributions to collective publications and anthologies.

Ackrill, J. L. *Aristotle the Philosopher* (Oxford: Clarendon Press, 1981)

Alcoff, L. M., 'Philosophy and Racial Identity', in P. Osborne and S. Sandford eds, *Philosophies of Race and Ethnicity* (London: Continuum, 2002)

Appiah, A. K. 'The Uncompleted Argument: Du Bois and the Illusion of Race', in *Race, Class, Gender and Sexuality: The Big Questions*, ed. C. Sartwell, L. Shrage and N. Zack (Oxford: Blackwell, 1998)

Appiah, A. K. and A. Gutmann. *Color Conscious: The Political Morality of Race* (Princeton, New Jersey: Princeton University Press, 1996)

Aristotle, *The Complete Works of Aristotle*, two vols, ed. J. Barnes (Princeton NJ: Princeton University Press, 1984)

Armour, E. T. *Deconstruction, Feminist Theology and the Problem of Difference: Subverting the Race / Gender Divide* (Chicago: University of Chicago Press, 1999)

Bainbridge, C. *Feminine Cinematics: Luce Irigaray, Women and Film* (Basingstoke: Palgrave MacMillan, 2008)

Bar On, B-A, ed. *Engendering Origins: Critical Feminist Readings in Plato and Aristotle* (New York: SUNY, 1994)

Battersby, C. *The Phenomenal Woman: Feminist Metaphysics and the Patterns of Identity* (Cambridge: Polity 1998)
——*The Sublime, Terror and Human Difference* (London: Routledge, 2007)
Bernasconi, R. 'Who invented the Concept of Race? Kant's Role in the Enlightenment Construction of Race', in Bernasconi, ed., *Race*
Bernasconi, ed., *Race*. Blackwell Readings in Continental Philosophy (Oxford: Blackwell, 2001)
Bolton, L. " 'But what if the object started to speak?': The Representation of Female Consciousness On-Screen", in Irigaray, *Teaching*
Bordo, S. *The Flight to Objectivity: Essays On Cartesianism and Culture* (New York: SUNY, 1987)
Bostic, H. 'Luce Irigaray and Love'. *Cultural Studies* 16 (5) 2002, 603–10
Braidotti, R. 'Of Bugs and Women: Irigaray and Deleuze on the Becoming-Woman', in Burke, Schor, and Whitford eds, *Engaging with Irigaray*
Brandhorst, K. *Descartes' 'Meditations on First Philosophy'* (Edinburgh: Edinburgh University Press, 2010)
Burke, C. 'Translation Modified', in Burke, Schor, and Whitford eds, *Engaging with Irigaray*
Burke, C., N. Schor, and M. Whitford, eds. *Engaging With Irigaray* (New York: Columbia University Press, 1994)
Butler, J. *Antigone's Claim: Kinship Between Life and Death* (New York: Columbia University Press, 2000)
——*Gender Trouble: Feminism and the Subversion of Identity* (London, New York: Routledge, 1990)
——*Bodies that Matter: On the Discursive Limits of 'Sex'* (London: Routledge, 1993)
Canters H. and G. Jantzen. *Forever Fluid: A Reading of Luce Irigaray's Elemental Passions* (Manchester: Manchester University Press, 2005)
Cavarero, *In Spite of Plato: A Feminist Rewriting of Ancient Philosophy*, trans. S. Anderlini-D'Onofrio and Á. O'Healy (Cambridge: Polity, 1995)
——*Relating Narratives: Storytelling and Selfhood*, trans. P. Kottmann (London: Routledge, 2000)
Chanter, T. *Ethics of Eros: Irigaray's rewriting of the Philosophers* (London, New York: Routledge, 1995)
Cheah, P. and E. Grosz, 'The Future of Sexual Difference: An Interview with Judith Butler and Drucilla Cornell'. *Diacritics*, vol. 28 no. 1 Spring 1998, 19–42

Cimitile, M. 'Irigaray in Dialogue With Heidegger', in Cimitile and Miller, eds, *Returning to Irigaray*.

Cimitile, M. and E. Miller, eds. *Returning to Irigaray* (New York: SUNY, 2007)

Constable, C. *Thinking in Images: Film Theory, Feminist Philosophy and Marlene Dietrich* (London: BFI, 2008)

Cooper, S. *Relating to Queer Theory: Rereading Sexual Self-Definition with Irigaray, Kristeva, Wittig and Cixous* (Bern: Peter Lang, 2000)

de Beauvoir, S. *The Second Sex*, trans. H. M. Parshley (New York: Vintage, 1997)

Descartes, R. *Oeuvres et Lettres*, ed. André Bridoux (Paris: Pléiade, 1953)

——*The Philosophical Works of Descartes*, vol. 1, trans. E. S. Haldane and G. R. T. Ross (Cambridge: Cambridge University Press, 1931, reprinted Dover, 1955)

——*The Philosophical Writings of Descartes: vol. 1*, trans. J. Cottingham, R. Stoothoff, and D. Murdoch (Cambridge: Cambridge University Press, 1985)

——*The Philosophical Writings of Descartes: vol. II*, trans. J. Cottingham, R. Stoothoff, and D. Murdoch (Cambridge: Cambridge University Press, 1984)

Deutscher, P. *A Politics of Impossible Difference: The Later Work of Luce Irigaray* (Ithaca, NY: Cornell University Press, 2002)

——'*Between East and West* and the Politics of "Cultural *Ingénuité*": Irigaray on Cultural Difference', in Cimitile and Miller, eds, *Returning to Irigaray*.

——'"Imperfect Discretion": Interventions into the History of Philosophy by 20th Century French Women Philosophers'. *Hypatia* vol. 15 (2) 2000, 160–80

Dover, K. ed. *Plato: Symposium* (Cambridge: Cambridge University Press, 1980)

Foucault, M. *The History of Sexuality: Volume 1*, trans. R. Hurley (Harmondsworth: Penguin, 1978).

Freeland, C. 'Nourishing Speculation', in Bar On, ed., *Engendering Origins*

Freud, S. *New Introductory Lectures on Psychoanalysis*, The Penguin Freud Library Volume II, general editor J. Strachey (Harmondsworth: Penguin, 1975)

——*On Metapsychology*, The Penguin Freud Library Volume XI, general editor J. Strachey (Harmondsworth: Penguin, 1991)

——*On Sexuality*, The Penguin Freud Library Volume VII, general editor J. Strachey (Harmondsworth: Penguin, 1977)

Frye, M. *The Politics of Reality: Essays in Feminist Theory* (Berkeley: The Crossing Press, 1983)

Fuss, D. *Essentially Speaking: Feminism, Nature and Difference* (New York: Routledge, 1989)

Gallop, J. *Feminism and Psychoanalysis: The Daughter's Seduction* (London: Macmillan, 1992)

Gatens, M. *Feminism and Philosophy: Perspectives on Difference and Equality* (Cambridge: Polity, 1991)

——*Imaginary Bodies: Ethics, Power and Corporeality* (London: Routledge, 1996)

Gelven, M. *A Commentary on Heidegger's 'Being and Time'*, revd edition (Dekalb, Illinois: Northern Illinois University Press, 1989)

Gerson, L. P., ed. *The Cambridge Companion to Plotinus* (Cambridge: Cambridge University Press, 1996)

Gilroy, P. *Black Atlantic: Modernity and Double Consciousness* (Cambridge, MA: Harvard University Press, 1993)

Grosz, E. 'The Hetero and the Homo: The Sexual Ethics of Luce Irigaray', in Burke, Schor, and Whitford, eds, *Engaging with Irigaray*

——*Sexual Subversions: Three French Feminists* (Sydney: Allen and Unwin, 1989)

——*Volatile Bodies: Towards A Corporeal Feminism* (Bloomington: Indiana University Press, 1994)

Guenther, L. *The Gift of the Other; Levinas and the Politics of Reproduction* (New York: SUNY, 2006)

Harth, E. *Cartesian Women* (Ithaca, NY: Cornell University Press, 1992)

Hegel, G. W. F. *Phenomenology of Spirit*, trans. A. Miller (Oxford: Oxford University Press, 1977)

——*Philosophy of Nature*, ed. and trans. M. Petry (London: Allen and Unwin, 1970)

——*Philosophy of Nature*, trans. A.V. Miller (Oxford: Clarendon Press, 2004)

——*System der Philosophie. Zweite Teil. Die Naturphilosophie*, vol.IX, dritte Auslage der Jubiläumsausgabe (Stuttgart: Frommanns Verlag, 1958)

Heidegger, M. *The Basic Problems of Phenomenology*, revised edition, trans. A. Hofstadter (Bloomington and Indianapolis: Indiana University Press, 1982)

——*Being and Time*, trans. J. Macquarrie and E. Robinson (Oxford: Blackwell, 1962)

——*The Essence of Truth*, trans. T. Sadler (London: Continuum, 2002)

264 Bibliography

—— *On the Way to Language*, trans. P. D. Hertz (New York: Harper and Row, 1971)
——*Pathmarks*, ed. W. McNeill, trans. F. A. Capuzzi (Cambridge: Cambridge University Press, 1998)
——*Poetry, Language, Thought*, trans. A Hofstadter (New York: Harper Collins, 2001)
——*Unterwegs zur Sprache* (Stuttgart: Klett-Cotta, 1959)
Hodge, J. 'Irigaray Reading Heidgger', in Burke, Schor, and Whitford, eds, *Engaging with Irigaray*
hooks, b. *Ain't I a Woman: Black Women and Feminism* (Cambridge, MA: South End Press, 1999)
Husserl, E. *Cartesian Meditations*, trans. D. Cairns (Dordrecht: Kluwer, 1995)
Hutchings, K. *Hegel and Feminist Philosophy.* (Cambridge: Polity, 2003)
Ingram, P. *The Signifying Body: Towards an Ethics of Sexual and Racial Difference* (New York: SUNY 2008)
Irigaray, L. *Between East and West; From Singularity to Community*, trans. S. Pluhácek (New York: Columbia University Press, 2002)
——*Ce sexe qui n'en est pas un* (Paris: Minuit, 1977)
——*Conversations* (London: Continuum, 2008)
——*Democracy Begins Between Two*, trans. K Anderson (London: Athlone, 2000)
——*Dialogues: Luce Irigaray presents Dialogues around her Work. Paragraph* 25 No. 3 (Edinburgh: Edinburgh University Press, 2002)
——*Elemental Passions*, trans. J. Collie and J. Still (London: Athlone, 1992)
——*An Ethics of Sexual Difference*, trans. C. Burke and G. Gill (London: Athlone, 1993)
——*Éthique de la différence sexuelle* (Paris: Minuit, 1984)
——*The Forgetting of Air in Martin Heidegger*, trans. M. B. Mader (Austin: University of Texas Press, 1999)
——*I Love to You; Sketch for a Felicity Within History*, trans. A. Martin (London: Routledge, 1996)
——*The Irigaray Reader*, ed. M. Whitford (Oxford: Blackwell, 1991)
—— '"Je – Luce Irigaray": a Meeting with Luce Irigaray'; Interview with E. Hirsch and G. Olson, trans. E. Hirsch and G. Brulotte, *Hypatia*, vol. 10 (2) Spring 1995, 93–114.
——*je, tu, nous: Towards a Culture of Difference*, trans. A. Martin (London: Routledge, 1993)
——*Key Writings* (London: Continuum, 2004)

——*Marine Lover: Of Friedrich Nietzsche*, trans. G. C. Gill (New York: Columbia University Press, 1980)

——*Sexes and Genealogies*, trans. G. Gill (New York: Columbia University Press, 1993)

——*Sharing the World* (London: Continuum, 2008)

——*Speculum de l'autre femme* (Paris: Minuit, 1974)

——*Speculum of the Other Woman*, trans. G. C. Gill (Ithaca, NY: Cornell University Press, 1985)

——*Teaching*, ed. L. Irigaray with M. Green (London: Continuum, 2008)

——*Thinking the Difference: For a Peaceful Revolution*, trans. K. Montin (London: Routledge, 1994)

——*This Sex Which is Not One*, trans. C. Porter with C. Burke (Ithaca, NY: Cornell University Press, 1985).

——*To Be Two*, trans. M. Rhodes and M. Cocito-Monoc (New York: Routledge, 2001)

——*To Speak is Never Neutral*, trans. G. Schwab (London: Continuum, 2002)

——*The Way of Love*, trans. H. Bostic and S. PluhÁcek (London: Continuum, 2002)

—— 'Women's Exile: Interview with Luce Irigaray'. *Ideology and Consciousness*, 1, 1977, 62–76

Kant, I. *Critique of Judgment*, trans. W. Pluhar (Indianapolis: Hackett, 1987)

——*Critique of Practical Reason*, ed. and trans. L. W. Beck (Chicago: University of Chicago Press, 1949)

——*Critique of Pure Reason*, trans. N. Kemp Smith (London: MacMillan, 1933)

——*Immanuel Kant: Practical Philosophy*, ed. and trans. M. Gregor (Cambridge: Cambridge University Press, 1999)

——*Observations on the Feeling of the Beautiful and Sublime*, trans. J. Goldthwait (Berkeley and Los Angeles: University of California Press, 1960)

——*Prolegomena to Any Future Metaphysics*, ed. and trans. G. Hatfield (Cambridge: Cambridge University Press, 2004)

——*Werke vol. 1: Vorkritische Schriften I 1747–1756* (Berlin: Walter de Gruyter, 1968)

——'What is Orientation in Thinking?', in Kant, *Critique of Practical Reason*

Kristeva, J. 'The Meaning of Parity', in *The Kristeva Critical Reader*, ed. J. Lechte and M. Zournazi (Edinburgh: Edinburgh University Press, 2003)

Lacan, J. *Écrits*, trans. Bruce Fink (New York: Norton, 2006)

—— *Encore: On Feminine Sexuality: The Limits of Love and Knowledge (1972–1973), The Seminar of Jacques Lacan XX*, ed. J-A Miller, trans. B. Fink (New York: Norton, 1998)

——*The Ethics of Psychoanalysis (1959–1960), The seminar of Jacques Lacan VII*, ed. J-A. Miller, trans. D. Porter (New York: Norton, 1997)

——*The Four Fundamental Concepts of Pyschoanalysis*, ed. J-A Miller, trans. A. Sheridan (Harmondsworth: Penguin, 1977)

——*Le Seminaire de Jacques Lacan, XX: Encore*, ed. J-A Miller (Paris: Éditions du Seuil, 1975)

Levinas, I. *Totality and Infinity*, trans. A. Lingis (Pittsburgh: Duquesne University Press, 1969)

Lloyd, G. *The Man of Reason: 'Male' and 'Female' in Western Philosophy*, 2nd edn (London: Routledge, 1993)

—— 'Feminism in History of Philosophy', in *The Cambridge Companion to Feminism in Philosophy*, ed. J. Hornsby and M. Fricker (Cambridge: Cambridge University Press, 2000)

Marks, E. and I. de Courtivron, eds. *New French Feminisms* (New York: Schocken, 1981)

McAfee, N. *Julia Kristeva*. Routledge Critical Thinkers (New York, London: Routledge, 2004)

Mills, P. 'Hegel's *Antigone*', in *Feminist Interpretations of G. W. F. Hegel*, ed. P. Mills (Pennsylvania: Pennsylvania State University Press, 1996)

Moi, T. *Sexual/Textual Politics*, 2nd edn (London: Routledge, 2002)

Mortensen, E. 'Woman's (Un)truth and *le féminin*: Reading Luce Irigaray with Friedrich Nietzsche and Martin Heidegger', in Burke, Schor, and Whitford eds, *Engaging with Irigaray*

Oliver, K. ed., *Ethics, Politics and Difference in Julia Kristeva's Writing* (New York, London: Routledge 1993)

——*Reading Kristeva: Unravelling the Double-Bind* (Bloomington: Indiana University Press, 1993)

O'Meara, D. J. 'The Hierarchical Ordering of Reality in Plotinus', in Gerson ed., *The Cambridge Companion to Plotinus*

Plaza, M. '"Phallomorphic" Power and the Psychology of "Woman"', *Gender Issues*, vol.1 no.1 March 1980, 71–102

Plato. *Collected Dialogues*, ed. E. Hamilton and H. Cairns (Princeton New Jersey: Princeton University Press, 1961)

——*Oeuvres Complètes*, trans. L. Robin (Paris: Gallimard, 1950)

——*Republic*, trans. G. Grube, revd C. Reeve (Indianapolis: Hackett, 1992)

——*The Symposium*, trans. R. Allen (New Haven: Yale University Press, 1991)

——*Timaeus*, trans. D. Lee (Harmondsworth: Penguin, 1977)

Plotinus. *Plotinus' Enneads*, trans. S. MacKenna, 2nd edn, revd B. S. Page (London: Faber and Faber, 1956)

Politis, V. *Aristotle and the 'Metaphysics'*, Routledge Philosophy Guidebook (London: Routledge, 2004)

Rawes, P. *Irigaray for Architects* (London: Routledge, 2007)

Robinson, H. *Reading Art, Reading Irigaray: The Politics of Art by Women* (London: I. B. Taurus, 2006)

Schwab, G. 'Reading Irigaray (and her Readers) in the Twenty-First Century', in Cimitile, M. and E. Miller, eds, *Returning to Irigaray*

—— 'Sexual Difference as Model: An Ethics for the Global Future', *Diacritics*, vol. 28 no. 1 Spring 1998, 76–92

Schor, N. 'Previous Engagements: The Receptions of Irigaray' in Burke, Schor, and Whitford eds, *Engaging with Irigaray*

—— 'This Essentialism Which Is Not One', in Burke, Schor, and Whitford eds, *Engaging with Irigaray*

Sellers, S. *Hélène Cixous: Authorship, Autobiography and Love* (Cambridge: Polity Press, 1996)

Shapiro, L., ed. and trans. *Princess Elisabeth of Bohemia and René Descartes: The Correspondence.* (Chicago: University of Chicago Press, 2007)

Sophocles, *Antigone*, in *Sophocles I*, ed. D. Grene and R. Lattimore, trans. D. Grene, 2nd edn (Chicago: University of Chicago Press, 1991)

Spivak, G. C. *In Other Worlds: Essays in Cultural Politics* (London, New York: Routledge, 1987)

——*A Critique of Postcolonial Reason: Toward a History of the Vanishing Present* (Cambridge, MA: Harvard University Press, 1999)

Stavrakakis, Y. *Lacan and the Political* (London: Routledge, 1999)

Still, J. 'Poetic Nuptials', in Irigaray, *Dialogues*

Stone, A. *An Introduction to Feminist Philosophy* (Cambridge: Polity, 2007)

——*Luce Irigaray and the Philosophy of Sexual Difference* (Cambridge: Cambridge University Press, 2006)

Taylor, A. E. *Plato: The Man and his Work* (London: Methuen, 1926)

Tuana, N. 'Aristotle and the Politics of Reproduction', in Bar On, ed., *Engendering Origins*

Vasseleu, C. *Textures of Light: Vision and Touch in Irigaray, Levinas and Merleau-Ponty* (London: Routledge, 1998)

Whitford, M. *Luce Irigaray: Philosophy in the Feminine* (London: Routledge, 1991)

——'Reading Irigaray in the Nineties', in Burke, Schor, and Whitford eds, *Engaging with Irigaray*

Index

otherness, 7, 30–1, 123, 161, 165,
   186, 212–14, 217, 219, 221,
   226–7
   irreducible, 7, 199, 214–16
   material, of matter, 108, 110,
     116
   within, 30–1, 98, 176, 193, 198,
     213, 225, 243n43
   see also alterity
Otherness, 146–7, 216

parler femme, 16, 30, 130, 179–80
see also speak (as a) woman
phallus, 86, 135, 137–9, 147–8,
   163–4
   as transcendental signifier,
     138
placental economy, 13, 83, 161–2,
   166, 176, 178, 231, 241n17
Plato,
   and western metaphysics, 12,
     38, 42–3, 46, 49, 52, 65, 81,
     88, 91, 94, 100
   Forms (Ideas), 12, 38, 45, 47–64,
     66–7, 69–84, 87–9, 95–8, 131,
     135, 147
   Myth of the Cave, 12, 38, 41,
     43–65, 66–75, 79–80, 82–5,
     87–91, 102, 112, 132, 137,
     142, 161
   Platonic metaphysics, 41, 47–8,
     52, 60, 68, 70, 74, 77–81, 84,
     87–8, 92, 94
   Timaeus, 12, 39, 66, 74–81, 83–4,
     96, 99, 140, 147
   see also Diotima; Freud; Lacan;
     mimesis; nature
Plotinus, 12, 36, 41, 95, 98–100, 111,
   128
poetics, 14, 178–9
pregnancy, 30, 47, 89, 92, 99–100,
   162, 193, 247n16
see also body, pregnant
projective announcement,
   178–80
psyche, *psychē*, 95, 128–9, 132

psychoanalysis, 2, 11, 13, 41,
   129–32, 136–8, 142, 145,
   172–3, 175, 244n18
see also Freud; Lacan

reason,
   as gender neutral (Irigaray's
     critique of), 28, 36,
     102–3
   gendering of, 24, 131, 167
race, 167, 217–28
   and cultural difference, 14,
     219–23
   and feminism, 167, 223–4
   and sexuate difference, 8,
     167–8, 183, 199, 217–19,
     221, 227–8
   ontological status of, 219,
     226–8
reproduction (sexual/biological),
   63, 97, 137–8, 192, 195,
   201
   reproductive function, 25, 91–2,
     137, 150, 195, 241n17

self, feminine / non–oppositional
   process of constitution, 31,
   159, 164–6, 168–9, 171–2,
   213, 230–1
sensible transcendental, 126,
   128–9, 219
sex/gender distinction, 4–6,
   249n40, 253n98
sexual difference, 2–4, 6–8, 10–12,
   14, 20–4, 26, 28–38, 42, 75–6,
   84–8, 94, 103, 109, 111–15,
   117, 119, 123, 126, 129–31,
   133, 142, 167, 169, 172,
   182–4, 186–7, 195–6, 208–10,
   212, 218, 221–3, 227–8, 231
   and alterity, 7, 14, 168, 183, 218,
     227
   and sexual orientation, 183,
     187–8, 198
   and the sexuate, 4
   as universal, 31, 208, 210, 218

symbolic, symbolic order, *see*
    Lacan
    female/feminine symbolic, 176,
        248n35

touch, 84, 92, 163–5, 185, 214–15,
    239n22
transcendence, 70, 113, 154,
    193, 197, 207, 212, 214,
    216
transcendental, 114, 116–23, 125–7,
    197, 218–19, 221–2, 227,
    243n2
see also sensible transcendental
two lips, *see* lips

unconscious, the, 131, 135, 141–3,
    150, 152, 204–8, 254n7
unconscious ethical being
    (woman as), 201–2

Whitford, M. 9–11, 170–4, 186,
    243n1, 248n18
Wollstonecraft, 27–9
womb, 51, 79, 81, 97, 102, 107, 128,
    140, 146, 162–3, 207, 238n8,
    243n43
    and Plato's cave, 47–52, 54–5,
        58–61, 63–5, 67, 70, 74–5, 79,
        82, 85, 171
wonder, 13, 112–13, 129, 198, 214